24·99

D0993613

Roxburgh's
Common
Skin
Diseases

Roxburgh's Common Skin Diseases

16th edition

R. Marks

Professor of Dertmatology
University of Wales College of Medicine
Cardiff, UK

CHAPMAN & HALL MEDICAL
London · Glasgow · New York · Tokyo · Melbourne · Madras

Published by Chapman & Hall, 2–6 Boundary Row, London SE1 8HN

Chapman & Hall, 2–6 Boundary Row, London SE1 8HN, UK

Blackie Academic & Professional, Wester Cleddens Road, Bishopbriggs, Glasgow G64 2NZ, UK

Chapman & Hall Inc., 29 West 35th Street, New York NY10001, USA

Chapman & Hall Japan, Thomson Publishing Japan, Hirakawacho Nemoto Building, 6F, 1-7-11 Hirakawa-cho, Chiyoda-ku, Tokyo 102, Japan

Chapman & Hall Australia, Thomas Nelson Australia, 102 Dodds Street, South Melbourne, Victoria 3205, Australia

Chapman & Hall India, R. Seshadri, 32 Second Main Road, CIT East, Madras 600 035, India

First edition 1932
Subsequent editions 1934, 1936, 1937, 1939, 1941, 1944, 1947, 1950, 1955, 1959, 1961, 1967, 1975, 1986
16th edition 1993

© 1961, 1967, 1975, 1986 H.K. Lewis & Co. Ltd., 1993 Chapman & Hall

Typeset in 10/12 pt Plantin by Falcon Graphic Art, Wallington, Surrey
Designed by Geoffrey Wadsley

Printed and bound in Hong Kong

ISBN 0 412 41130 X   0 412 59980 5 (Special edition)

A catalogue record for this book is available from the British Library

Library of Congress Cataloging-in-Publication data available

Contents

Preface

Recognition and treatment of skin disease is an important part of the practice of medicine. These skills should form an essential part of the undergraduate curriculum because skin disorders are common and often extremely disabling in one way or another. Apart from the fact that all physicians will inevitably have to cope with patients with rashes, itches, skin ulcerations, inflamed papules, nodules and tumours at some point in their careers, skin disorders themselves are intrinsically fascinating. The fact that their progress both in development and in relapse can be closely observed, and their clinical appearance easily correlated with their pathology, should enable the student or young physician to obtain a better overall view of the way disease processes affect tissues.

The division of the material into chapters has been pragmatic, combining both traditional clinical and 'disease process' categorization. After much thought it seems to the author that no one classification is either universally applicable or completely acceptable. A detailed description of the structure and function of the skin has been omitted as a separate section but included when applicable in the various chapters.

It is planned that the book fulfil both the educational needs of medical students and young doctors as well as being of assistance to general practitioners in their everyday professional lives. Hopefully it will also excite some who read it sufficiently to want to know more so that they consult the appropriate monographs and larger, more specialized works.

R. Marks
Cardiff

Structure of the Book

Besides the typical features that make up a book of this nature – text, illustrations, tables and so on – *Roxburgh's Common Skin Diseases* makes use of boxed summaries throughout the book.

These summaries are used to reinforce important points and to indicate areas where important research is being done at present. Key clinical points are indicated by *green* boxes; *yellow* boxes indicate growth areas in research and development.

> Boxes are used to bring out of the text points that are vital to the reader's understanding of the topic, giving them the emphasis they deserve.

> Yellow boxes indicate growth areas in research and development.

Boxes that appear in the margin bring together a number of points where importance needs to be stressed collectively. Boxes that appear in the text emphasise a key point that has just been made.

It is hoped that these boxed summaries will guide the reader through the book, highlighting important topics and features, and making the book easier to use and refer to.

> Key clinical points are highlighted throughout the book by placing them in green-coloured boxes.

> The boxed summaries will guide the reader through the book.

Introduction: prevalence and significance

Skin is an extraordinary structure. We are absolutely dependent on this 1.7 m² of barrier separating the potentially harmful environment from the body's vulnerable interior. It is a composite of several types of tissue that have evolved to work in harmony one with the other, each of which is modified regionally to serve a different function (Figure 1.1, Table 1.1). The large number of cell types (Figures 1.2 and 1.3) and functions of the skin and its proximity to the numerous potentially

Figure 1.1 Overall plan view of skin.

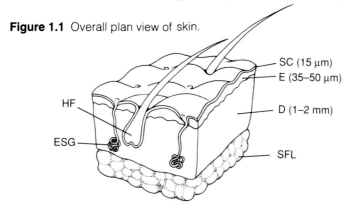

SC (15 µm)
E (35–50 µm)
D (1–2 mm)
HF
ESG
SFL

Table 1.1 Functions of skin

(1)   Protection against water loss – stratum corneum (SC); water gain – stratum corneum; penetration by toxic substances – stratum corneum; microbial attack – stratum corneum; mechanical injury – dermis (D) and stratum corneum.

(2)   Thermal regulation through heat loss via (a) sweat evaporation – eccrine sweat glands (ESG); (b) vasomotor regulation – vasculature; and through heat conservation via (a) body hair; (b) insulation from body fat.

(3)   Communication via sensory messages and sensory nerves and end organs, and display – secondary sex characteristics.

(4)   Immune function with a role in protection against foreign antigens from epidermal antigen presenting cells (Langerhans cells). It is an incompletely characterized role in priming some types of T-lymphocytes.

(5)   Metabolic function with an important role in synthesis of vitamin D after solar ultraviolet radiation. HF = hair follicle. E = epidermis. SFL = subcutaneous fat layer.

Figure 1.2 Epidermis. DC = desquamating horn cell. SC = stratum corneum. GCL = granular cell layer. MCL = Malpighian cell layer. Me = melanocyte. LC = Langerhans cell. MiC = cell in basal layer of epidermis undergoing mitosis. BL = basal lamina.

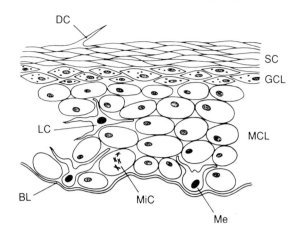

Figure 1.3 Diagram to show corneocytes in stratum corneum and diminishing binding force between them as the surface is reached. This enables the corneocyte to be shed from the surface in the process of desquamation.

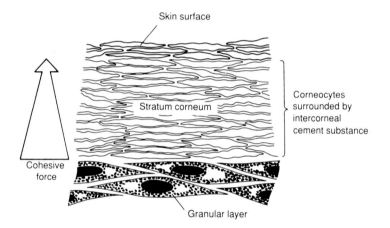

damaging stimuli in the environment result in two important consider-ations. The first is that the skin is frequently damaged because it is right in the 'firing line' and the second is that each of the various cell types that it contains can 'go wrong' and develop its own degenerative and neoplastic disorders. This last point is compounded by the ready visibility of skin so that minor deviations from normal give rise to a particular set of signs. The net effect is that there seems to be a large number of skin diseases.

Skin disease, its recognition, treatment and prevention are in the province of the dermatologist who is generally trained in a similar manner and with a similar philosophy to specialists in internal medi-cine. In recent years, however, dermatologists have taken increasing interest and had increasing involvement in surgical treatments for some skin disorders. This is partially in response to the increase in the incidence of the various types of skin cancer.

Hair and nails are the products of specialized skin structures and their care and their disorders are also in the province of the dermatolo-gist. The epithelium of skin is in direct continuity with the oral, nasal and genital mucosae and these areas should also be inspected in the course of examination of the skin. In most countries diseases contracted from sexual contact (venereal diseases) are also considered to be within the professional ambit of the dermatologist. This has not been the case in the UK and Ireland but is likely to change in the near future.

Dermatologists overlap with rheumatologists and internists when it comes to diagnosis and treatment of the connective tissue disorders such as lupus erythematosus (Chapter 6). Dermatologists and vascular surgeons share an interest in caring for patients with chronic leg ulcers. There are many examples of disorders in which two or more specialist groups share special knowledge and skill in management. Whether the dermatologist or another specialist becomes involved in the care of a particular patient will depend on many local factors, including the facilities available and the interest and the propensities of the individual physicians concerned.

Skin disease is very common. However 'healthy' we think our skin is, it is likely that we will have suffered from some degree of acne and maybe one or other of the many common skin disorders. Atopic eczema and the other forms of eczema affect some 5 or 6% of the population, psoriasis affects 1 to 2%, while viral warts, seborrhoeic warts and solar keratoses affect large segments of the population. It should be noted that 10–15% of the general practitioner's work is with skin disorders, and that skin disease is the second commonest cause of loss of work.

Although skin disease is not uncommon at any age it is particularly frequent in the elderly. Skin disorders are not often dramatic but cause considerable discomfort and much disability. The disability caused is physical, emotional and socioeconomic, and patients are much helped by an appreciation of this and attempts by their physician to relieve the various problems that arise.

CHAPTER

2

Signs and symptoms of skin disease

Skin disorders may either be generalized, affecting all parts of the integument, localized to one or several sites of abnormality known as 'lesions', or they may be eruptive (or exanthematic) in which large numbers of lesions appear spottily over the skin. It is important to note that skin which appears normal to the naked eye may have structural abnormalities when inspected microscopically and may also demonstrate functional abnormalities. For example, the skin around a psoriatic plaque shows slight epidermal thickening and minor inflammatory changes; similarly there are quite marked alterations in blood flow and vascular reaction in the normal appearing skin nearby inflamed and eczematous skin.

Any widespread abnormality of the skin may also affect the scalp, the mucosae of the mouth, nose, eyes and genitalia, and the nail-forming tissues of the digits (nail matrix). For this reason it is important to inspect these sites whenever practically possible in the course of an examination of the skin.

Alterations in skin colour

The colour of normal skin is for the most part dependent on the degree of melanin pigment production (page 298) and the blood supply. Other factors may influence it including the optical qualities of the stratum corneum and the presence of other pigments in the skin. One of the most common accompaniments of skin disease is redness or erythema.

> One of the most common accompaniments of skin disease is redness or erythema.

Erythema
The degree of erythema depends on the degree of oxygenation of the blood that travels through the cutaneous vasculature, the rate of movement of blood through the skin, the number and size of the small cutaneous blood vessels and depth of the blood vessels in the skin. There is a tendency for different disorders to be associated with particular shades of red. Psoriatic plaques, for example, are characterized by a dark red colour rather than a pink, a bright red or a bluish red colour (Figure 2.1). Amongst other well-known examples in which diseases are associated with specific colours are lichen planus and

dermatomyositis. Lichen planus has a well known mauve hue which is often helpful in reaching a diagnosis. Dermatomyositis characteristically has the colour of the heliotrope flower associated with the periocular swelling that frequently occurs in this disease (Figure 2.2). The reasons for the specific shades of red are not always known, but the shading of melanin pigment from damaged epidermis into the dermis, thickening of the epidermis and the presence of inflammatory cells around the blood vessels may all contribute to the particular colour of lichen planus.

Measurement of the degree of erythema may be helpful in assessing the effects of treatment on an erythematous skin disease. There are now two types of device that can do this, one is based on the comparator principle and the other uses reflectance spectroscopy. Both employ complex electronics, are packed and available commercially, and are easy to use.

> Measurement of the degree of erythema may be helpful in assessing the effects of treatment on an erythematous skin disease.

Brown-black pigmentation

The degree of brown-black pigmentation depends on the activity of the pigment producing cells – the melanocytes – not the number of cells. It also depends on the size of the granules and the distribution of the pigment particles within the epidermal cells. Shedding of the pigment from the epidermis, where it is produced, is known as pigmentary incontinence and causes a kind of tattooing in which the dusky pigment produced hangs on for many weeks or months.

> The degree of brown-black pigmentation depends on the activity of the pigment producing cells – the melanocytes – not the number of cells. It also depends on the size of the granules and the distribution of the pigment particles within the epidermal cells.

Brown pigmentation is also caused by a breakdown product of blood – haemosiderin – when this has leaked into the tissues (Figure 2.3). It is very difficult to tell this apart from melanin pigment, both clinically and in tissue sections microscopically. In the latter case, special stains can help.

> Brown pigmentation is also caused by a breakdown product of blood – haemosiderin.

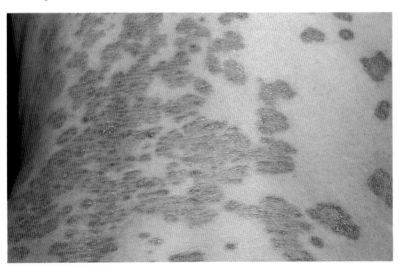

Figure 2.1 Plaques of psoriasis with typical red colour.

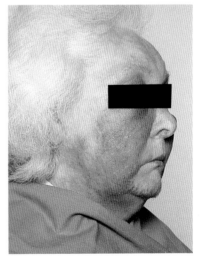

Figure 2.2 Reddened areas on the face in dermatomyositis showing typical heliotrope discolouration.

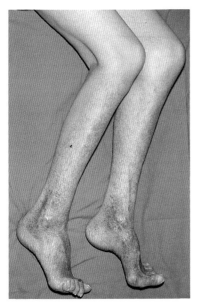

Figure 2.3 Lower legs of patient with chronic venous hypertension and brown pigmentation due to haemosiderin deposits.

> When the process of formation of the stratum corneum (keratinization) is disturbed, the horn cells can no longer separate from their neighbours and they tend to separate in clumps or scales rather than as single cells.

A brown-black discolouration of the skin over cartilaginous structures (ears and nose) and to a lesser extent at other sites is seen in the inherited disorder known as alcaptonuria, due to the deposition of homogentisic acid. A dark brown pigmentation of acne scars or of areas on the limbs is sometimes observed as an uncommon side effect of the tetracycline-type drug minocycline.

Generalized darkening of the skin, more pronounced in the flexures, is observed in Addinson's disease and seems to be due to increased secretion of melanocyte-stimulating hormone and the consequent activation of the melanocytes to produce more pigment. Nelson's syndrome following adrenalectomy is another cause of generalized pigmentation which can be startlingly intense in some patients. This is also thought to be due to the action of melanocyte-stimulating hormone. Darkening of the palmar creases and mucosae may be seen in both these endocrine disorders.

Disorders of pigmentation are also discussed in Chapter 17.

Alterations in the skin surface

The sensation experienced by touching or stroking normal skin is due in part to the normal skin surface markings which vary to some extent in different areas of the body (Figures 2.4 and 2.5). It is also dependent on the presence of hair, sweat and sebum at the skin surface and to the overall mechanical properties of the skin at that site. Horn cells are constantly being shed from the skin surface (desquamation) at a rate that approximates to the rate that the epidermal cells are being produced. The replacement time (turnover time) of the normal stratum corneum is approximately 14 days, but varies with different body sites and lengthens in old age. Normally, horn cells are shed singly, and the process is imperceptible. When the process of formation of the stratum corneum (keratinization) is disturbed, the horn cells can no longer separate from their neighbours and they tend to separate in clumps or scales rather than as single cells. Sometimes the process is so disturbed

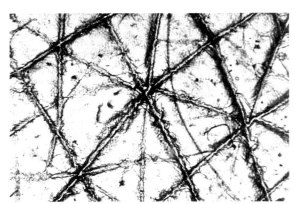

Figure 2.4 Skin surface of forearm showing typical romboidal pattern.

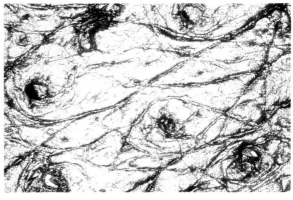

Figure 2.5 Skin surface of beard area in a man with accentuation of the follicular orifices.

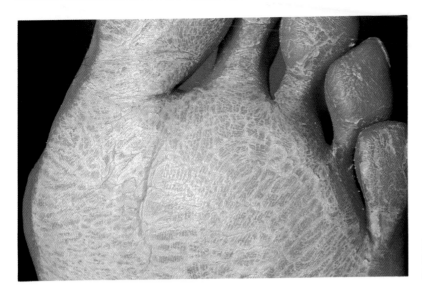

Figure 2.6 Plantar hyperkeratosis in patient with a congenital disorder of keratinization.

that shedding of any type is impossible and the horny layer builds up into a thickened horny patch of hyperkeratosis (Figure 2.6). When the skin surface is scaly and roughened it looks dry, and scaling skin disorders are sometimes known colloquially as 'dry skin disorders'. Water placed on scaling skin makes the surface less scaly temporarily and this reinforces the view that the scaling is due to a water deficiency. However, this is mixing up cause with effect, and the causes of scaling are many and various without true water deficiency figuring amongst them.

As mentioned above, scaling is due to disturbances in the process of keratinization and these may be primary or secondary. In the primary disorders of keratinization there is some metabolic abnormality that prevents full and complete differentiation of the stratum corneum ending in the release of intact single keratinocytes. These disorders are generally (but not always) congenital in origin – the ichthyoses being the best examples.

Scaling is also seen when keratinization is affected secondary to some other pathological process affecting the epidermis. For example, the scaling seen in psoriasis and eczema is due to the inflammation that affects the epidermis in these disorders. In psoriasis, and probably in some patients with chronic eczema, epidermal cell production is greatly increased and the rapid movement of the epidermal cells upwards results in immature cells within the stratum corneum.

Damage to the epidermal cells also distorts the process of keratinization.

The causes of scaling are summarized in Table 2.1. There are no simple ways to quantify scaling although there are established methods for assessing skin surface contour, in which the contour of the skin surface is tracked with a very sensitive stylus from replicas, and recorded electronically. Skin surface contour may also be recorded optically by measuring the reflection of light from the skin surface.

Scaling is due to disturbances in the process of keratinization and these may be primary or secondary. In the primary disorders of keratinization there is some metabolic abnormality that prevents full and complete differentiation of the stratum corneum ending in the release of intact single keratinocytes.

Table 2.1   Causes of scaling

Mechanism	Examples
High rate of epidermal cell production with decreased opportunity for complete differentiation.	Psoriasis, lichenified eczema, some uncommon ichthyotic disorders.
Primary disorder of keratinization or desquamation. There is a failure in a metabolic step for the process of epidermal differentiation leading to failure in the usual loss of binding forces between horn cells.	Most of the common ichthyotic disorders.
Damage to the upper epidermis leading to simultaneous shedding of the stratum corneum and this part of the epidermis.	Scarlet fever, and some unusual conditions such as pityriasis lichenoides.

The size, shape and thickness of skin lesions

When a localized lesion no more than discolours the skin surface, the lesion is known as a macule. If the abnormal area is raised up above the skin surface it is said to be a plaque. The mild fungal disorder known as pityriasis versicolor (page 32) causes macules over the chest and back (Figure 2.7) but the lesions of psoriasis (page 128) are thickened and easily palpable and are called plaques. Sometimes lesions are very considerably proud of the skin and are known as nodules or tumours. If the tumours are connected with the skin surface by a stalk they are said to be pedunculated. Nodules and tumours and pedunculated tumours are all present in the congenital condition called neurofibromatosis (Von Recklinghausen's disease).

The edge of lesions can give some diagnostic help, well-defined edges are especially characteristic of psoriasis and ringworm. Different areas

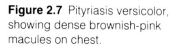
Figure 2.7 Pityriasis versicolor, showing dense brownish-pink macules on chest.

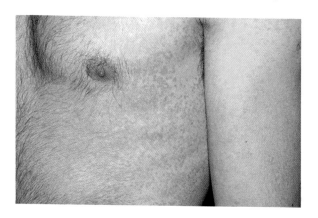

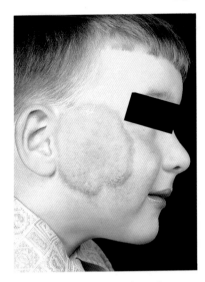

Figure 2.8 Annular lesion of ringworm.

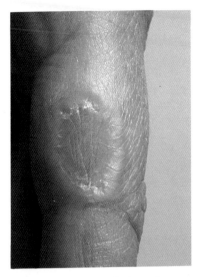

Figure 2.9 Annular lesion of granuloma annulare.

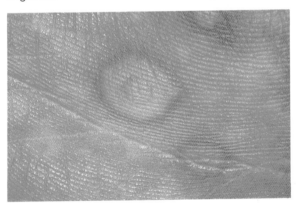

Figure 2.10 Lesion of erythema multiforme showing annular form.

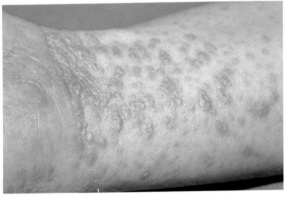

Figure 2.11 Typical lesions of lichen planus on the front of the wrist. The individual papules have a roughly polygonal outline and are mauvish in colour.

where it is difficult to discern where the abnormality ends are characteristic of eczematous disorders.

The shape of skin lesions can also guide one to the correct diagnosis. Some skin disorders start off as macular but clear in the centre, making ring-like or annular lesions. Ringworm, granuloma annulare (page 268) and erythema multiforme (page 69) are three conditions in which the developed lesions tend to be annular (Figures 2.8–2.10). Some skin disorders often produce oval lesions, pityriasis rosea being the best example of this tendency. Occasionally lesions assume bizarre patterns on the skin surface that almost seem to be representing a particular pattern or symbol. This is termed figurate, and many disorders, including psoriasis, may produce such lesions. For the most part skin lesions are not usually angular and do not form squares or triangles. One condition, however, lichen planus (page 142), does produce small

> Some skin disorders start off as macular but clear in the centre, making ring-like or annular lesions. Ringworm, granuloma annulare and erythema multiforme are three conditions in which the developed lesions tend to be annular.

9

lesions that seem to have a roughly polygonal outline (Figure 2.11).

In some instances lesions such as plaques or tumours infiltrate into the substance of the skin and in the case of such malignant lesions as basal cell carcinoma, squamous cell carcinoma or malignant melanoma, the presence of deep extensions of the lesion is important to recognize in order to plan the most appropriate form of treatment. Clinically it is possible for experienced observers to form some impression of the degree of infiltrate present by palpation but the clinical impression gained has to be validated by histological support before any major surgical decision is made. There is some hope that noninvasive assessment techniques such as ultrasound will be better able to guide the surgeon than clinical examination alone.

> Clinically it is possible for experienced observers to form some impression of the degree of infiltrate present by palpation but the clinical impression gained has to be validated by histological support before any major surgical decision is made. There is some hope that non-invasive assessment techniques such as ultrasound will be better able to guide the surgeon than clinical examination alone.

Oedema, fluid-filled cavities and ulcers

When a tissue contains excess water both within and between its constituent cells it is said to be affected by oedema. Oedema fluid may collect because of inflammation, when it is protein rich and known as an exudate, or as a result of haemodynamic abnormalities, when it is known as a transudate. Oedema is a common feature of inflammatory skin disorders and accounts for the swelling seen in such conditions as acute allergy, contact dermatitis or erythema multiforme. Oedema may be the predominant clinical feature in the conditions of urticaria and dermographism (page 67) in which localized areas of pink, swollen skin, known as weals, occur, lasting for several hours (Figure 2.12).

> Oedema is a common feature of inflammatory skin disorders and accounts for the swelling seen in such conditions as acute allergy, contact dermatitis or erythema multiforme. Oedema may be the predominant clinical feature in the conditions of urticaria and dermographism.

> Blisters may form within or beneath the epidermis. Small intra epidermal blisters (vesicles) are characteristic of eczema.

Oedema fluid collects within tiny tissue cavities within the epidermis known as vesicles (Figure 2.13); these lesions are characteristic of eczematous disorders and are usually 1 mm in diameter or less. Larger

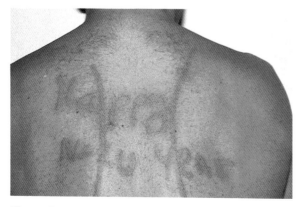

Figure 2.12 Dermographic wheals.

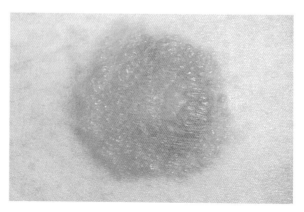

Figure 2.13 Vesicles in eczema from patch test.

Figure 2.14 (a) Bullous lesion in senile pemphigoid. (b) Numerous bullae in groin in patient with pemphigus.

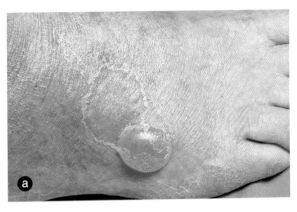

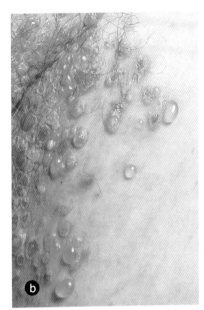

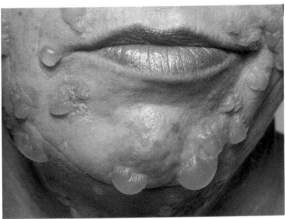

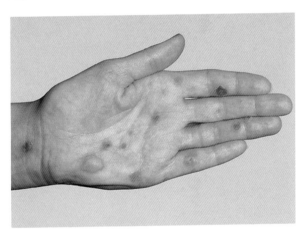

Figure 2.15 Vesicles in dermatitis herpetiformis.

Figure 2.16 Bullae of palm in erythema multiforme.

fluid-filled cavities are called bullae (blisters). These may form by fluid collecting beneath the epidermis (subepidermal) in which case their walls tend to be tough and the captured blister fluid may be blood-stained, or they may form by separation or breakdown of epidermal cells (intraepidermal) when the walls tend to be thin, flaccid and fragile. Subepidermal bullae form in bullous pemphigus, dermatitis herpetiformis and erythema multiforme (Figure 2.14–2.16) (Chapter 6). Intradermal bullae form in the different types of pemphigus (page 87) and herpes virus infections (page 45) (Figure 2.17 and 2.18).

An erosion is any breach of the epidermis. The term ulcer is used to denote a broad and deep erosion that persists. Erosions may be covered by serous exudate or crust; ulcers tend not to be covered.

11

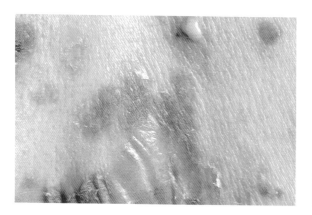

Figure 2.17 Flacid bullae in pemphigus.

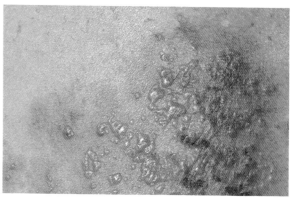

Figure 2.18 Vesicles in herpes zoster.

Secondary changes

> Secondary changes are superimposed on primary spontaneously arising skin lesions and are due to scratching and infection.

Secondary changes are superimposed on primary spontaneously arising skin lesions. They include (1) impetiginization – due to a bacterial infection of the affected skin resulting in exudation and golden-yellow crusting (Figure 2.19), (2) lichenification – the result of constant rubbing and scratching causing thickening of the affected skin with exaggeration of the skin surface markings (Figure 2.20) (page 102), and (3) prurigo papules – these are also the result of scratching, but for some reason the skin's response differs and instead of producing lichenification, variably sized inflamed papules and even quite large nodules appear (Figure 2.21).

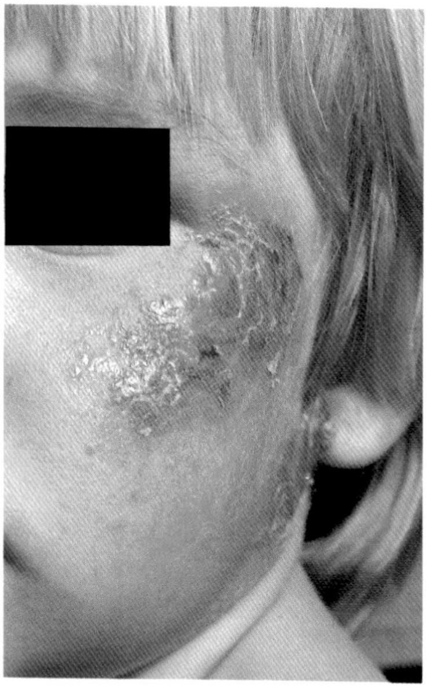

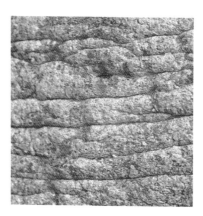

Figure 2.19 Impetigo contagiosa showing exudation and golden-yellow crusting.

Figure 2.20 Lichenification showing scaling and accentuation of skin markings.

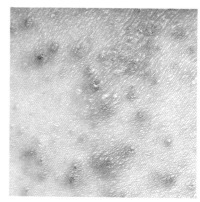

Figure 2.21 Excoriated papules in prurigo.

Symptoms of skin disorder

Skin disease causes pruritus (itching), pain and soreness and discomfort, difficulty with movements of the hands and fingers, and cosmetic disability.

Pruritus

Itching is the classic symptom of skin disorders but it may occur in the apparent absence of skin disease (page 297). Any skin abnormality can give rise to irritation, but some seem particularly able to cause severe pruritus. Scabies is also characterized by severe and persistant irritation. Some patients complain of a 'burning' sensation to their irritation quite unlike other types of itching that they have experienced. Most scabies patients complain that their symptom of itch is much worse at night, but this is probably not specific to this disorder as many patients with itching from numerous other conditions complain that it is worse at night when they get warm. Itching in atopic dermatitis, senile pruritus, senile xerosis and several other eczematous disorders are made worse by repeated bathing and vigorous towelling afterwards, as well as by central heating and air conditioning with low relative humidity. If pruritus is worsened by aspirin or food additives such as tartrazine, sodium benzoate or the cinnemates it is quite likely that urticaria is to blame. Uncommonly urticaria may be induced and pruritus develop after exposure to a variety of physical stimuli such as cold, pressure, the sun and water.

Determining the cause of pruritus is usually only a problem when there is no obvious skin disorder present. Unfortunately, providing relief from this symptom is much less straightforward than reaching a diagnosis, and persistent severe pruritus can be the most disabling and distressing symptom to have. The act of scratching provides partial and transient relief from the symptom and it is fruitless to ask or even demand that the patient stop scratching. Scratching itself causes damage to the skin surface visible as scratch marks (excoriations). In some patients the repeated scratching and rubbing causes lichenification and in others prurigo papules occur (see above). Occasionally the scratch marks become infected. Uncommonly the underlying disorder occurs at the site of the injury from the scratch. The phenomenon is found in patients with psoriasis and lichen planus and is known as the isomorphic response or the Koebner phenomenon.

> Itching is the classic symptom of skin disorders but may occur in the apparent absence of skin disease.

> Persistent severe pruritus can be the most disabling and distressing symptom to have.

> In some patients the repeated scratching and rubbing causes lichenification and in others prurigo papules occur.

Painful skin disorders

The large majority of skin disorders do not give rise to pain. The notable exception to this is shingles (herpes zoster) which may cause pain and distorted sensations in the nerve root involved (page 47). The pain may be present before the skin lesions appear, while they are there, and occasionally for some considerable time afterwards in the skin innervated by the affected sensory nerve root. Pain and tenderness are characteristic of acutely inflamed lesions, especially if tissue tension is rapidly increased. Boils, acne cysts, cellulitis and erythema nodosum (page 71) are examples of localized inflamed painful lesions that are tender to palpation. Most skin tumours are not painful, at least until they enlarge and infiltrate nerves. However, there are some uncommon benign tumours which cause pain, including the benign vascular tumour known as the glomus tumour (page 198) and the benign tumour of plain muscle known as the leiomyoma.

Chronic ulcers are often 'sore' and the cause of a variety of other discomforts, but they are not often the cause of severe pain. When they do give rise to severe pain ischaemia is usually the cause. Pain is also the result of chronic eczema or psoriasis affecting the palms, soles or fingers. The abnormal horny layer produced by the diseased epidermis is not as flexible as normal and cracks, causing fissures, when the area is moved. These fissures are very painful and are themselves the cause of considerable disability.

Disabilities from skin disease

> A very major cause of disability is the abnormal appearance of the affected skin. For reasons that are not altogether clear there is a primitive fear of diseased skin which even amounts to feelings of disgust and repulsion.

The degree of disability experienced by subjects with skin disease is rarely appreciated by others unless they have first-hand knowledge of the many problems that may affect such patients. A very major cause of disability is the abnormal appearance of the affected skin. For reasons that are not altogether clear there is a primitive fear of diseased skin which even amounts to feelings of disgust and repulsion. The idea of touching skin that is scaling or exudative seems inherently distasteful and something that one tries to avoid. These attitudes appear universal and inherent, and it is difficult to prevent them. It is little use pointing out that there is no rational basis for these attitudes and all that can be hoped for is that a mixture of comprehension, compassion and common sense eventually supplants the primitive revulsion felt by all. It has been suggested that the origins of the inherent fear described above are the contagious nature of leprosy and the infestations of scabies and lice. Indeed the problem is sometimes referred to as the 'leper complex'. Regardless of the origins it is only too abundantly evident that individuals with obvious skin disease do not do well where the choice of others is concerned. They suffer more unemployment overall but in addition find great difficulty in obtaining positions which require any kind of interpersonal relationships. Young patients with acne have particular problems because the disease is only too visible as it usually affects the face. Psoriasis quite often affects the hands, nails and scalp margin, also causing difficulty for those whose occupation takes them into contact with the public. The disorder of leprosy may cause severe visible deformities and although patients are at a safe and inactive phase they suffer discrimination.

Numerous other skin disorders put the affected individual at an economic and social disadvantage. Vascular birth marks, for example, and pendulous, large, benign neurofibromata are disfiguring and tend to isolate the bearers of these congenital malformations. Chronic inflammatory skin disorders of the face also fall within this category and

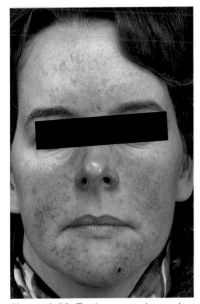

Figure 2.22 Erythema and papules of the cheek in rosacea.

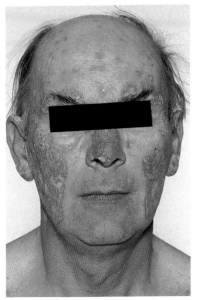

Figure 2.23 Plaques of erythema, scaling and hyperkeratosis in a man with discoid lupus erythematosus.

rosacea (Chapter 10) and chronic discoid lupus erythematosus (Chapter 6) (Figures 2.22 and 2.23) are two such conditions. To summarize this point, individuals with visibly disordered skin are disabled because of society's inherent tendency to fear, isolate and even ostracise such persons. One other aspect of this same problem is the sufferer's own perception of the impact he or she is making on all with whom they come in contact. In most subjects who have persistent 'unsightly' skin problems, the affected individuals become depressed and isolated. It is especially damaging for those in their late 'teens and twenties who are desperately trying to make relationships. Self confidence is anyway not at a high point at this time in their emotional development and a disfiguring skin disorder lowers their self esteem incalculably. Many youngsters with acne and psoriasis find it difficult to conquer their embarassment sufficiently to have 'girl-' or 'boyfriends' and that aspect of their development may become stunted. It was once thought that many skin disorders were caused by neurotic traits, 'stress' and personality disorders. It is now increasingly appreciated that skin disorder often causes depression, anxiety and stress, so that the wheel has turned full circle.

> Individuals with visibly disordered skin are disabled because of society's inherent tendency to fear, isolate and even ostracize such persons.

> Inflammatory skin conditions of the palms and soles prevents full use of these areas and can be extremely disabling.

Skin disease can be enormously disabling when it affects the palms or soles. Although the areas only occupy some 1 to 2% of the body's skin surface, when the skin of these sites is affected it may prevent the patient concerned from walking and using their hands for anything but the simplest of tasks, i.e. they are virtually completely disabled. Psoriasis and eczema are the usual causes of this form of disablement. As mentioned previously the abnormal horn produced by these chronic inflammatory skin disorders is less flexible than the normal stratum corneum and when attempts are made to move the affected parts, splitting occurs, producing painful fissures (Figure 2.24). Occasionally patients with a severe atopic dermatitis may develop similar painful fissures around the popliteal and antecubital fossae, so that movements of the arms and legs become extremely painful (Figure 2.25). Patients with severe congenital disorders of keratinization are often severely troubled by this disordered mobility.

Patients with generalized skin disorders are also prone to a variety of functional problems, but these are dealt with in Chapter 19. Suffice it to say at this point that patients with universal erythroderma or whose skin disorder occupies more than 75% of the body surface may suffer from severe systemic consequences.

From what has been said so far it will be appreciated that contrary to popular belief, patients with quite complex skin disorders are often appreciably disabled. They are disabled on account of society's and their own reaction to the disease and because of the physical limitations that the skin disease puts on them. Skin disease infrequently kills, but often produces unhappiness, usually loss of work and social deprivation as well as considerable physical discomfort.

> Skin disease infrequently kills, but often produces unhappiness, usually loss of work and social deprivation as well as considerable physical discomfort.

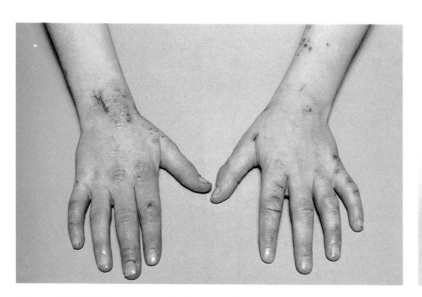

Figure 2.24 Skin fissures in atopic dermatitis.

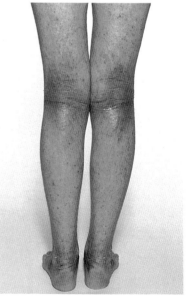

Figure 2.25 Painful fissures in popliteal fossae in atopic dermatitis.

3

Skin damage from environmental hazards

A major function of skin is its capacity to protect against damage from the environment to the vulnerable tissues of the body. All parts of the skin contribute to its role as protector. The stratum corneum is a remarkably efficient barrier, protecting against water loss from the body's tissues to a dry exterior as well as preventing flow in the reverse direction when body parts are immersed in water. The same structure prevents (or at least greatly impedes) the passage of toxic substances from the environment into the body. It also contributes to protection against solar ultraviolet irradiation and against heat injury. In addition it contributes to the mechanical protectivity of the skin as a whole (see later).

> The stratum corneum is a remarkably efficient barrier, protecting against water loss from the body's tissues, preventing the entry of toxic substances and giving mechanical protection.

The vasculature is vital to the maintenance of a constant body temperature. Vasodilatation and vasoconstriction enable body heat to be lost to the environment or conserved, respectively. The sweat glands, the hair, and the subcutaneous fat are other parts of the skin which assist in the maintenance of a constant body temperature in the face of an environment with a widely variable ambient temperature. The evaporation of sweat cools the skin and causes heat loss. The subcutaneous fat and body hair helps insulate the skin and conserve heat.

Protection against ultraviolet radiation (UVR) from the sun is provided by melanin pigment generated by melanocytes (Chapter 22) (Figure 3.1). Synthesis of melanin is stimulated by exposure to sunlight

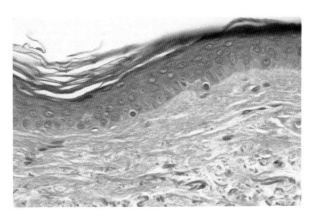

Figure 3.1 Photomicrograph of normal skin showing melanocytes, identifiable as so-called 'clear cells' in the basal layer.

so that exposed skin develops a brownish 'sun tan'. The pigment produced by this mechanism absorbs the ultraviolet radiation and protects the keratinocytes and other cells in the skin from the damaging effects of this type of radiation. Some protection against UVR is also given by the stratum corneum.

We are subjected to a constant barrage of mechanical stimuli of all types. They vary widely in intensity, direction and rate of delivery as well as in area of skin contact over which the stimulus is delivered. The dermis contains a connective tissue network of orientated tough collagenous fibres, the interstices of which are filled with a viscid proteoglycan containing ground substance, elastic fibres and fibroblasts. This dermal connective tissue confers important biomechanical characteristics to skin, in fact most of the way in which skin responds to mechanical stimuli is on account of this dermal connective tissue. Overall, the mechanical properties can be described as 'viscoelastic', signifying that skin both extends in response to a linear force and will tend to regain its original length after release of this force (elastic), and 'flows' and 'creeps' with some mechanical stimuli (viscous). Skin is also said to be anisotropic, as its mechanical properties vary according to the orientation to the body axis in which the mechanical stimulus is made. This anisotropy results from the anatomical arrangement of the collagenous bundles, which varies according to the body part under discussion. The different arrangements result in different resting tensions and the fact that scars tend to be broad and ugly if incisions are made across the main orientation of the collagen fibres rather than parallel to it. Langer's lines were an early attempt at portraying the directions of resting tension in skin. It is now recognized that there are additional local considerations specific to the anatomical region as to where to position a surgical incision.

The responses to a mechanical stimulus are also 'time dependent', that is, they vary with the rate of delivery of the stimulus. Mechanical function also depends on the 'stress history' of the part – recent stress history being more important than distant events.

The most superficial layer of skin – the stratum corneum – also has a mechanical protective function. Without its comparatively tough covering we would be much more vulnerable to the attentions of biting and stinging arthropods as well as a multitude of other minor scratches and pricks.

> The dermis contains a connective tissue network of orientated tough collagenous fibres, the interstices of which are filled with a viscid proteoglycan containing ground substance, elastic fibres and fibroblasts.

> Most of the way skin responds to mechanical stimuli is on account of dermal connective tissue. Overall, the mechanical properties can be described as "viscoelastic". They are also time-dependent and anisotropic.

Damage caused by toxic substances

Skin comes into contact with an enormous variety of chemical substances, some of which are more or less innocuous, and others frighteningly damaging. We will not spend much time here discussing the problem of systemic absorption of toxic agents but it should be noted that some substances used in treatment, when applied to the skin, such as corticosteroids, podophyllin and salicylic acid, can penetrate the stratum corneum barrier in sufficient amounts to cause

> Some substances used in treatment, when applied to the skin, such as corticosteroids, podophyllin and salicylic acid, can penetrate the stratum corneum barrier in sufficient amounts to cause systemic toxicity.

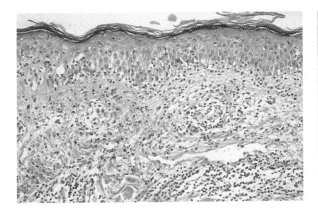

Figure 3.2 Photomicrograph showing inflammation, with inflammatory cells in the dermis and epidermis and oedema (spongiosis) of the epidermis.

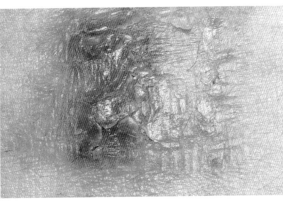

Figure 3.3 Severe irritant dermatitis caused by sodium lauryl sulphate, showing crusting.

systemic toxicity. Detergents, alkaline soaps and lubricating oils and greases are some of the substances that, by repeated contact, may cause damage to the skin. They damage and penetrate the stratum corneum and then irritate the epidermis, causing a dermatitis (Chapter 8). Some of the damage to the horny layer is due to the removal of complex lipids and glycoproteins from between the constituent horn cells of this structure.

Although toxic substances are capable of injuring all who come into contact with them, there are some who are very sensitive to their effects and others who are relatively resistant. In general, more heavily pigmented subjects are more resistant to this form of injury by irritants. Fair-skinned subjects, especially those with reddish hair, blue eyes and pinkish skin (people of Celtic origin in particular), tend to be much more sensitive. The basis of these differences is not clear but it is interesting to note that sensitivity to chemical irritants parallels the sensitivity to solar ultraviolet irradiation. The dermatitis that results is an inflammatory response to the mild injury produced and is characterized by oedema and the presence of inflammatory cells (Figure 3.2).

More vigorous injury from corrosive substances such as acids and alkalis may cause superficial erosions (Figure 3.3) and even deep ulcers.

> In general, more heavily pigmented subjects are more resistant to injury by irritants. Fair-skinned subjects – especially those with reddish hair, blue eyes and pinkish skin (people of Celtic origin in particular) – tend to be much more sensitive.

> Apart from dermatitis contact with chemical agents may cause erosion and/or blistering, a form of acne or an abnormality of pigmentation.

Less common toxicities

Corrosive injury

Some agents cause blistering when they come into contact with the skin and are sometimes called vesicants on account of this. One source of 'vesicant' is from 'blister beetles' which when crushed release a highly

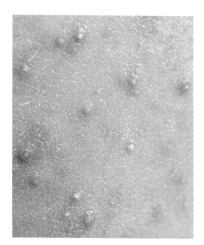

Figure 3.4 Acne lesions induced by cosmetic preparations.

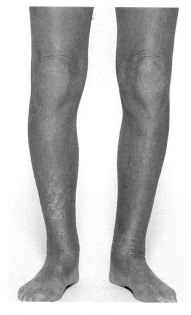

Figure 3.5 Postinflammatory hyperpigmentation from irritant dermatitis.

The ultraviolet portion of radiation (UVR) runs from 250–400 nm and is of great importance biologically.

irritant group of chemicals. One of these is cantharidin, sometimes known as 'Spanish fly', which has unjustifiably (and dangerously) gained the folk reputation of being an aphrodisiac. One other major category of vesicants is the category of chemical agents known as the mustards. These are alkylating agents having the property of cross-linking DNA and so preventing cell division. Unfortunately blisters, erosions and burns are still seen from contact with these chemicals as they have been used recently as chemical warfare agents.

Acneiform response

Thick oily materials sometimes have the property of irritating hair follicle canals, causing the production of a plug of sticky horn (blackhead or comedo) (page 147) which may result in an acne type of inflammation in the follicle. Cocoa butter and paraffin waxes are amongst such 'comedogenic' substances; lubricating and cutting oils can also be responsible. These special forms of acne seem to occur mainly in predisposed individuals after the use of cosmetics containing these materials and in workers (machine, tool workers, mechanics) who come into contact with oils industrially. The response that develops differs from ordinary acne only by virtue of the site in which it occurs (the sites of contact only in oil or cosmetic acne) and the comparative uniformity of lesions in the oil-induced condition (Figure 3.4).

Pigmentary disorders from toxic substances

Some materials have the ability to injure the pigment-producing cells (melanocytes), causing depigmentation. The white patches that result closely resemble spontaneously occurring vitiligo (page 300). Substances used in the rubber industry are notorious in this respect – particularly one known as *para*-tertiary butyl-phenol, which is used as a rubber additive. Depigmentation can also occur as a temporary phenomenon after an area of irritant dermatitis or other inflammatory dermatosis has subsided. More commonly, hyperpigmentation develops following skin inflammation, and this may be long lasting (Figure 3.5). This is on account of the hyperpigmentation resulting from the melanin pigment being released from injured keratinocytes and dropping off into the dermis where it is engulfed by macrophages as in a tattoo.

Injury from solar ultraviolet irradiation

The sun emits a continuous band of energy over a wide range of wavelengths, but only the radiation on either side of the visible part of the spectrum interests us in this chapter (Figure 3.6). The ultraviolet portion of radiation (UVR) runs from 250 to 400 nm and is of great importance biologically. It is conventionally divided into three wavebands, UVA (320–400 nm), UVB (280–320 nm) and UVC (250–280 nm) – the long, medium and short wave portions of UVR, respectively. The short wave portion is of little biological importance at the moment

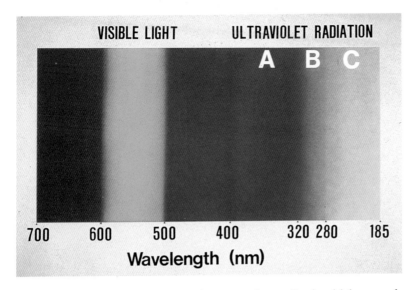

VISIBLE LIGHT   **ULTRAVIOLET RADIATION**

A B C

700   600   500   400   320 280   185

Wavelength (nm)

Figure 3.6 Solar spectrum to show visible light and ultraviolet radiation (UVR). The UVR is divided into three portions: (a) long wave UVR, (b) medium wave UVR, and (c) short wave UVR.

as most of it is filtered out by the ozone layer. It should be noted, however, that if the ozone becomes seriously depleted, as it seems likely to do because of the increasing concentrations of ozone-destroying manmade chlorofluorocarbons and other gases, UVC could cause very considerable harm to the environment.

> Decreasing ozone concentrations will become more important as increasing amounts of UVR will reach the earth's surface.

The medium wave part of the spectrum (UVB), especially radiation around 290 nm, is mainly responsible for sunburn as well as the much sought-after sun tan type of pigmentation after the acute reaction has subsided. The UVB waveband penetrates the skin only to the bottom of the epidermis and the initial burn reaction is confined to the epidermis, where scattered dead cells can be found, known as 'sunburn cells' (Figure 3.7). The injured epidermal cells release mediators which diffuse into the adjoining dermis causing oedema, vasodilatation and both polymorphonuclear leukocytes and mononuclear cells to collect around the blood vessels. A day or two after the UVR injury the

> Radiation around 290 nm is mainly responsible for sunburn, as well as the much sought-after sun tan.

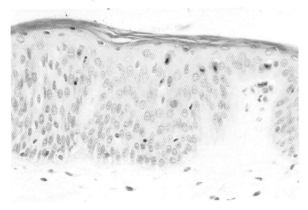

Figure 3.7 Photomicrograph to show epidermis injured by ultraviolet irradiation. There are isolated pink cells in the upper epidermis which show degenerative change known as 'sunburn cells'.

21

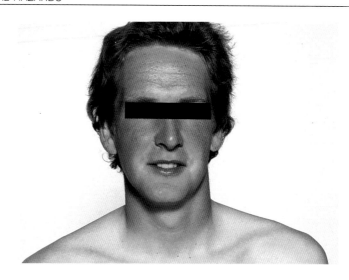

Figure 3.8 Uniform redness of exposed facial skin after sunburn.

Sensitivity to solar UVR depends mostly on the degree of skin pigmentation.

melanocytes respond to the stimulus and start to synthesize more melanin, which is then donated to epidermal cells and causes the well-known golden brown tanned appearance. It is probably not possible to stimulate the tan without sustaining a degree of UVR-induced epidermal damage.

Clinically acute sunburn is easily recognized by the redness confined to the area of skin exposed (Figure 3.8). It is unexplained but interesting to note that the line between the burnt area and the unaffected skin is quite sharply defined. When severe, the affected area may become blistered and swollen. It is often very sore and uncomfortable and when extensive may make the victim feel generally unwell, and if blistered and very extensive may require management as for any sort of severe burn.

An individual's sensitivity to solar UVR depends mostly on the degree of skin pigmentation but to some extent on inherent metabolic factors. Sensitivity is conventionally graded as follows in answer to the question, 'Do you burn or tan in the sun?':

Type I Always burns, never tans
Type II Always burns, sometimes tans
Type III Sometimes burns, always tans
Type IV Never burns, always tans
Type V Brown-skinned individuals of Asian descent
Type VI Black-skinned individuals of African descent

UVA penetrates down into the dermis. It is biologically less effective at causing erythema (by about 1000-fold!) but there is a lot of UVA in sunshine. It is thought that UVA may be important in causing damage to the dermal connective tissue known as solar elastotic degenerative change which is associated with the appearance of aging. UVA is also important because most of the photosensitivity reactions are caused by wavelengths in the UVA part of the spectrum. In addition, UVA contributes to the production of neoplastic disease of skin alongside UVB.

Chronic photodamage (photoaging)

The wrinkling and other changes in exposed skin that are commonly believed to be due to the effects of age are for the most part the results of chronic damage to the skin from solar UVR. They are seen especially but not exclusively in those who spend most of their time outdoors in such occupations as farming, building or military service. These skin changes are also much more intense in the fair-skinned, blue-eyed subjects of north west Europe (types I and II) who sunburn easily. Clearly, fair-skinned individuals who work outdoors in hot sunny climates are especially likely to become extensively sun damaged. However, with the advent of cheap travel, package holidays, glorification of 'the great outdoors' and the obsession with obtaining a sun tan in the post-Second World War years excess sun exposure is commonplace, resulting in unnecessary photodamage.

> The wrinkling and other changes in exposed skin that are commonly believed to be due to the effects of age are for the most part the results of chronic damage to the skin from solar UVR.

> Persistent sun exposure causes normal dermal connective tissue to be replaced by degenerate mechanically inefficient tissue that stains for elastic tissue.

Persistent sun exposure results in both dermal and epidermal damage.

Dermal damage

A particular change takes place in the dermal connective tissue in which the normal fibrillar collagenous dermis is replaced in part by 'chopped up' looking or 'homogenous' looking elastic tissue staining material. This is known as solar elastotic degenerative change and starts in the subepidermal region, progressing to involve the mid dermis (Figure 3.9). The dermal vasculature in the damaged dermis becomes dilated. This abnormal connective tissue has abnormal mechanical qualities which results in wrinkling and the lines around the mouth and eyes (known as 'crow's feet') (Figure 3.10). The abnormal dermal connective tissue also imparts a curious pasty yellow appearance to the skin. The dilated vasculature also accounts for the telangiectasia seen at the skin surface (Figure 3.11) and because of its vulnerability is often damaged, causing purpura ('senile purpura').

In recent years it has been recognized that these degenerative changes in the skin can be improved by the topical use of preparations of al *trans*-retinoic acid – tretinoin, (0.025–0.05%) over some months. Topical isotretinoin and other topical retinoids may also be useful for this purpose. In some way as yet uncharacterized the topical retinoids stimulate the production of new dermal connective tissue.

Epidermal damage

The epidermal damage is the more serious aspect of the condition because it results in precancerous lesions (solar keratoses, page 207; Bowen's disease, page 211) as well as frank invasive basal cell carcinomata, potentially metastasizing squamous cell carcinoma and life-threatening malignant melanomata (page 222).

Figure 3.9 Photomicrograph to show solar elastotic degenerative change. The dermis has lost its normal fibrillar quality and is more basophillic than usual.

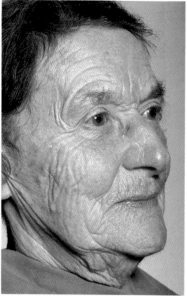

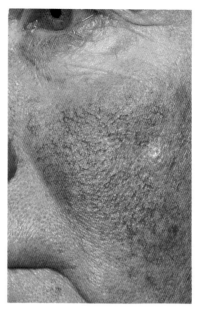

Figure 3.10 Clinical changes of solar elastotic degenerative change, showing marked wrinkling around the mouth and eyes.

Figure 3.11 Solar elastotic degenerative change of the cheek, showing marked telangiectasia.

Prophylaxis

Avoidance of exposure is the best form of prevention but some form of exposure is usually unavoidable in those with outdoor occupations and in those whose recreational pursuits take them outside. The next best aim is to reduce the UVR dose as much as possible in the following ways:

1. avoidance of direct exposure between the hours of 11 a.m. and 2 p.m.;
2. seeking shade wherever possible;
3. the use of 'protective' clothing, including broad brim hats, light but opaque long-sleeved blouses and shirts, and trousers;
4. the use of sunscreens.

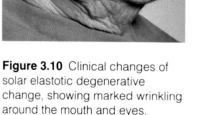

Sun screens now contain substances that protect against UVA as well as UVB.

Sunscreens are creams or lotions that filter out or reflect off the damaging UVR. The older sunscreens only contained substances such as the esters of *para*-amino benzoic acid, the salicylates, the benzphenones and the cinnamates which were primarily designed to absorb and filter out the sunburning 290 nm UVB segment of the UVR, although some do offer slight protection against UVA. The newer sunscreens also contain substances which protect against the longer UVA wavelengths, as it is thought that these longer wavelengths contribute to long-term damage resulting in both the appearance of aging (photoaging) and the development of skin cancer (photocarcinogenesis) (see later). Reflectant substances such as titanium dioxide and zinc oxide reflect off the UVR energy instead of filtering off specific wavelengths, and are designed to protect against both UVA and UVB.

The efficiency of sunscreens is measured in terms of their ability to inhibit UVB-induced sunburn as 'sun protection factor' (SPF) which is a number that expresses the relationship between the time to skin burning without sunscreen protection to that with sunscreen protection, for example, if a cream permits exposure to a UVR source 15 times longer to burning than without the cream, the SPF is 15.

Protection against UVA is more difficult to measure and express. It is thought that UVA protection is best expressed as a ratio of the protection against UVB. This is embodied in a relatively new 'star system', in which four stars expresses the most desirable ratio to one star which is the least desirable.

Further points concerning exposure include:

1. UVR is readily reflected from whitish surfaces such as sand, snow and white walls, and this increases the dose of UVR sustained.
2. A certain amount of UVR 'diffuses' through overcast and cloudy skies, so that it is possible to be burnt on even dull days.
3. The nearer the equator, the more direct the UVR and the easier it is to burn. The higher the altitude of exposure the greater the UVR exposure, so that skiing (with the reflecting snow) can be dangerous.
4. Lighter skinned subjects are more at risk, i.e. ginger or flaxen-haired, blue-eyed, pink-skinned individuals 'who never tan and always burn' – type I subjects – and to a lesser extent, type II individuals. A Celtic ancestry, even in comparatively darker complexioned subjects, usually signifies a marked sensitivity to solar UVR, and there are other exceptions too.

Inflammatory skin disorders caused by ultraviolet radiation (Table 3.1)

Dermatoses precipitated and/or caused by solar exposure

Photosensitivity reactions

Skin may become exquisitely sensitive to a part of the solar spectrum (often long wave UVR) after exposure to a chemical substance that reaches the skin after systemic administration or after topical application. The sensitizing molecule becomes damaging to the tissues after absorbing UVR at a particular wavelength. Such a reaction is termed a phototoxic reaction. Occasionally a molecule may become allergenic after exposure to UVR (photoallergen) and this type of reaction is known as a photoallergic response. Common photosensitizing agents,

Skin may become exquisitely sensitive to a part of the solar spectrum (often long wave UVR) after exposure to a chemical substance that reaches the skin after systemic administration or after topical application.

Table 3.1   Skin disease precipitated, caused or aggravated by sunlight

Disorder	Wavelengths responsible	Comment
Porphyrias	400 nm	Photosensitivity usually visible, mostly active LPP which causes erythema or urticarial patches
Polymorphic light eruption	Mostly the UV part of the spectrum but visible light may be involved	Papular or eczematous rash on exposed areas
Actinic prurigo	Uncertain	Excoriations rash on exposed areas
Photosensitivities	Mostly the long wave part of the UV spectrum	Many drugs and chemicals may cause this
Lupus erythematosus	Varies with patient	Acute attack may be precipitated by exposure
Chronic actinic dermatitis (persistent light reaction or actinic reticuloid)	Variable. Mostly the long wave part of the UV spectrum	May be acutely sensitive to light exposure
Eczema/psoriasis	Unknown	Some patients improve, some are aggravated
Rosacea	Unknown	Most are aggravated

UV = ultraviolet.

Table 3.2   Examples of common photosensitizing agents

Systemically administered drugs
Tetracylines
Phenothiazines
Amiodarone
Nalidixic acid
Psoralens

Topically administered drugs
Halogenated salicylanilides
Psoralens
Tars

both phototoxic and photoallergic, are set out in Table 3.2. The reaction produced is mostly confined to the exposed skin but not necessarily so in the photoallergic type. Phototoxic rashes mostly look like bad sunburn but may become eczematous or start off with blistering.

> The reaction may be due to the toxic effect of the chemical when energized by light (phototoxic) or a hypersensitivity response to a chemical altered by light (photoallergic).

Phytophotochemical reactions are photosensitivity responses that result from contact with plants or their products on areas exposed to the sun. The psoralens and coumarins are the most frequent plant sensitizers. Giant hogweed and meadow grass contain coumarins and psoralens are found in some fruits such as the bergamot.

Chronic actinic dermatitis (persistent light reaction: actinic reticuloid syndrome)

There are a group of patients who appear to start off with a 'photoallergic dermatitis' but who are severely affected and don't seem to be greatly improved by routine methods of light avoidance. Sometimes photosensitivities can be identified, to plant extracts, for example, or to halogenated salicylanilides (e.g. tribromosalicylanilide) used as antimicrobial, but some patients do not improve after all contact with such

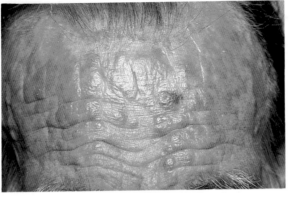

Figure 3.12 Clinical photograph to show thickening and inflammation of the skin of the forehead in actinic reticuloid.

substances has been avoided. The condition is so severe in one small group of subjects that the condition is not restricted to the light exposed areas but affects all parts of the skin. When this is accompanied by severe inflammation and thickening of the skin the condition is known as actinic reticuloid (Figure 3.12)

MANAGEMENT
Some patients are completely disabled in that they cannot go outdoors at all and need to be nursed in a darkened room. Topical agents generally do not help greatly. Some improvement with azathioprine (50–150 mg daily) may be expected.

Polymorphic light eruption
This is a quite common disorder most often seen in young and middle-aged women.

> Polymorphic light eruption and Hutchinson's summer prurigo are uncommon photodermatoses of unknown cause.

CLINICAL FEATURES
Papules and papulovesicles and more uncommonly plaques occur on exposed sites within a day of sun exposure (Figure 3.13). It causes irritation and considerable discomfort. In some patients the sun sensitivity is so marked that they suffer from the disorder throughout the spring and summer months.

PATHOLOGY AND PATHOGENESIS
Patients are sensitive to long wave UVR but the ultimate cause is unknown. Histologically there is quite marked perivascular inflammation in the dermis and eczematous change (Chapter 8).

TREATMENT
Mildly affected patients improve when they keep out of the sun and when using sunscreens to block UVA. Weak topical corticosteroids provide some relief when the rash is present. Severely affected individuals may need systemic treatment with the antimalarial compound hydroxychloroquine (100 mg b.d.) or even azathioprine (50 mg b.d.).

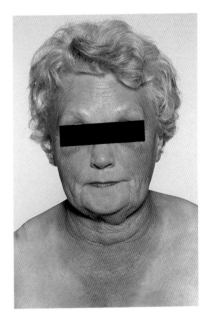

Figure 3.13 Polymorphic light eruption with erythematosus affecting the face and the light exposed part of the neck and upper cheek.

Desensitization with photochemotherapy with ultraviolet radiation of the 'A' type (PUVA) treatment (page 318) for short periods is helpful in some patients.

Hutchinson's summer prurigo (actinic prurigo)

This is an uncommon photosensitivity in prepubertal children and adolescents.

CLINICAL FEATURES
The rash in the light exposed areas looks just like atopic dermatitis (Figure 3.14).

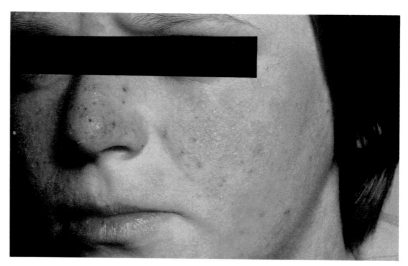

Figure 3.14 Hutchinson's summer prurigo.

TREATMENT
This is similar to polymorphic light eruption.

Porphyria cutanea tarda, variegate porphyria and erythropoietic protoporphyria

These are described in Chapter 17.

The diagnosis of the photodermatoses

There are special tests available to confirm the clinical suspicion of a photodermatosis:

1. **Photopatch tests**: Substances that are suspected of being the photosensitizing agents responsible are placed on sites of the skin of the back and irradiated with broad-spectrum UVR. Control patches without the substances but with irradiation, and patches with the substances but without irradiation are simultaneously applied. The patches are examined for signs of eczema for up to 72 hours after irradiation.
2. **Photoprovocation tests**: These are somewhat specialized and only available at a few centres. A very important test is performed using a monochromator which can supply radiation over very

small parts of the spectrum so that the wavelength dependency of the disorder can be determined.

Sweat rash

Sun exposure is also responsible for 'sweat rash' as a consequence of the heating infrared component of solar irradiation. Actually the term 'sweat rash' is quite nonspecific, and signifies to the lay public any skin disorder associated with heat and sweating. Dermatoses as diverse as intertrigo and folliculitis are sometimes known as sweat rashes.

A common form of sweat rash is that caused by blockage of the sweat gland openings (sweat pores) or the upper parts of the ducts near the skin surface. The most frequently observed is known as miliaria crystallina because of the appearance of numerous tiny delicate vesicles due to blockage of the pore right at the surface. If the pores are more extensively blocked an inflammatory response is produced, with the eruption of red papules ('miliaria rubra'). Rarely, there is deep inflammation within the skin with considerable systemic disturbance (miliaria profunda). The most effective treatment for miliaria is to cool the patient to prevent further sweating, using air conditioning, fans and cold water bandaging if required. For the inflammatory types of miliaria systemic antibiotics and anti-inflammatory agents may be required.

Dermatoses aggravated by solar exposure

Lupus erythematosus is the disorder par excellence that may be aggravated by being exposed to the sun. Rosacea, atopic dermatitis and psoriasis are other skin diseases that are not infrequently made worse by sun exposure. This latter group are particularly difficult to understand because a proportion of patients in each of these disease categories are 'improved' by exposure to UVR.

Cold injury

Injury from the cold is well known as 'frost bite' and chilblains. The former is a form of acute tissue necrosis of fingers, toes, nose, ears or, rarely, elsewhere, which is luckily quite uncommon in times of peace. Chilblains are quite often seen in the UK, but less often in other parts of Europe and the USA, where they can cause diagnostic difficulty. A particular form of damp cold and subsequent warming seems responsible, but all the factors involved in the cause of chilblains are unknown.

Clinically, chilblains afflict anyone but seem particularly to favour plump young women and the elderly. The tips of the fingers and toes are commonly affected but other odd sites such as the thighs, calves and flanks may also develop lesions.

The lesions themselves are raised and dusky red or mauve, and painful and itchy. There are 'traditional' remedies but no certain method to guarantee the elimination of these annoying lesions. Keeping the affected part warm and use of a weak topical corticosteroid is the best one can offer.

Raynaud's phenomenon

This is a common distinctive reaction of the digital arteries to the cold. It is caused by a host of diseases as well as occurring for no discernible reason (Table 3.3). Classically the fingers suddenly go a deathly white when exposed to the cold. After a variable period they go pink and then develop a bluish discolouration – the whole sequence lasting up to 30 minutes or so. The disorder is painful and disabling. It usually recurs every winter for a number of years. If severe it can lead to nutritional changes in the skin and soft tissues with 'tapering' of the fingers and paronychial infections.

The treatment of this disorder should be directed to the underlying cause. If no cause is found ('idiopathic Raynaud's phenomenon') or the cause cannot be removed, symptomatic treatment is required. This entails keeping the hands as warm as possible with the use of gloves (there are special electrically heated gloves available) and the use of drugs. Many drugs have been advocated but few seem to provide major relief. Inositol nicotinate (1.5 g b.d.), Nifedirine (5–10 mg t.d.s.) and oxypentifylline (400 mg 2–3 times daily) are amongst those for which benefit is claimed.

Table 3.3   Some common causes of Raynaud's phenomenon

Systemic sclerosis

Systemic lupus erythematosus

Use of vibratory tools

Carpal tunnel syndrome

Cervical rib

Atherosclerosis

Polycythaemia rubra vera

But in the majority of cases no precipitating cause can be found

Heat injury

The effects of acute burns on the skin are well known and will not be described here.

Chronic heating also causes injury to the skin. Persistent sitting in front of focal sources of heat cause the condition known as erythema ab igne. This is marked reticulate reddish discolouration and brown pigmentation (Figure 3.15). Biopsy shows elastotic degenerative change of the dermal connective tissue. Sometimes keratoses and squamous cell carcinoma arise in these areas (page 207). Chronic heat injury from hot water bottles or from heating pots also causes these problems.

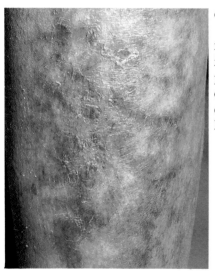

Figure 3.15 Erythema ab igne, showing a brownish reticular network on the leg.

Infection of the skin

The skin surface is an effective barrier against potentially lethal micro-organisms in the environment. It is, however, itself vulnerable to microbial attack and this chapter is concerned with the clinical features of skin infections and the ways of treating such disorders.

The skin surface and its adnexal structures harbour a stable microflora which lives in symbiosis with human skin and may indeed be beneficial to humans. Gram-positive cocci (*Staphylococcus epidermidis*) and Gram-positive lipophilic microaerophilic rods (*Propionibacterium acnes*) live in the follicular lumina and although the use of antimicrobial substances may cause some reduction in numbers it is impossible to remove the normal microflora completely.

The follicles also contain a Gram-positive yeast-like micro-organism – *Pityrosporum ovale* (also known as *Malassezia furfur*). This yeast is for the most part quite harmless, but causes pityriasis versicolor and seborrhoeic dermatitis when conditions are particularly favourable to it.

Infection only takes place when (1) the skin encounters a pathogen and (2) the skin's defences cannot eliminate or control the pathogen. The skin's defences are compromised because of local factors, for example, when the skin becomes hydrated for long periods of time such as during occlusion and the barrier ceases preventing the entry of pathogenic micro-organisms, or because of systemic factors as in acquired immune deficiency syndrome (AIDS), when effective immunological defence is not possible.

> The skin surface and its adnexal structures harbour a stable microflora that lives in symbiosis with human skin and may indeed be beneficial to us. Gram positive cocci – Staphylococcus epidermidis – and Gram positive lipophilic microaerophilic rods (Propionibacterium acnes) live in the follicular lumina.

Fungal disease of the skin

Fungal disease of the skin is divided into the superficial mycoses and the deep mycoses.

The superficial mycoses

Infections with ringworm fungi (dermatophyte infections)
These infections are restricted to invasion of horny structures: the stratum corneum, the nails and the hair.

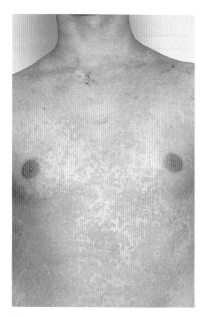

Figure 4.1 Brownish pink macules on the trunk due to infection with pityriasis versicolor.

Pityriasis versicolor

This is caused by the yeast-like micro-organism *Pityrosporum ovale* (*Malassezia furfur*), a normal microaerophilic and lipophilic denizen of the hair follicles and only occasionally pathogenic.

> Pityriasis versicolor causing brownish scaling macules is caused by yeast like microorganisms (Pityrosporum ovale) normally present in hair follicles.

CLINICAL FEATURES

Pityriasis versicolor is a common disorder often seen in young adults. It causes brownish, slightly scaly macules over the front and back of the upper trunk (Figure 4.1). In dark-skinned individuals the affected areas usually appear hypopigmented. The lesions are sometimes prolific and may 'spill over' to involve other areas such as the abdomen and upper arms and thighs. When the disorder resolves, pale patches are left at the sites of the lesions. The disorder is reputedly more common in patients with Cushing's syndrome.

DIAGNOSIS

Skin scrapings should be taken with a blunt scalpel and examined microscopically after treatment for 20 minutes with 20% potassium hydroxide. When positive, a characteristic meshwork of pseudohyphae and clusters of grape-like spores are seen (Figure 4.2). A more elegant and permanent preparation may be made by removing a strip of stratum corneum with a cyanoacrylate adhesive ('crazy glue'). A drop of the adhesive is placed on the slide which is then pressed on to the skin. The slide is 'rolled off' the skin after about 30 seconds and the resulting skin surface biopsy is then stained with periodic acid–Schiff reagent (Figure 4.3). Cultures of the scrapings are pointless because the yeast is difficult to grow and because the significance is unclear as the same

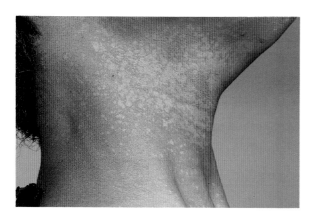

Figure 4.2 Hypopigimented macules on neck of black-skinned subject.

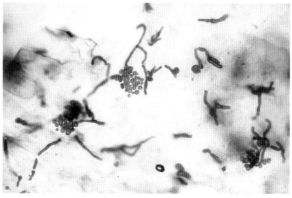

Figure 4.3 Periodic acid–Schiff-positive spores and pseudomycelium on pityriasis versicolor in skin surface biopsy.

micro-organism is also found in normal skin. The patches often fluoresce an apple green under long wave ultraviolet radiation (UVR) (Wood's light).

The disorder is insidious in onset and persistent. After successful treatment recurrences are common.

TREATMENT

The majority of patients respond to a topical imidazole drug such as miconazole, clotrimazole or econazole in a cream formulation. The treatment should be applied once daily for a six-week period. Ketoconazole shampoo can also be used to wash the affected areas daily for a period of five days. Older treatments which are sometimes effective include Whitfield's ointment (a mixture of 6% benzoic acid and 3% salicylic acid in emulsifying ointment), selenium disulphide shampoo and 20% sodium thiosulphate solution. An oral agent itraconazole (100–200 mg per day for 7–15 days) has revently been introduced.

Tinea (ringworm) infections

Three species are responsible for this group of dermatophyte infections: *Trichophyton*, *Epidermophyton* and *Microsporon* species. *Microsporon* species are mainly caught from infected dogs (*M. canis*) or cats or from children infected with this fungus. They cause tinea capitis in children. The common ringworm infections in humans are caused by *Trichophyton* species, particularly *T. rubrum* and *T. mentagrophytes*, and *Epidermophyton* species, particularly *E. floccosum*. Less commonly infections are contracted from farm animals caused by species such as *T. verrucosum* (cattle) or *T. equinium* (horse) and these tend to be much more inflammatory diseases.

> Three species are responsible for dermatophyte infections – Trichophyton, Epidermophyton and Microsporon species.

> Dermatophyte infection is confirmed by direct microscopy or culture of skin scrapings.

Whenever a dermatophyte infection is suspected, skin scrapings should be both sent for culture and examined by direct microscopy. The scrapings for examination by direct microscopy need to be soaked in 20% potassium hydroxide solution for 20 or 30 minutes prior to inspection so as to make the scale more transparent. The thin hyphal forms of the fungus are not always easy to distinguish from debris and practice is required. The skin surface biopsy technique with cyanoacrylate adhesive (as for pityriasis versicolor) is also suitable (Figure 4.4).

Culture may be positive when direct microscopy is not because of the inherent sampling error of microscopy, but it takes at least two weeks before the fungus grows sufficiently to be identified.

Nail clippings and hair samples should be examined in the same way as skin scrapings.

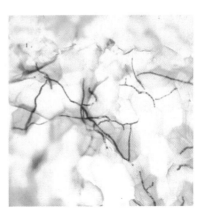

Figure 4.4 Periodic acid–Schiff-positive fungal mycelium hyphae in skin surface biopsy.

CLINICAL FEATURES

Tinea corporis

This is ringworm of the skin of the body and of the limbs. Pruritic, round, red, scaling, well-marginated patches are typical (Figure 4.5). Tinea corporis has to be distinguished from eczema and psoriasis by the history and by the presence of fungal mycelium in the scale. Any of the dermatophyte species may cause the disorder but when an animal species such as *T. verrucosum* is responsible the patch tends to be very inflamed, with pustules, and to clear up spontaneously after a month or so.

> Dermatophyte infections cause red sometimes annular scaling patches. Vesicular and pustular lesions may also be seen.

Tinea cruris

Tinea cruris or groin ringworm is very itchy and is for the most part a disorder of young men. Well-defined, itchy, red scaling patches occurring assymmetrically on the medial aspects of both groins are typical (Figure 4.6). These gradually extend down the thigh and on to the scrotum unless treated. *Trichophyton rubrum* and *E. floccosum* are the causative fungi. Differential diagnoses include seborrhoeic dermatitis or intertrigo (page 110) where the rash is symmetrical and does not have a well-defined border, and flexural psoriasis in which there are usually lesions elsewhere (page 125).

Tinea pedis

Ringworm infection of the feet may be.

1. vesicular, with itchy vesicles occurring on the sides of the feet on a background of erythema;
2. plantar, in which the sole is red and scaling; or
3. interdigital, in which the skin between the fourth and fifth toes in particular is scaling and macerated.

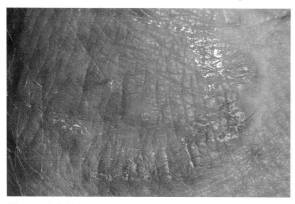

Figure 4.5 Well demarcated scaling patch due to ringworm.

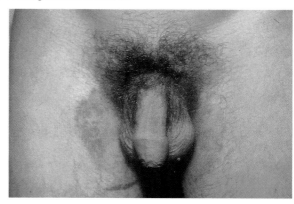

Figure 4.6 Ringworm of the groins (tinea cruris).

Tinea pedis is very common and particularly so in young and middle-aged men who often seem to contract it from communal changing rooms. It tends to be itchy and is often very persistent. *Trichophyton rubrum* in particular, but also *T. mentagrophytes* and *E. floccosum* cause the infection.

Tinea manuum

This less common, chronic form of ringworm usually involves one palm only. The affected palm is usually a dull red and dry, and there are silvery scales in the palmar creases (Figure 4.7). *Trichophyton rubrum* is usually to blame.

Tinea capitis

Ringworm of the scalp occurs in children exclusively and is mainly due to *M. canis*. It invades the scalp stratum corneum and the hair cuticle (ectothrix infection) causing pink scaling patches on the scalp skin and areas of hair loss caused by the breakage of hair shafts (Figure 4.8). It is easily spread by, for example, the sharing of hair brushes. Infected areas sometimes fluoresce a light green under long wave UVR (the so-called 'Wood's light').

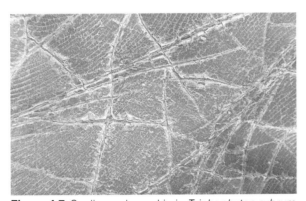

Figure 4.7 Scaling palmar skin in *Trichophyton rubrum* infection of the palm.

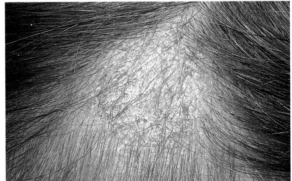

Figure 4.8 Scaling area with hair loss in tinea capitis.

In another variety of ringworm of the scalp, caused by a fungus known as *T. schoenleini*, the fungus invades the interior of the hair shaft (endothrix) and causes an area of intense inflammation on the scalp with swelling and pus formation with eventual scarring.

Tinea unguium

This condition is due to ringworm infection of the nail plate and the nail bed. The fungi responsible are usually *T. rubrum*, *T. metagrophytes* or *E. floccosum*. Infected nail plates are usually discoloured a yellowish white and thickened. Onycholysis (page 293) is often seen and subungual debris collects (Figure 4.9). The condition is much more frequent in the toe nails than the finger nails. Tinea unguium has to be distinguished from psoriasis of the nails (page 139) and from the yellow nail syndrome (page 282).

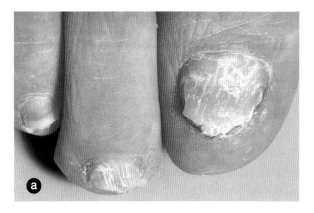

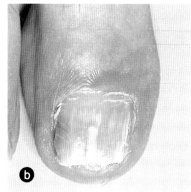

Figure 4.9 (a,b) Thickened irregular toe nails in ringworm infection of the nails (tinea unguium).

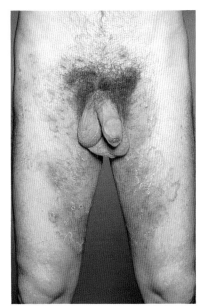

Figure 4.10 Tinea unguium showing extensive and unusual looking infection due to tinea incognito.

Tinea incognito

This is the name given to extensive ringworm with an atypical appearance due to the inappropriate use of topical corticosteroids (Figure 4.10). The corticosteroids suppress the protective inflammatory response of the skin to the ringworm fungus allowing it to spread and altering its appearance.

TREATMENT

For ordinary ringworm of the hairy skin, one of the imidazole-containing preparations (miconazole, econazole and clotrimazole) used twice daily for a two- or three-week period is usually adequate. Topical allylamines such as the recently introduced terbinafine are also very effective. Older preparations such as 'Whitfield's ointment' are not quite as effective and are more irritating.

When multiple areas are affected in tinea unguium or tinea capitis and when topical treatment has for some reason failed, systemic drugs need to be used. These are:

1. Griseolfulvin (500 mg b.d.) which is only active in ringworm infections and which has a low incidence of serious side effects but may occasionally cause gastrointestinal disturbances and photosensitivity.
2. Ketoconazole (200 mg daily) which is active in both yeast and dermatophyte infections. This drug should be reserved for patients with severe and resistant disease because of the possibility of serious hepatotoxicity and the occurrence of other side effects including rashes, thrombocytopaenia and gastrointestinal disturbances.
3. Itraconazole (100 mg daily). As with ketoconazole, this is effective in both yeast and dermatophyte infections. Serious side effects are uncommon.
4. Terbinafine (250 mg daily). This is mainly indicated for dermatophyte infections. Serious side effects are uncommon.

These agents are administered for two to six weeks except for griseofulvin which, when given for tinea unguium of the toe nails, may need to be given for 6–12 months.

Candidiasis (moniliasis, thrush)

This frequent infection is due to a yeast pathogen (*Candida albicans*) that may also reside in the gastrointestinal treact and the orifices as a commensal. It is a not infrequent cause of vulvovaginitis in pregnant women, in women taking oral contraceptives and those on broad-spectrum antibiotics for acne. It is also responsible for some cases of stomatitis in infants and the cause of infection of the gastrointestinal tract and elsewhere in the immunosuppressed. It may contribute to the clinical picture in the intertrigo seen in the body folds of the obese and in the napkin area in infancy. *Candida albicans* may also invade the nail plate and may contribute to the inflammation in patients with chronic paronychia. Treatment with the imidazole preparations, topical and systemic, is effective. Oral and vaginal moniliasis responds to preparations of nystatin and amiphenazole as well as the imidazoles. Serious Candida infections respond to systemic fluconazole.

> *Candidiasis* is due to a yeast pathogen (Candida albicans) that may also reside in the gastrointestinal tract and the orifices as a commensal.

Deep fungus infection

There are several fungal species that cause deep and sometimes life-threatening infection. They are much more common in immuno-compromised patients including those with AIDS, transplant patients, those on corticosteroids or immunosuppressive agents and those with congenital immunodeficiencies. Some, such as histoplasmosis, crypto-coccosis and coccidioidomycosis, are widespread systemic infections which only occasionally involve the skin.

Actinomycosis, sporotrichosis and blastomycosis infect the skin and subcutaneous tissues causing chronically inflamed hyperplastic and sometimes eroded lesions. Sporotrichosis may produce a series of inflamed nodules along the line of lymphatic drainage. Deep fungus infections of this type produce a granulomatous type of inflammation with many giant cells and histiocytes as well as polymorphs and lymphocytes. There is often considerable necrosis in the lesion.

Madura foot is a deep fungus infection of the foot and is seen in various countries of the African continent and India. It is caused by various fungal micro-organisms including forms of Actinomycetes, *Nocardia*, *Madurella* and Phialophora. The affected foot is swollen and infiltrated by inflammatory tissue with many sinuses. The infection spreads throughout the foot, invades bone and is very destructive and disabling.

Bacterial infection of the skin

Acute bacterial infection

> Impetigo is a superficial infection caused by staphylococci mainly. Ecthyma is a deeper infection caused by streptococci which can provoke glomerulonephritis. Erysipelas is an acute severe infection due to streptococcus.

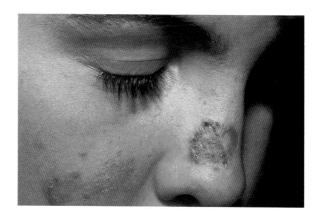

Figure 4.11 Patch of impetigo on the nose.

Impetigo contagiosa

Impetigo is a contagious superficial skin infection caused by *Staphylococcus aureus* in most instances and perhaps by the haemolytic streptococcus in a few cases.

CLINICAL FEATURES

Red sore areas that may blister appear on the exposed skin surface (Figure 4.11). Yellowish gold crust surmounts the lesions which appear and spread within a few days. It is mostly a disorder of prepubertal children. It is, however, not uncommon for the signs of the lesions to appear over an area of eczema (page 107) or other skin disorder such as Darier's disease. The condition is then said to be 'impetiginized'. Impetigo may persist for long periods unless the condition is adequately treated.

In tropical and subtropical areas an impetigo-like disorder is spread by flies and biting arthopods. This disorder is more destructive than ordinary impetigo and produces deeper, oozing and crusted sores and is caused mostly by beta haemolytic streptococci. It is sometimes known as *ecthyma*. There have been several outbreaks of acute glomerulonephritis following episodes of this infective disorder.

TREATMENT

There is controversy as to whether 'ordinary' impetigo needs treatment with systemic as well as local drugs. It is the view of the author that local treatment with some kind of antibacterial wash solution to remove the crust and debris, as well as a topical antimicrobial compound such as betadine or mupiricin is needed in all cases, and that unless the area is solitary and very small (e.g. 1 cm^2) a systemic antibiotic such as penicillin V (250 mg 6-hourly for seven days) is also required. Patients usually respond within a few days.

Erysipelas

Erysipelas is a severe infective disorder of the skin caused by the beta haemolytic Streptococcus.

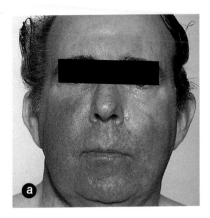
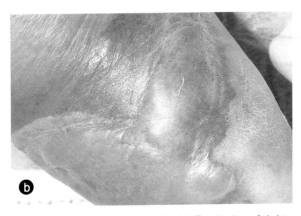

Figure 4.12 (a) Erysipelas of right cheek showing swelling and erythema now resolving following treatments. (b) Severely inflamed erythematous area on the thigh due to erysipelas.

CLINICAL FEATURES

Now an uncommon disorder, this was a common 'killer' in the pre-antibiotic era. There is a sudden onset of a well-marginated, painful and swollen erythematous area usually on the face or lower limbs (Figure 4.12a and b). The inflammation may be very intense and the area may become haemorrhagic and even blister. There is usually an accompanying pyrexia and malaise.

TREATMENT

Treatment with antibiotics by mouth (penicillin V, 250 mg 6-hourly) should be rapidly effective.

Cellulitis

This is a diffuse inflammatory disorder of the subcutis and skin caused by several different micro-organisms and is of variable severity.

CLINICAL FEATURES

It is relatively common, seen particularly on the limbs and often occurs on legs affected by venous ulceration (page 173) or by lymphoedema. There is pain, tenderness, slight swelling and a variable degree of diffuse erythema at the involved sites.

TREATMENT

Broad-spectrum antibiotics are indicated as the micro-organisms may be Gram-negative in type (e.g. *Escherichia coli*) as well as Gram-positive. Cephradine and flucloxacillin (250 mg of each 6-hourly) is one suitable combination.

Furuncles (boils) and carbuncles

Both these lesions result from *S. aureus* infection of hair follicles.

CLINICAL FEATURES

These lesions are much less common now than 30 or even 20 years ago, presumably because of improved levels of hygiene. Nonetheless, there are still families and individuals who are troubled by recurrent boils. In many instances the pathogenic Staphylococcus colonizes the external nares, the perineum or other body sites and is difficult to dislodge. The lesions are localized, red, tender and painful swellings. Furuncles are relatively small and represent the infection of one follicle; carbuncles may be quite large, perhaps 3 or 4 cm in diameter, and represent the infection of several follicles. They may develop pus centrally and when large often produce a pyrexia and toxaemia.

TREATMENT
When there is pus centrally, surgical drainage is indicated. Systemic antibiotics are required but as the Staphylococcus responsible may have multiple resistances the choice is limited and whenever possible should be guided by the pattern of sensitivities found by culture.

Anthrax
Anthrax is due to a rare, potentially fatal infection with a Gram-positive bacillus (*Bacillus anthracis*) causing black scabbed sores and septicaemia. It is spread by farm animals and because the micro-organism has a resistant spore form it can stay on infected land for years.

TREATMENT
The disease responds well to penicillin.

Diphtheria
There is a cutaneous form of this serious, usually pharyngeal infection. It causes large superficial ulcers in tropical zones and is one variety of 'tropical sore'.

TREATMENT
The disorder responds well to penicillin.

Tuberculosis
Tuberculosis is a multisystem disease caused by varieties of the waxy-enveloped bacterium *Mycobacterium tuberculosis*. Several types of skin tuberculosis were once commonly seen but are now quite rare in developed countries. It is now, unfortunately, once again becoming quite common because of the appearance and spread of AIDS. The bacillus can be cultured in special media *in vitro* but grows very slowly. Special stains are needed to detect it in tissue. The Ziehl-Nielsen is the most famous of these and the red stain resists alcohol and acid reagents, giving rise to the colloquial term for tuberculosis of 'acid fast infection'. There are also fluorescent and immunocytochemical techniques which can detect the micro-organism. In addition, extremely light infections can now be detected by a polymerase chain reaction.

> Mycobacterium tuberculosis infections of the skin include lupus vulgaris, tuberculosis verrucosa cutis and tuberculosis ulcers.

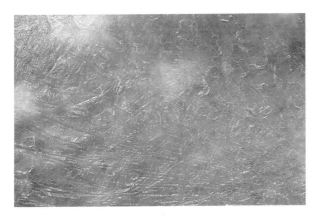

Figure 4.13 Brownish-red plaque due to lupus vulgaris.

Lupus vulgaris

Lupus vulgaris (LV) is a rare, slowly progressive, granulomatous plaque on the skin caused by the tubercle bacillus. It may be present, slowly increasing in size, over one, two or three decades. It often has a thickened psoriasiform appearance (Figure 4.13) but blanching with a glass microscope slide ('diascopy') will reveal grey-green foci ('apple jelly nodules') due to the underlying granulomatous inflammation. There may be (but not invariably) underlying pulmonary, renal or some other form of tuberculosis. Clinical diagnosis is sustained by biopsy showing tuberculoid granulomas. Culture of the Mycobacterium from the lesions is possible but difficult.

TREATMENT
Treatment is initially with 'triple therapy' of rifampicin, pyrazinamide and isoniazid over a two-month period followed by a 'continuation' treatment phase with isoniazid and pyrazinamide.

Tuberculosis verrucosa cutis (warty tuberculosis)

This is seen on the backs of the hands, knees, elbows and buttocks whenever abrasive contact with the earth and expectorated tubercle bacilli has been made. It is not uncommon now in south-east Asia.

CLINICAL FEATURES
Thickened warty plaques are present which are sometimes misdiagnosed as viral warts. Diagnosis is confirmed by biopsy showing tuberculoid granulomata and caseation necrosis. Appropriate staining may also demonstrate the bacilli.

TREATMENT
Treatment is as for lupus vulgaris.

Other forms of cutaneous tuberculosis

1.   A persistent ulcer may arise at the site of inoculation as a 'primary' infection.
2.   An eroded weeping area with bluish margins often develops

where a tuberculous sinus drains on to the skin from an underlying focus of tuberculous infection.

3. Multiple lesions may develop as a hypersensitivity to the tubercle bacillus. These are known as 'tuberculides' and are now very rare. *Papulonecrotic tuberculide* is one of these, in which papules arise over the limbs particularly and develop central necrosis with a black crust. *Erythema induratum* is an uncommon odd disorder whose exact status has been hotly debated and which in many cases appears to fulfil the criterion of being a response to tuberculous infection. It is characterized by the development of plaque-like areas of induration and necrosis on the lower calves and occurs predominantly in young and middle-aged women.

> All forms of tuberculosis and other mycobacterial infections are more common in AIDS patients.

Some other mycobacterial infections

Swimming pool granuloma

Mycobacterium marinum which lives in water causes infection either sporadically or in small epidemics. It is sometimes caught from swimming pools and fish tanks, with a three-week incubation period. It causes plaques, abscesses and erosions on elbows and knees in particular.

TREATMENT

The condition responds to minocycline or a trimethoprim–sulphamethoxazole combination.

Buruli ulcer

Mycobacterium ulcerans is responsible for this disorder occurring in Uganda and south-east Asia. Large undermined ulcers form quite rapidly and persist.

TREATMENT

Drugs are ineffective. Surgical removal is currently the best treatment.

Sarcoidosis

It is a moot point whether this belongs in a chapter on skin infections or not, but recent data suggest that the disorder is in many patients an unusual reaction to *M. tuberculosis*, so there is some justification for its inclusion here. Sarcoidosis is a multisystem disease with manifestations in the respiratory system commonly, the reticuloendothelial system often, the skin not infrequently, and occasionally the bony skeleton, the central nervous and cardiovascular systems. In the skin there are several types described. Multiple reddish purple papules are one of the commonest varieties (Figure 4.14). Deeper nodules and plaques are also seen as are bluish chilblain-like swellings of the fingers, nose and

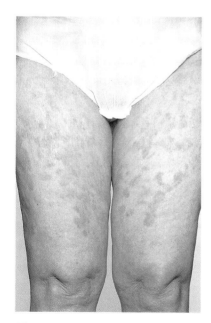

Figure 4.14 Multiple papules and nodules of the skin of the thighs due to cutaneous sarcoidosis.

ears (lupus pernio). These types are infiltrated by typical sarcoid tissue (see below) but another manifestation, erythema nodosum (page 71), is not.

PATHOLOGY

The typical lesion is the 'naked' tubercle which contains foci of macrophages and giant cells without many surrounding lymphocytes. The diagnosis is sustained by signs of sarcoidosis elsewhere and by the presence of depressed delayed hypersensitivity.

TREATMENT

Treatment may not be required if the lesions are not troublesome as they are self-healing, but when large they may leave scarring. For these, systemic corticosteroids or nonsteroidal anti-inflammatory agents may be required.

Leprosy (Hansen's disease)

This is caused by a slow-growing bacillus of the mycobacterial type (*M. leprae*) which cannot be grown *in vitro* although it can be passaged in armadillos and small rodents. As with the tubercle bacillus it is detected in tissue by the Ziehl-Nielsen stain or by an immunocytochemical test. The disease is spread by droplet infection and maybe otherwise by close contact with an infected individual. It is still a serious problem globally, with 1–2 million people affected, mostly in the poor and underprivileged of Africa and Asia, although there are also foci of infection in the USA and Europe.

> Leprosy is still a serious problem globally, with 1–2 million people affected – mostly in the poor and underpriviledged of Africa and Asia, although there are also foci of infection in the USA and Europe.

CLINICAL FEATURES

The pattern of involvement is much dependent on the immune status of the individual. The two extremes are the lepromatous form seen in 'anergic individuals' and the tuberculoid form seen in individuals with a high resistance. Because there are many gradations between these polar types, the range of clinical signs and the corresponding nomenclature has become very complicated. Where the changes are near tuberculoid the term 'borderline tuberculoid' is used; similarly 'borderline lepromatous' is used for lesions that are close to the other type. 'Dimorphic' refers to both types of lesion being present. In tuberculoid lesions nerves are infected which become thickened. The affected areas are well-defined, macular and hypopigmented, as well as being anaesthetic because of the nerve involvement. The anaesthesia results in injury, deformity and disability. In lepromatous leprosy the infection is much more extensive, with thickening of the affected tissue as well as surface changes with some hypopigmentation. On the face the thickening gives rise to the characteristic leonine facies with accentuation of the soft tissues of the nose and supraorbital areas. Where there is resistance few bacteria can be detected in the lesions (paucibacillary types of leprosy). Types in which many bacteria are found and where the patients are anergic are known as 'multibacillary'.

In general the disease can produce dreadful deformity and disability

> The lepromatous form is seen in 'anergic individuals' and the tuberculoid form seen in individuals with a high resistance.

> In tuberculoid lesions the infection infects nerves which become thickened.

> In lepromatous leprosy the infection is much more extensive, with thickening of the affected tissue as well as surface changes with some hypopigmentation.

unless skilfully treated and still evokes great fear in primitive communities. Because the disorder causes patchy hypopigmentation the differential diagnosis includes vitiligo and pityriasis versicolor. Pityriasis alba, a form of patchy eczema of the face in children, and post inflammatory hypopigmentation from psoriasis or other diseases can also give rise to difficulties, especially in districts where leprosy is common.

PATHOLOGY

In tuberculoid types there is a striking granulomatous inflammation with many giant cells and only a few *M. leprae* to be found. In the lepromatous types there are many macrophages that are stuffed with *M. leprae* (causing the appearance of foamy macrophages).

TREATMENT

The treatment of choice is with dapsone (100 mg daily, for periods of a minimum of six months) with rifampicin (600 mg monthly) for paucibacillary types of leprosy. During treatment the patient's condition may flare and deteriorate, causing curious appearances in some, including an erythema nodosum-like reaction and an ichthyosis-like reaction. Multibacillary types should also be treated with dapsone (100 mg daily) and in addition rifampicin (600 mg once monthly) and clofazimine (50 mg daily). Drug resistance is becoming a major problem. If any of the drugs are not well tolerated other drugs, such as prothionomide, may be substituted.

Lyme disease

Lyme disease is caused by the *Borrelia burgdorfii* micro-organism which is spread by the bite of a tick, and has been described in several areas of Europe including the UK, and in the USA. The disorder is multisystem in that there may be arthropathy, cardiovascular and central nervous components, as well as systemic upset. The skin may be involved in the early stages and show an erythematous ring which expands outwards (erythema chronicum migrans). In the later stages of the disease, skin atrophy may be seen (acrodermatitis chronica atrophicans), or fibrosis in a morphoea-like condition. Diagnosis is made by identification of the organism in the tissues or by detection of antibodies in the blood.

TREATMENT

Treatment is with antibiotics – penicillin preferably.

Leishmaniasis

The term refers to a group of diseases caused by a genus of closely related protozoal parasites with complex life cycles which include a time spent in small rodents. They are spread by biting arthropods (mostly sandflies) in tropical and subtropical areas. Some forms cause severe systemic disease and are prevalent in some areas of Africa and South America and the Indian subcontinent: *visceral leishmaniasis*. Others cause predominantly cutaneous or mucocutaneous disease.

44

Cutaneous forms are found around the Mediterranean littoral and North Africa and in South America. The 'Mediterranean' type is caused by *Leishmania major* and *L. tropica*. After an incubation period of about two months a boil-like lesion appears, usually on an exposed site ('Baghdad boil'). Later this breaks down to produce a sloughy ulcer ('oriental sore') (Figure 4.15). This persists for some months before healing spontaneously with scarring and the development of immunity.

Mucocutaneous forms occur mainly in South America (New World leishmaniasis), and are due to *L. mexicana* and *L. brasiliensis*. Small ulcers develop (Chiclero's ulcer) that seem more destructive than the Old World types but also more persistent, and later in the disease destructive lesions appear, affecting nasal mucosa in about half of the patients. The lips, tongue and pharynx may also be involved.

A *cutaneous component to visceral forms* is less common but more extensive and includes a diffuse cutaneous form with many plaques and nodules resembling lepromatous leprosy, a recidivans form with persistent plaques resembling lupus vulgaris, and post kala-azar – dermal leishmaniasis – occurring after the visceral disease and marked by the appearance of numerous small papules.

DIAGNOSIS

This is made with the help of biopsy which shows mixed granulomatous inflammation. The parasites can be identified by special stains and also by culture in specialized media. There is also an intracutaneous skin test (leishmanin) which becomes inflamed after injection in most patients.

TREATMENT

The localized small ulcers heal spontaneously but can be treated by freezing or curettage. Infiltration with sodium stibogluconate has been used. Systemic sodium stibogluconate or pentamidine may also be used for severe and resistant cases.

> *Cutaneous forms* of Leishmaniasis are found around the Mediterranean littoral and North Africa and in South America. The 'Mediterranean' type is caused by Leishmania major and Leishmania tropica.

> *Mucocutaneous forms* occur mainly in South America (New World leishmaniasis), and are due to Leishmania Mexicana and Leishmania Brasiliensis.

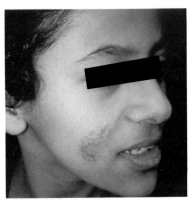

Figure 4.15 Cutaneous leishmaniasis in boy, showing persistent plaque and papules on the skin of the cheek.

Viral infection of the skin

Herpes simplex

This is caused by a small DNA virus of two antigenic types, I and II. Type II herpes simplex infects the genitalia and type I is responsible for the common herpetic infection of the face and oropharynx and less commonly elsewhere.

> Herpes simplex is caused by a small DNA virus of two antigenic types – Type I causing lesions of face and oropharynx and Type II producing genital lesions.

CLINICAL FEATURES

The initial infection may be quite unpleasant with severe stomatitis, systemic upset and pyrexia in infants mostly. Resolution takes place in about ten days. Reactivation of the herpes infection occurs in a proportion of the population at intervals that vary tremendously in different individuals, from annually to monthly. Up to 20% of the population suffer from recurrent 'cold sores', so named because the disorder is often precipitated by minor pyrexial disorders. It may also be precipitated by sun exposure – and this seems to be the explanation for its frequent appearance in skiers. Commonly the lesions occur around the mouth or on the lip. They start as grouped tender and/or painful papules of papulovesicles (Figure 4.16). Vesicles become more prominent and then coalesce to form a crusted erosion. The sequence takes some 7–14 days from initial discomfort to final pink macule marking where lesions have been.

Genital herpes affects the glans penis commonly but the shaft of the penis is another common site. In women the vulval region or labia minora are usually involved but lesions may occur elsewhere on the buttocks or mons pubis. It may occur cyclically with the menses.

The disorder is caught venereally and because of the 'sexual revolution' that has occurred in the past 25 years it has become an extremely common disorder. It is painful and inhibits sexual activity.

PATHOLOGY
The lesion occurs within the epidermis, the vesicle resulting from epidermal cell degeneration (Figure 4.17). Smears taken from the lesion showing degenerate cells may help in diagnosis. The diagnosis can also be made by identifying the virus using an immunofluorescent method with antibodies to the herpes virus.

TREATMENT
Most patients are not troubled sufficiently to request treatment and keeping the area clean is mostly sufficient. Dabbing with surgical spirit or a weak antiseptic will make it sting and is of doubtful efficacy. Idoxuridine is a viral metabolic antagonist which as a 5% lotion can

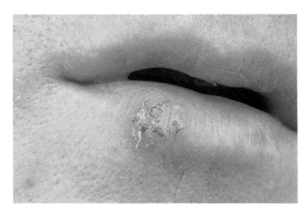

Figure 4.16 Herpes simplex (cold sore) on the lip, with a crust and vesicles.

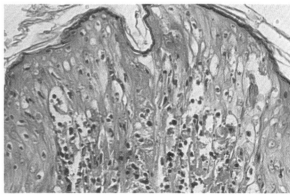

Figure 4.17 Photomicrograph to show extensive vacuolar degenerative cells in the epidermis due to early lesion of herpex simplex.

shorten the disorder if used four to six times per day if the treatment is started on the first day. Acyclovir (5% cream) is the most effective agent for shortening the attack if started early and used five or six times per day. Acyclovir can also be used orally, (200 mg five or six times per day) in severe infections.

Herpes zoster (shingles) and chicken pox (varicella)

The same small DNA virus causes both these disorders which differ only as to the extent of the disease, the symptoms caused and the immune status of the individual affected. Most (but not all) children develop chicken pox (varicella) during infancy or childhood. Reactivation of the virus occurs in a proportion of those previously affected.

> Chicken pox and shingles are caused by the same DNA virus. Shingles is due to reactivation of the virus in someone who had chicken pox previously.

Varicella

This common childhood ailment which is spread by droplets and by the debris from the lesions has an incubation period of about 17 days (14–21 days). There is generally an accompanying fever and malaise. Lesions are common on the face and trunk but less common on the limbs. Papules and papulovesicles give way to pustules which become crusted. After some 7–14 days these drop off, leaving pock type scars in many instances.

Herpes zoster (shingles)

This mostly afflicts those past the age of 50 years but also affects immunosuppressed individuals such as patients with AIDS. It is not 'caught' but is due to the reactivation of a virus that has been 'sitting' latent in a posterior root ganglion of a spinal nerve. Although shingles is not caught from patients with shingles, chicken pox is. If someone without immunity to chicken pox contacts a patient with shingles they may well develop chicken pox.

The disorder often starts with paraesthesiae or pain in the distribution of one or more dermatomes. Involvement of one of the branches of the trigeminal ganglion with lesions in the distribution of the maxillary, mandibular or ophthalmic sensory nerves is common as is involvement of dermatomes of the cervical and thoracic regions. Lumbosacral areas are not commonly affected. The systemic upset, fever and lesions are similar to those seen in varicella but the lesions tend to be more inflamed and are confined to the skin innervated by the dorsal primary root(s) infected (Figure 4.18) although there may be a small number of lesions elsewhere. About 25–30% of patients with shingles continue to suffer from pain and paraesthesiae in the area long after the skin lesions have disappeared. This post herpetic neuralgia can be extremely distressing and disabling.

Figure 4.18 (a) Herpes zoster of axillae and chest wall showing clusters of vesicles and pustules. (b) Herpes Zoster affecting ophthalmic branch of trigeminal nerve involving right side of forehead and eye.

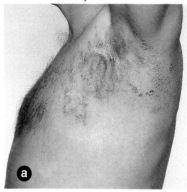

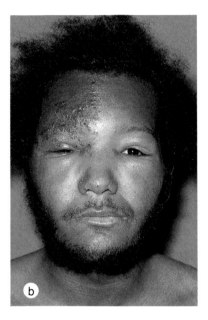

Herpes zoster may occur where there is immunosuppression as in AIDS or a lymphoma. When this occurs the disorder is often very severe and may involve several dermatomes.

TREATMENT
For most children with varicella and most adults with zoster no specific treatment is required apart from keeping the lesions clean and if necessary application of antimicrobial preparations to prevent or combat secondary infection. The drug acyclovir administered by mouth in a dose of 800 mg five times daily (or by infusion) on day one of the disorder shortens the disease and decreases its severity.

Viral warts

Warts are caused by a member of the papilloma virus family, the human papilloma virus, of which there are many antigenic types (Table 4.1). Particular clinical types of wart are caused by particular antigenic types. It is likely that they are caught by direct contact of skin with wart virus-containing horny debris. Genital warts are caught mostly (but not exclusively) by venereal contact. Some perianal warts may be transmitted by homosexual contact or by 'child abuse' but this is by no means invariable.

> Warts are caused by a member of the papilloma virus family, the human papilloma virus, of which there are many antigenic types.

CLINICAL FEATURES
These lesions are so common that they hardly require description! The different varieties are illustrated in Figure 4.19a–g showing hand warts, paronychial warts, plantar warts, mosaic warts, plane warts on the face, perianal warts and genital warts. There are usually little black dots near the surface of the wart representing thombosed capillaries in elongated dermal papillae.

Table 4.1   Human papilloma visus (HPV) types and the common clinical varieties of warts with which they are associated

Clinical type	Most frequent antigenic type of HPV associated
Common warts of hands and fingers (verruca vulgaris)	2, 4
Deep plantar warts ('Myrmecia warts')	1
Plane warts	3, 10
Mosaic warts	2
Epidermodysplasia verruciformis	5, 8 (but many others isolated on occasion)
Genital warts (condyloma acuminatum)	6, 11. (N.B. types 16 and 18 also responsible occasionally, and these are known to be associated with carcinoma of the cervix)
Laryngeal papilloma	6, 11

Plantar warts are painful, some warts are irritating, and all warts are unsightly and 'get in the way' but give rise to no other symptoms. They are a particular problem in immunosuppressed patients (Chapter 7) particularly renal transplant recipients. In one congenital condition plane warts spread extensively on the arms, face, trunk and limbs and some lesions can transform to squamous cell carcinoma. This rare disorder, known as epidermodysplasia verruciformis, seems to have its basis in a disorder of delayed hypersensitivity.

PATHOLOGY
There is epidermal thickening with particular increase in the granular cell layer which also shows a characteristic basophilic stippled appearance (Figure 4.20).

TREATMENT
All warts disappear spontaneously, but may take their time doing so. They may persist for many months or some years. Treatment is in general not very satisfactory and relies on some form of local tissue destruction. The techniques mostly used are cryotherapy (tissue freezing with liquid nitrogen or solid carbon dioxide), curettage and cautery or chemical destruction with topical preparations containing salicylic acid, lactic acid, podophyllin or glutaraldehyde. Popular preparations contain high concentrations of salicylic acid (12–20%) and lactic acid (4–20%) or podophyllin (up to 15%). Podophyllin is a plant extract containing potent cytotoxic alkaloids, one of which, podophyllotoxin, is

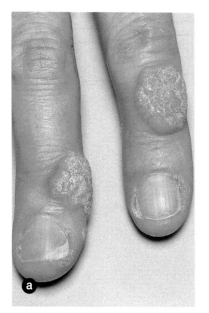

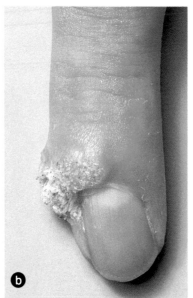

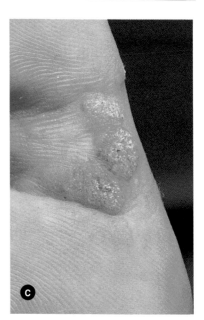

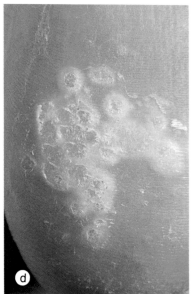

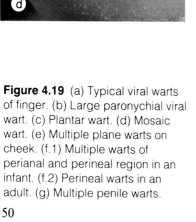

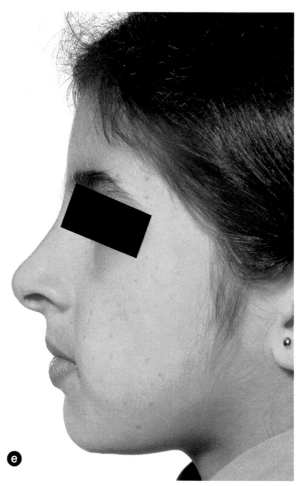

Figure 4.19 (a) Typical viral warts of finger. (b) Large paronychial viral wart. (c) Plantar wart. (d) Mosaic wart. (e) Multiple plane warts on cheek. (f.1) Multiple warts of perianal and perineal region in an infant. (f.2) Perineal warts in an adult. (g) Multiple penile warts.

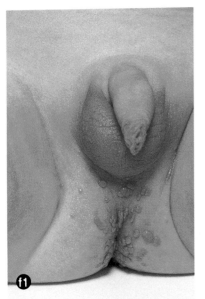

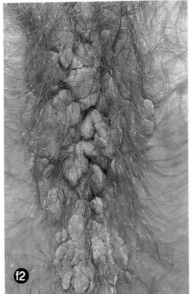

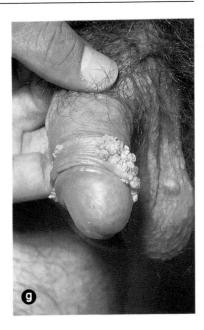

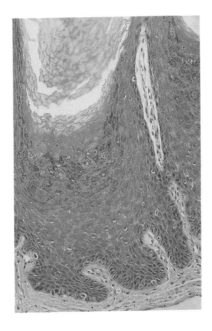

Figure 4.20 Photomicrograph of viral wart showing marked hypergranulosis and vacuolar change in thickened epidermis.

51

also available as a pure preparation (0.5%). Other methods that have been used include intracutaneous injections of cytotoxics such as bleomycin and injections of recombinant interferon.

Molluscum contagiosum

Molluscum contagiosum is a common infection of the skin caused by a virus of the pox virus group. It is transmitted by skin-to-skin contact.

CLINICAL FEATURES

The typical molluscum lesion is a pink- or skin-coloured umbilicated papule containing a greyish central plug (Figure 4.21 and 4.22). There may be one or many lesions. The face and genital regions are commonly involved areas but anywhere on the trunk or limbs may bear lesions.

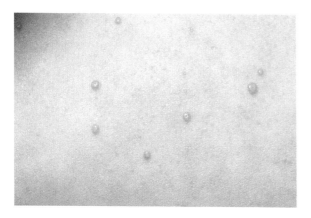

Figure 4.21 Perianal lesions of molluscum contagiosum.

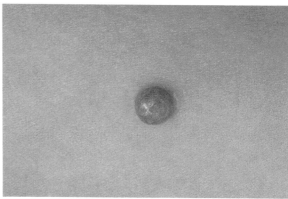

Figure 4.22 Single lesion of molluscum contagiosum showing central plug.

PATHOLOGY

There is cup-shaped epidermal thickening with a characteristic degenerative change in the granular cell layer in which the cells become converted to globular eosinophilic bodies (molluscum bodies) (Figure 4.23).

Figure 4.23 Photomicrograph of molluscum contagiosum showing thickened epidermis with central degenerative change and formation of molluscum bodies.

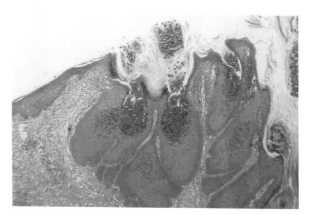

TREATMENT

Mollusca spontaneously resolve within months, but to prevent spread of the lesions to others in the community treatment is helpful. Curettage and cautery, strong salicylic acid preparations as for warts or just plain squeezing the soft centre out (e.g. with a paper clip) will do the trick.

Orf (contagious pustular dermatitis of sheep)

This disorder is caused by a pox-type virus that mostly affects sheep but also cattle. The lesions are solitary, acute, inflammatory and blistering and are mostly on the fingers (Figure 4.24). Following the attack a surprisingly high proportion of patients develop erythema multiforme (page 69).

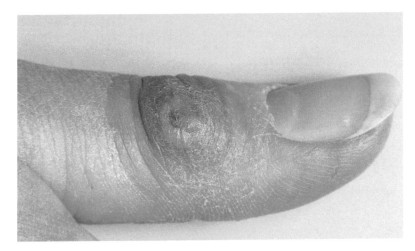

Figure 4.24 Area of orf infection on thumb.

5

Infestations, insect bites and stings

In this chapter we will deal with some of the effects on human skin of the hostile attentions of arthropods such as insects and arachnids as well as some other small invertebrates. It should be noted that the way that the skin reacts depends partially on the extent and severity of the attack and particularly on the immune status of the individual attacked.

Each geographical region has its own spectrum of skin problems due to the local fauna. Although some disorders such as scabies are the same the world over, the pattern and incidence of infestations and bites differs markedly from place to place. In general terms the extent of skin problems due to arthropods and like creatures is directly related to the sophistication and wealth of the society in question. This is explained by the effects of personal hygiene, education, effective waste disposal and prophylaxis on the opportunities for attack.

Scabies

Scabies is due to infestation with the human scabies mites (*Acarus hominis, Sarcoptes scabiei*). The mite is an obligate parasite and has no separate existence off the human body.

> Scabies is caused by Acarus hominis, an obligate parasitic mite, spread by close bodily contact the female of which lives in the stratum corneum.

AETIOLOGY AND EPIDEMIOLOGY

The female mite burrows into the human stratum corneum and lays eggs within the burrow made. The male is smaller than the female and dies shortly after impregnating the female. The symptoms of itch and the characteristic eczematous rash caused by invasion of the scabies mite is the result of the affected individual becoming sensitive to the waste products of the scabies mites within the intracorneal burrows. This generally doesn't happen before one month after the initial invasion of the mite: subsequent infestations cause symptoms and signs within a few days as the individual is already sensitized.

Infestation occurs after close skin-to-skin contact with an infested individual, sexual contact being the most frequent but not the only cause of infestation.

There have been several notable pandemics of scabies in recent history. The most recent of these started in the mid 1960s and ended in the early 1970s, although between peaks of incidence the disorder continues to appear sporadically and in localized mini-epidemics – such as within families or in nursing homes.

CLINICAL FEATURES

The disorder is notorious for the intensity of itch that it causes, even in the presence of relatively minor physical signs. The physical signs are essentially those of eczema with a predominance of the effects of scratching. Vesicles are seen but excoriations are much more frequently observed (Figure 5.1). Prurigo-like papules are also present (Figure 5.2). Scaling, oozing and crusting may also be present in some sites as secondary infection is often present. But the primary lesion is that of the scabies 'burrow' or run, which is a tiny raised linear white mark (Figure 5.3).

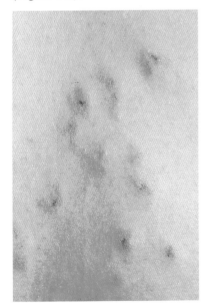

Figure 5.1 Papules and excoriations in scabies.

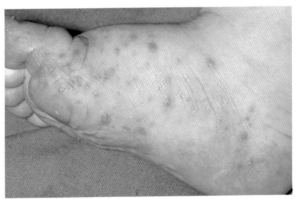

Figure 5.2 Multiple papules and vesicles due to scabies.

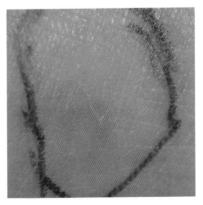

Figure 5.3 Scabies burrow on foot.

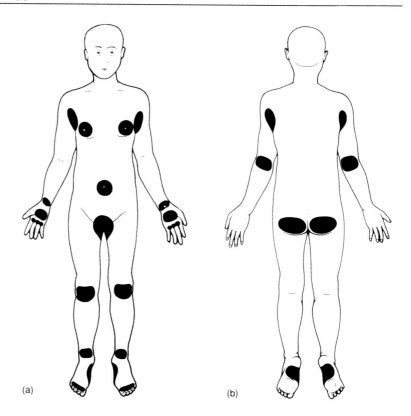

Figure 5.4 Diagrams showing sites of predilection for scabies infestation on (a) the front of the trunk and limbs, and (b) the back of the trunk and limbs.

(a) (b)

The favourite sites for lesions are portrayed in Figure 5.4. It is odd that they should be symmetrical and concentrated in certain sites consistently. The best sites on which to find scabies burrows are the palms and the interdigital areas of the fingers, the flexural creases and over the elbows. Scabies lesions also commonly occur around the anterior axillary fold, the areolae of the breast, the buttock folds, the lower abdomen, the genitalia, the knees and ankles and the soles. Lesions are observed on the head and neck in infants only.

The severity of the eruption depends on the numbers of mites present and this is in large part dependent on the immune status of the individual. In severely immunosuppressed individuals, such as those with acquired immune deficiency syndrome (AIDS) or patients receiving immunosuppressive drugs for renal transplants, the infestation is very heavy and the resulting eruption correspondingly severe. Norwegian scabies is the term used to describe a very severe and extensively crusted version of the infestation seen in the frail elderly and congenitally immunodeficient population (Figure 5.5).

DIAGNOSIS

The diagnosis of scabies is not always easy. It is much helped by finding the burrows of the female scabies mite. This is pathognomonic of the disease and it is important that they can be recognized. They are grey-white linear, slightly raised marks, some 1–4 mm long, and are present on the favoured sites shown in Figure 5.4. The number of

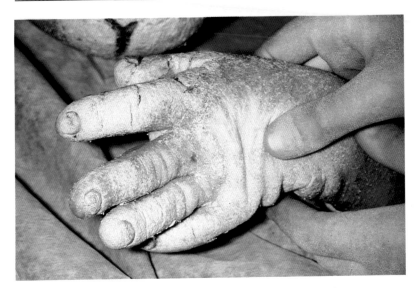

Figure 5.5 Severely crusted eruption due to scabies in immunosuppressed child.

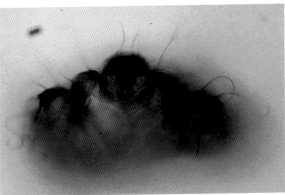

Figure 5.6 Scabies mite seen on microscopic examination of skin surface biopsy.

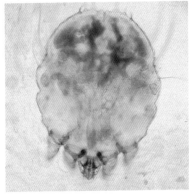

Figure 5.7 Scabies mite seen by microscopy in skin scrapings treated with potassium hydroxide.

burrows present is variable – myriads in severe infestations in the elderly but few in the fastidiously hygienic young.

The diagnosis is confirmed by removal of the mite either with a pin, or by scraping the area with a blunt scalpel to obtained skin surface debris, or by the technique of skin surface biopsy using a rapidly bonding cyanoacrylate adhesive (Figure 5.6). The presence of the mite should then be confirmed microscopically (Figure 5.7). The presence of scabies mite eggs is as important in reaching a diagnosis.

What should be done if the burrows and mites can't be seen? Unfortunately identification of the tell-tale burrows or mite is not always easy, even for the experienced! Perhaps this may apply to 20% of patients in the UK with scabies. In this case a positive family or social history with itching contacts is helpful evidence and in the presence of a compatible clinical picture, treatment should be instituted. Differential diagnosis is set out in Table 5.1.

Table 5.1 Differential diagnosis of scabies

Disorder	Comment
Canine scabies	Different distribution – not transmitted between humans
Eczematous diseases	Particularly atopic dermatitis – usually a history of eczema in the patient or family is present
Dermatitis herpetiformis	Similar distribution! Vesicles and urticarial lesions more prominent – biopsy discriminates
Mechanical irritation by fibreglass	The glass fibres can be found microscopically in clothes
Pediculosis	Presence of lice and nits

TREATMENT

Treatment should be instituted as soon as the diagnosis has been made to prevent the infestation spreading. It should also be offered to all who live with the patient and all other sexual contacts who should use the treatment at the same time as the patient.

The treatments employed are applied to the whole skin surface apart from the head and neck, and are for this reason usually lotions, but creams are also sometimes employed. The patient should be instructed to have a hot bath before applying the treatment. After the treatment no further application or bathing is permitted for 24 hours. A second bath and all-over treatment is advised for benzyl benzoate and Lindane applications. The particular agents used are set out in Table 5.2

Table 5.2 Treatments used for scabies

Agent	Percentage	Comment
Benzyl benzoate	25.0	Irritant to young children
Lindane (gammexane)	1.0	Occasionally irritates
Malathion	0.5	
Permethrin	1.0	New effective agent
Crotamiton	10.0	Claimed to be antipruritic as well
Monosulfiram	25.0	May cause Antabuse (disulfiram) like alcohol reaction

Dog scabies

The mite causing dog scabies is very similar to that causing human scabies but there is marked species specificity and the dog scabies mite does **not** cause the same clinical picture as human scabies. The rash of eczema in the patient or family only occurs at the site on the skin with which the dog has been in contact. Scabies burrows are not found. The correct treatment is to treat the dog and to give any topical anti-itch preparation to the patient for the affected site.

Pediculosis

Pediculosis is the result of infestation with one of the varieties of the human louse. The different varieties cause different patterns of infestation.

Pediculosis capitis (head lice)

Infestation with *Pediculus capitis* is extremely common and seems to be becoming even more common. Although once more often seen in the poorer sections of society, the head louse is now no respecter of social barriers and is seen in long-haired young schoolchildren regardless of the social background. It is nonetheless more common during times of social upheaval. The louse is passed between children by casual contact and by sharing combs and brushes.

CLINICAL FEATURES
Itching is the predominant complaint. The scratching that results can cause secondary infection with exudation and crusting, but if this does not occur all that may be seen are excoriation and red papules on the skin surface.

Examination of the hair will reveal the louse eggs (nits) stuck to the hair shaft (Figure 5.8). Careful inspection will also detect the adult louse itself which on being observed may scuttle off to another hair shaft or disappear 'into the forest'. The louse is less than 1 mm in diameter and greyish, or after feeding, reddish in hue. When it moves it deserves the description of 'mobile dandruff'.

> Pediculosis is the result of infestation with one of the varieties of the human louse. The different varieties cause different patterns of infestation. Head lice are recognized by louse eggs stuck to the hair (nits). It occurs in all social groups.

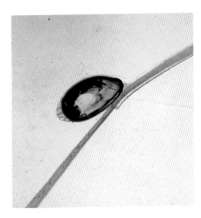

Figure 5.8 Louse egg (nit) on hair.

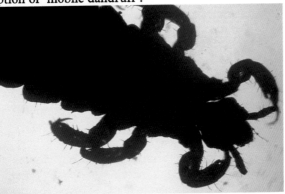

Figure 5.9 Hair louse seen microscopically.

Table 5.3 Treatments for pediculosis capitis

Agent	Percentage	Comment
Lindane (gammexane)	1.0	Resistance to this agent is now common
Malathion	0.5	Both lotion and shampoo
Carbaryl	0.5	Both lotion and shampoo
Phenothrin	0.2	Lotion

Confirmation of the diagnosis is the microscopic identification of the louse (Figure 5.9) or the nits stuck on to the hair shafts.

TREATMENT

The pediculicides used are set out in Table 5.3. The recommended regimen is application to the scalp of malathion or carbaryl lotion for a 12-hour period followed by shampooing with shampoo containing the same pediculicide. Care must be taken to ensure that all close friends and family are also treated. A further treatment one month later is also necessary to kill off all the young lice that may have hatched from nits that remained alive after the initial treatment.

Pediculosis corporis (body lice)

Infestation with body lice is uncommon in modern developed societies but may reach epidemic proportions in times of war or natural disaster. It also occurs sporadically in poor, socially deprived communities where there is poor hygiene. Transmission is via infested clothes or bedding or by close contact with the infested subject. The body louse is responsible for transmission of epidemic typhus which is due to *Ricketessia prowazeki*, as well as trench fever and relapsing fever due to *Borrelia recurrentis*.

The body louse resembles the head louse. It spends most of its time attached to the fibres of clothing, where it and its eggs should be sought if the disorder is suspected.

CLINICAL FEATURES

Itching without a great deal to see to account for the symptom is usual in the early stages. Some excoriations, blood crusts and bluish marks on the skin where the louse has fed may also be seen. Later in the disease, lichenification and eczema complete the picture of 'vagabond's disease'.

TREATMENT

Destruction and/or disinfestation of all clothes and bedding of the infested individual, the individual's family, friends and close contacts must be organized and effected. In many countries there are 'disinfestation centres' where this essential task is preformed. Treatment with one of the pediculicides in Table 5.3 is mandatory. A further treatment after one month is advised.

Pediculosis pubis (pubic lice, crab lice)

The pubic louse (*Phthirus pubis*) looks different to the head and body louse as it is broader, with crab-like rear legs (Figure 5.10). It is mostly spread by sexual contact. The crab lice cling tenaciously to pubic hair, nipping down to skin level every so often to have a blood meal. In heavy infestations the lice spread to body hair and even to the eyebrows and eyelashes! Diagnosis is confirmed by finding the louse and/or its nits.

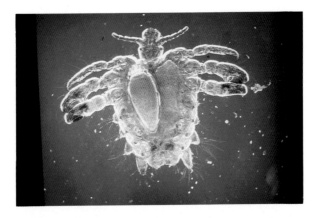

Figure 5.10 Pubic louse.

> Pediculosis pubis (crab lice) looks more crab-like than a body or hair louse and is mostly spread by sexual contact.

TREATMENT

One of the pediculicides in Table 5.3 should be used, with a repeat treatment in one month. Shaving of pubic hair is sometimes advised but is not really necessary. All sexual contacts should be treated.

Insect bites and stings

A vast number of flying, jumping and crawling arthropods are capable of causing injury to human skin. Some are capable of transmitting disease and some important examples of this are given in Table 5.4. The ways in which the arthropods injure the skin varies (see Table 5.5).

Bites from mosquitoes, blackflies, bedbugs and fleas may be quite difficult to recognize and even more difficult to eradicate.

> Bites and stings are usually on exposed areas and are painful or itchy. Diagnosis can be difficult as the possibility of insect bite is often denied and the typical control 'puncture' is not always easily seen.

Table 5.4   Examples of important arthropod-spread disease

Disease	Arthropod	Micro-organism
Malaria	Mosquitos (anopheline species)	Malaria parasite (plasmodium species)[c]
Trypanosomiasis (sleeping sickness)	Tsetse fly	Trypanosoma brucei

Leishmaniasis
  Visceral
  Cutaneous[a]
  Mucocutaneous
	Sandfly (phlebotomus species)	
		Leishmania donovani[c]
		Leishmania tropica[c]
		Leishmania braziliensis[c]

Onchocerciasis	Blackfly (similium species)	Onchocerca volvulus[d]
Bubonic plague	Rat flea	Pasteurella pestis[e]

c) Protozoon
d) Thread-like nematode worm
e) Bacterium

Table 5.5 Examples of methods of injury to the skin from arthropods

Mechanism	Arthropod
Bites from piercing and cutting mouthpieces — injection of saliva	Mosquitos, ticks, sandflies, blackflies
Stings from 'purpose built' structures with injection of toxic materials	Wasps, bees, scorpions, jellyfish
Release of toxic body fluids after being crushed on the skin surface, causing blistering	'Blister beetles' — cantharidin

Mosquitos

Mosquito bites tend to be on exposed areas but as they are much more prevalent in warm climates and in summer time there is more skin exposed than just the face, neck and hands. Some varieties of mosquito (e.g. the culicine mosquitoes) tend to cause blisters when they bite. The bites may be extremely itchy and prominent (Figure 5.11). They may become infected after being scratched.

Fleas

Flea bites are mainly sustained from cat and dog fleas that live on their respective hosts but occasionally temporarily 'visit' a human host. They drop off their original hosts and live on carpets and rugs, as do their young, and jump up when they feel the vibration of footsteps. The bites, which are small and itchy, are often, but not exclusively, on the legs.

Figure 5.11 Mosquito bites on leg.

62

Ticks

Ticks stay stuck to the skin for some time after biting and are found mainly in agricultural communities as the principal host is mostly sheep.

Mites

A large variety of mites may occasionally bite humans. Most of these, like bird-mites or cheyletellia mites living on cats, dogs and rabbits (amongst others) cause small red itchy papules and are quite difficult to identify (Figure 5.12).

Bedbugs (*Cimex lectularius*)

This primitive creature lives in the woodwork of old houses and comes out at night to bite its sleeping victims. The bites are often quite large and inflamed and arranged in straight lines where the creature has taken a 'stroll' over the skin surface.

Wasps and bees

The stings of wasps and bees are usually quite painful. The stung part may become very swollen a short time after the sting and when hypersensitivity is present the individual may develop a widespread reaction. Rarely such a reaction can cause anaphylactic shock and even death.

Papular urticaria

Papular urticaria is a term used to describe a recurrent disseminated itchy papular eruption due to either insect bites or hypersensitivity to them.

DIAGNOSIS
The lesions themselves should be compatible, i.e. they should be papules or, less commonly, blisters, and it helps if puncture marks can be found in the lesion. It is commonplace for the patients (or their parents) to deny the possibility of insect bites being responsible for the lesions as there seems to be a social stigma attached to being the recipient of insect bites. A detailed history is necessary with particular attention being given to the presence of domestic animals, proximity to farms, the occurrence of similar lesions in other family members, and the periodicity of lesions.

Biopsy may occasionally be helpful in that it may well rule out other disorders. The presence of a mixed inflammatory cell infiltrate in the upper and mid dermis is typical but the pattern and density of cellular infiltrate is variable (Figure 5.13).

Searching for the biting arthropod in the home may be fruitless unless the assistance of trained personnel is sought. Examination of 'brushings' from the coats of dogs by veterinarians may be successful in identifying the culprit – cheyletellia, for example.

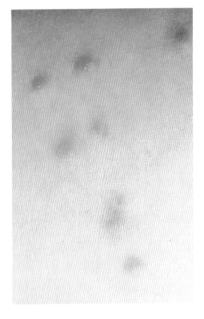

Figure 5.12 Multiple small papules due to mite bites.

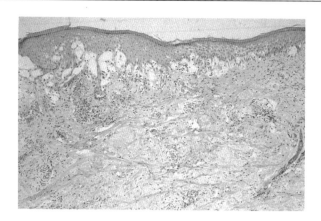

Figure 5.13 Pathology of insect bite showing marked inflammation and subepidermal oedema.

TREATMENT

For the most part treatment is not required, other than to identify the creature responsible and prevent further attack. Uncommonly when there is evidence of hypersensitivity (as in a bee or a wasp sting) systemic antihistamines may be required, and when the local hypersensitivity is accompanied by a severe systemic reaction then systemic steroids and even adrenalin may be needed.

A major problem with insect bites is their intense itchiness. Occasionally this may result in infection in the excoriated skin, when treatment is required for this complication (page 312). Topical antihistamines (e.g. diphenhydramine, promethazine, dimentidine) are often prescribed and may have a slight antipruritic effect, but all that is usually required is a calamine or mentholated calamine preparation.

PROPHYLAXIS

Dependent on the prevalence of potential 'biters' and the climate, long-sleeved shirts, trousers, bed 'nets' and veils may be used to prevent access. Creams and lotions containing dimethyl phthalate, dibutyl phthalate or diethyltoluamide are extensively used as insect repellants but are only partially effective.

Helminthic infestations of the skin

Onchocerciasis

This is caused by the parasite *Onchocerca volvulus* and is found in equatorial West Africa. The disorder is spread by the bite of the blackfly *Simulium damnosum* which is found around rivers. The larval forms, known as microfilariae, are injected into the skin by the blackfly and develop after some years into adult onchocercal worms. These are extremely long (up to 1 m) but very thin (1–2 mm diameter) creatures that live curled up in the subcutis surrounded by a palpable host-supplied fibrous capsule. The adult worm procreates by producing enormous numbers of microfilariae that invade the subcutis of large areas of truncal skin.

Microfilariae from onchocerca volvulus cause itching and lichenified areas while the adult worms produce skin modules in the condition of onchocerciasis.

CLINICAL FEATURES

The disorder is characterized by severe and persistent irritation of affected skin. Affected areas become thickened, lichenified (page xx), slightly scaly and often hyperpigmented (Figure 5.14). The microfilariae may also invade the superficial tissues of the eye and cause blindness ('river blindness').

DIAGNOSIS

The disorder should be suspected in anyone who has been resident in an endemic area and who a few years later complains of persistent itch. Skin nodules should be sought by palpation. Biopsies usually only show a nonspecific inflammation but occasionally demonstrate portions of the microfilariae. A more successful way of identifying the larval forms is by taking a series of skin 'snips' with a needle and scalpel. The tiny portions of skin are then immersed in saline and observed microscopically to watch for the emergence of microfilariae from the edges of the skin.

There is usually a marked eosinophilia and there is also a complement fixing test for antibodies that is available in some centres.

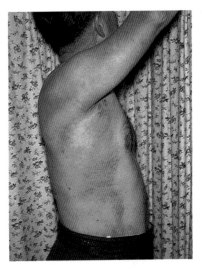

Figure 5.14 Skin changes of onchocerciasis, with marked thickening and discolouration.

TREATMENT

The microfilarial rash and pruritus are much improved with Hetrazan (diethyl carbamazine). The drug must be given cautiously because of the possibility of a severe systemic reaction as a result of the liberation of toxic products from the dead and dying microfilariae. Hetrazan has no effect on the adult worm and it is necessary to treat with the potentially toxic drug Suramin to kill off the worm and prevent further production of microfilariae. Newer drugs have been produced but their advantage is as yet not clear cut. The drug Invermectin certainly appears quite effective and of low toxicity.

CHAPTER

6

Immunologically mediated skin disorders

This chapter will describe several disorders with a strong immuno-pathogenic component. Convenience has dictated, however, that some 'nonimmunological' disorders are included, and others, that are clearly due to 'allergy', are placed elsewhere in the book.

Urticaria and angioedema

Urticaria and angioedema are the result of histamine release from mast cells in the skin and are often, though not invariably, caused by allergic hypersensitivity.

These common disorders are the result of histamine release from mast cells in the skin and are often, though not invariably, caused by allergic hypersensitivity.

CLINICAL FEATURES

Urticaria is extremely common ('nettlerash' or 'wheals' or 'hives' are popular names for this disorder) and there are few individuals who do not experience the disorder in one form or another during their life time. Urticarial lesions are itchy red papules and plaques of variable size (Figure 6.1) that arise suddenly, often within a few minutes, and last 6–24 hours. They may assume odd polycyclic annular and geographic forms.

An important characteristic of urticaria is its transience, but very occasionally urticarial lesions stay for days rather than hours and leave a brownish stain. This type of urticaria is due to involvement of small blood vessels and is known as urticarial vasculitis.

In many patients with urticaria and in a few people without, firm pressure over a track with a blunt object such as a key or the 'wrong' end of a pen or pencil over the skin of the back will produce first blanching, then redness, then a wheal. This phenomenon, which is an exaggeration of the normal 'triple response' is known as dermographism. It causes itching and discomfort and is itself a reason for patients presenting.

In angioedema the lesions are deeper and the swelling much more extensive than in urticaria (Figure 6.2). Angioedema may accompany urticaria or may occur independently. The face and the tissues of the oropharynx are sometimes affected by the angioedema which can lead to life-threatening difficulties in swallowing and breathing.

Urticaria and angioedema can last for a few days or some years. A

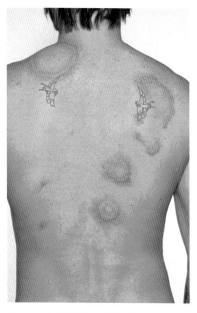

Figure 6.1 Urticarial lesions on the back of a young man.

common pattern is for the disorder to recur in a series of attacks. 'Chronic urticaria' is a common and sometimes disabling disorder which in most cases is of unknown origin.

CAUSES

The ultimate cause of urticaria and angioedema is release of histamine from mast cell granules but there are a large number of stimuli that can do this. Many of these are in the broadest sense immunological but some appear purely 'pharmacological' and others are physical. Type I immunological reactions are involved in the production of urticarial lesions. Table 6.1 has some of the known causes and notes on some of the special varieties of urticaria are given at the end of this section. Although the cause(s) of urticaria can be identified in some patients it has to be admitted that the reason for the urticaria remains mysterious in most patients with the disorder.

> The reason for the urticaria remains mysterious in most patients with the disorder.

Table 6.1 Some causes of urticaria

Sensitivity to exogenous antigens
Foods, e.g. fish, prawns, crabs, milk, etc.
Drugs, e.g. penicillin
Pharmacological provocation
Aspirin, opioids
Systemic disorders
Lupus erythematosus
Henoch Schönlein purpura
'Physical' causes
Cholinergic urticaria
Light pressure (dermographism)
Persistent pressure
Cold

The 'physical' urticarias

Cold urticaria

Urticarial swelling of the hands, the face and elsewhere may occur after exposure to the cold. The reaction can be elicited by an ice block (Figure 6.3). There is a familial form.

Pressure urticaria

Urticarial lesions develop some time (up to several hours) after pressure on the skin, for example, from belts or other tight clothing, or from the rungs of a ladder.

Dermographism

Many patients with urticaria mark easily when their skin is rubbed firmly, for example, with a key or the blunt end of a pen. This is an exaggerated 'triple response' and is quite troublesome to some patients (Figure 6.4).

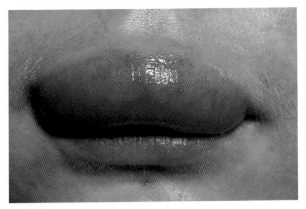

Figure 6.2 Marked swelling of the upper lip in angiodema. It seemed to be due to fish hypersensitivity in this patient.

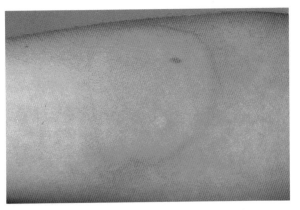

Figure 6.3 Cold urticaria elicited by a block of ice.

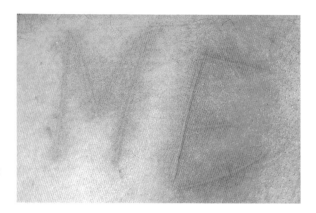

Figure 6.4 Dermographic response to firm stroking of the skin with the 'blunt' end of a pencil.

Solar urticaria

Urticarial spots develop on exposed skin a few minutes after exposure to the sun. Various wavelengths may be responsible (Figure 6.5).

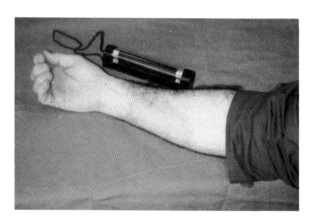

Figure 6.5 Solar urticaria. This patient was so sensitive that he developed an urticarial response to the minimal ultraviolet radiation of the 'A' type (long wave) (UVA) energy emitted by a battery driven hand-held fluorescent lamp.

> Common causes of urticaria include penicillin, aspirin, food hypersensitivies and physical stimuli.

Cholinergic urticaria

Irritating small urticarial spots develop after exercise or hot baths – stimuli that evoke sweating from the postganglionic cholinergically ennervated sweat glands. This very common disorder can be very disabling in a few patients as it effectively prevents them doing any kind of physical activity.

Drug-induced urticaria

Penicillin hypersensitivity is a common cause of urticaria. Attacks vary from the life-threatening acute anaphylactic type to crops of small urticarial papules. Opioid drugs can cause urticaria, probably by directly stimulating histamine release. Aspirin also causes urticaria in some. Up to one-third of patients with urticaria develop lesions after 'challenge' with aspirin but whether this is entirely due to pharmacological stimulation of histamine release, involvement in prostanoid metabolism, or due to hypersensitivity is not certain.

Stings
Nettles, jellyfish tentacles and some insect stings elicit histamine release at the site of skin contact, producing painful local histamine reactions.

Urticaria can also be a sign of an underlying systemic disorder such as lupus erythematosus and amyloidosis. It is also one component of some generalized skin disorders including dermatitis herpetiformis (page 85) and allergic vasculitis (page 80).

TREATMENT
Any identifiable cause or aggravating factor should if possible be removed. Antihistamines of the H_1 receptor blocker type are the most effective agents to relieve symptoms in this disorder. There are large numbers of these and it is better to become really familiar with just a few than try to memorize the whole range available. The 'older' antihistamines such as promethazine, chlorpheniramine and diphenhydramine are quite effective but have a hypnotic effect and must not be taken if the patient intends driving or using machinery. The suppressive effects last a few hours only, and regular dosing is required to maintain relief. Newer antihistamines such as terfenadine, astemizole, cetirizine and loratidine are also effective, with less hypnotic effect. A suitable regimen with which to start is terfenadine 60 mg twice daily. A few patients obtain increased benefit by adding an H_2 antagonist such as cimetidine to the H_1 antagonist already being administered.

Acute severe urticaria and angioedema may require oral corticosteroids. Where the condition is life-threatening intravenous hydrocortisone should be used.

Erythema multiforme

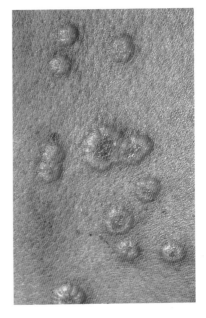

Figure 6.6 Vesiculobullous lesions of erythema multiforme. Some seem 'target-like'.

DEFINITION
An acute and relatively short-lived inflammatory reaction of skin and mucosae occurring in response to a variety of antigenic stimuli resulting in scattered lesions at the dermoepidermal junction.

CLINICAL FEATURES
The individual lesions are red to purple maculopapules, some of which become annular or target-like and may blister (Figures 6.6 and 6.7). There may be just a few or large numbers of them. The face and upper limbs are preferentially involved. The buccal mucosa is often involved in severely affected patients. In the worst cases there is severe systemic upset. The front of the mouth is eroded and sloughy in severely affected patients (Figure 6.8). The conjunctivae and genital mucosae are affected in a few. The disorder starts acutely and is usually over in less than two weeks, although crops of new lesions often develop in the first few days.

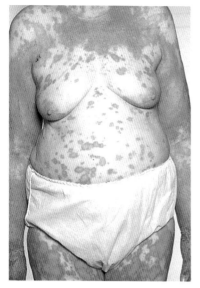

Erythema multiforme lasts 10–14 days causes multiple inflamed target lesions on the skin and mucosal erosions and is provoked by many stimuli.

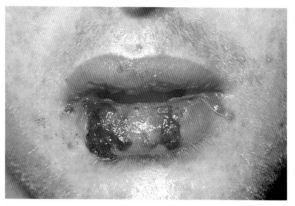

Figure 6.7 Widespread lesions of erythema multiforme.

Figure 6.8 Eroded mucosa of labial mucosa in erythema multiforme. This patient's mouth was also affected.

Table 6.2   Causes of erythema multiforme

Drugs, e.g. Nonsteroidal anti-
inflammatory drugs
Psychotropic drugs
Sulphonamides,
other antimicrobial
drugs

Infections, e.g. Herpes simplex
Orf (vacania)
Mycoplasma
Histoplasmosis
Coccidioidomy-
cosis

Ultraviolet irradiation

Ulcerative colitis and Crohn's
disease

AETIOLOGY AND PATHOGENESIS

The details of the immunological causation are not known. The disorder may be precipitated by infections including herpes simplex, orf, coccidioidomycosis and histoplasmosis, drugs such as phenylbutazone, piroxicam, indomethacin and other nonsteroidal anti-inflammatory compounds, sulphonamides and thiazide diuretics, amongst others. It is also precipitated by sun exposure. In a proportion of patients it recurs for no very obvious reason (Table 6.2).

PATHOLOGY

Mononuclear inflammatory cells collect at the dermoepidermal interface. There are some degenerative changes in the epidermis and in a few cases blister formation by fluid collecting beneath the epidermis (Figure 6.9).

Figure 6.9 Pathology of erythema multiforme. There are degenerative changes at the dermoepidermal junction, epidermal oedema and an inflammatory cell infiltrate.

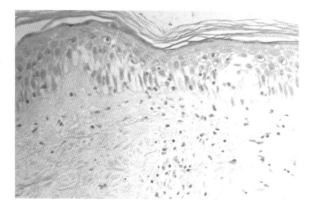

TREATMENT

The disorder is self-limiting and only symptomatic treatment is required. Where there is serious systemic disturbance systemic steroids may be given.

Erythema nodosum

DEFINITION

A painful inflammatory disorder in which crops of tender nodules occur in response to antigenic stimuli.

CLINICAL FEATURES

Individual lesions are red, raised and tender and vary in size from 1 to 3 cm in diameter. They occur in crops on the shins (Figure 6.10) and less commonly on the forearms and, rarely, elsewhere. There may be malaise, fever and an accompanying arthralgia of the ankles and even the knees. The lesions take two to six weeks to resolve and when they do they leave a bruised appearance. Crops of lesions may continue to appear over some months.

AETIOLOGY AND PATHOGENESIS

Nothing is known of the immunological cause of the disorder. There are numerous causes including infections, drugs and systemic illnesses (Table 6.3). The most important are sarcoidosis (page 42) and pulmonary tuberculosis. It is also rarely seen in ulcerative colitis and leprosy. A cause is identified in some 50% of patients with the disorder.

PATHOLOGY

The disorder is essentially a panniculitis with inflammation and bleeding occurring in the fibrous septa between fat lobules.

TREATMENT

Treatment for the disorder is mainly rest and mild analgesics and/or anti-inflammatory agents. But treatment directed to the underlying disorder will be required if any is detected.

Annular erythemas

There are several disorders which are marked by the appearance of erythematous rings and whorls on the skin surface which usually gradually enlarge and then disappear. For the most part their significance is uncertain but one known as *erythema gyratum repens* signifies the presence of an underlying visceral neoplasm (page 285) and another, *erythema chronicum migrans*, indicates the presence of Lyme disease.

> Erythema nodosum is a painful inflammatory disorder in which crops of red tender nodules occur in response to various antigenic stimuli.

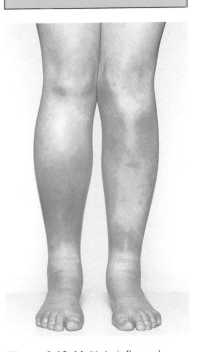

Figure 6.10 Multiple inflamed lesions of erythema nodosum.

Table 6.3 Causes of erythema nodosum

Tuberculosis

Sarcoidosis

Brucellosis

Ulcerative colitis and Crohn's disease

Leprosy

Autoimmune disorders

These disorders are also known as 'autoaggressive diseases', the 'collagen vascular disorders' and the 'connective tissue diseases'. In general terms the immune system of an individual with autoimmune disease fails to 'recognize' the individual's own tissues and mounts an attack on these. In most of the disorders in this group the inflammatory process seems to involve the small blood vessels in particular (vasculitis) and in some the vascular component is the major part of the disease.

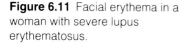
In general terms the immune system of an individual with autoimmune disease fails to 'recognize' the individual's own tissues and mounts an attack on these.

Lupus erythematosus

This is divided into systemic and cutaneous forms, although there is some overlap.

Systemic lupus erythematosus

Systemic lupus erythematosus (SLE) often involves the skin as well as many other organ systems but in one type of SLE – subacute SLE – the skin is prominently affected. Antibodies to nuclear DNA occur in 80–90% of patients with SLE and antibodies to other nuclear components are present in subgroups of the population of patients with SLE. These 'antinuclear factors' may be intimately involved in the pathogenesis of the disease.

Common components of SLE include a rheumatoid-like arthropathy, a glomerulonephritis, inflammatory disorder of the pulmonary and cardiovascular systems, a polyserositis, central nervous system involvement and skin disorder. The skin components of SLE include facial erythema across the cheeks and nose (butterfly erythema) (Figure 6.11) and on the hands, and discoid lupus erythematosus (DLE) as occurs in the pure cutaneous form (see below).

Figure 6.11 Facial erythema in a woman with severe lupus erythematosus.

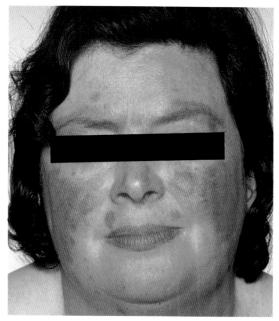

Systemic lupus erythematosus may affect anyone but attacks young women disproportionately frequently. The pace of the disease is variable but can be acute and devastating or so insidious that its effects are only barely noticeable. The five-year mortality has been variously estimated between 15 and 50% dependent on the organ systems affected and the pace of the disease.

Lupus erythematosus may be due to alteration of nuclear constituents by infection or drugs and is associated with antinuclear factors in 80–90% The disease is multisystem but skin lesions are common.

PATHOLOGY AND LABORATORY FINDINGS

Affected skin shows oedema, degenerative change in the basal epidermal cells and a tight cuff of mononuclear cells around the small blood vessels (Figure 6.12). Unexposed uninvolved skin has deposits of immunoprotein (IgG or IgA) in about 60% of patients at the dermo–epidermal junction detectable by direct immunofluorescent methods. Circulating antibodies to DNA or other nuclear components are found in the large majority of patients. An increase in the level of serum gamma-globulin is a frequent finding. Haematological findings include a normochromic, normocytic anaemia, a neutropaenia, a lymphopaenia and a thrombocytopaenia.

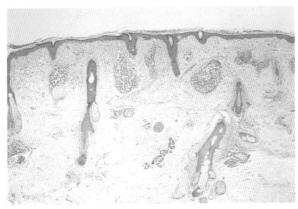

Figure 6.12 Pathology of skin lesion in systemic lupus erythematosus. There are collections of lymphocytes perivascularly.

AETIOLOGY

It has been suggested that infections may spark off the autoimmunity. Virus infections have been suggested as the initiating agency. Some drugs (e.g. hydrallazine, penicillamine) are known to set off an SLE-type disease.

TREATMENT

Patients with active progressive disease may require systemic steroids to suppress the inflammatory process. Immunosuppressive agents such as methotrexate, azathioprine and cyclosporin may also be needed.

Chronic discoid lupus erythematosus

Lesions of chronic discord lupus erythematosus (CDLE) can occur in the course of SLE or may be the only manifestation of the disorder. Frequently patients with CDLE have minor haematological changes of the sort described in SLE but no other features of SLE. Some 5% of patients with CDLE transform to SLE.

CLINICAL FEATURES

Irregular red plaques appear on light exposed skin of the face, scalp, neck, shoulders, hands or arms (Figure 6.13). The plaques develop patchy atrophy with patchy hypo- and hyperpigmentation (Figure 6.14) while other areas are thickened and warty. On the scalp, scarring alopecia occurs in the affected areas (Figure 6.15). The disorder is very light sensitive and may be aggravated or initiated by exposure to the sun.

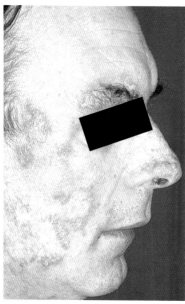

Figure 6.13 Multiple irregular red plaques due to discoid lupus erythematosus.

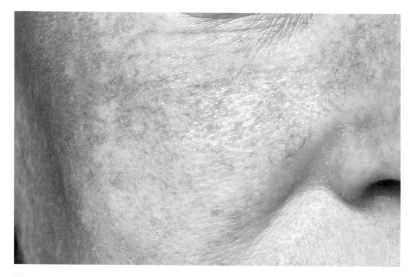

Figure 6.14 Hypopigmentation of facial skin due to lesion of discoid lupus erythematosus.

PATHOLOGY

The changes are similar to those described for SLE but the epidermal degenerative changes are more marked, with scattered cytoid body formation and patchy epidermal atrophy and thickening. Mononuclear inflammatory cell infiltrates around blood vessels and hair follicles are present (Figure 6.16).

TREATMENT

Patients must be advised to avoid the sun and to use sunscreens. Individual lesions sometimes respond to potent topical corticosteroids. Where these do not cope with the disease, hydroxychloroquinine (200–400 mg per day) is often helpful. Caution must be exercised concerning the possible although rare toxic effects of this drug on the

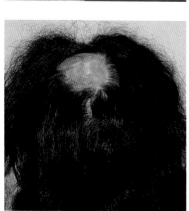

Figure 6.15 Patch of discoid lupus erythematosus causing alopecia.

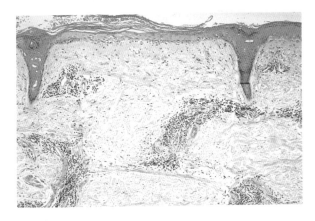

Figure 6.16 Pathology of discoid lupus erythematosus with collections of lymphocytes around the small blood vessels and degenerative change in the basal layer of epidermis.

retina. Systemic steroids, the oral gold compound auranofin, and the retinoid drugs etretinate and acitretin (page 316) are other drugs that have been used successfully.

Systemic sclerosis

Scleroderma is an important component of systemic sclerosis. In this autoimmune disorder the fibroblast is stimulated to produce new collagen by factors released in the course of the immunological response. When other organ systems are involved the disorder affects the vasculature as well as fibroblasts and Raynaud's phenomenon, renal involvement with glomerular disease, gut involvement with dysphagia, and gut hypomobility with its consequences, a rheumatoid type of polyarthropathy and skin stiffening are all seen (Table 6.4). As with SLE the disease is mostly seen in young women, and the pace of the disorder is extremely variable. At one end of the spectrum the disorder starts insidiously over some months or even years, with progressively worsening Raynaud's phenomenon and increasing nutritional changes of the fingers as a result of this and gradual thickening and stiffening of the skin of the hands and face. This causes a characteristic facial appearance with a beak-like appearance and narrowing of the mouth (Figure 6.17). Telangiectatic macules appear over the face (Figure 6.18) and deposits of calcium develop in the skin. The term CRST syndrome is used for this constellation of problems (calcinosis cutis, Raynaud's, sclerosis and telangiectasia). When there is also dysphagia due to oesophageal involvement the term CREST is more appropriate. Although relatively benign, this disorder can produce considerable disability because of the limitation of movements of the hands.

In more rapidly progressive systemic sclerosis there may be more serious vascular disease affecting the fingers, resulting in tissue necrosis and even the loss of portions of the digits (Figure 6.19). In addition serious renal or pulmonary disease may eventually cause the death of the patient – the five-year mortality rate of this disease being 30% or more.

Table 6.4 Manifestations of systemic sclerosis

Raynaud's phenomenon
Skin thickening and stiffness
Ischaemic necrosis of digits
Dysphagia
Glomerulosclerosis and renal insufficiency
Hypertension
Malabsorption; constipation
Pulmonary fibrosis

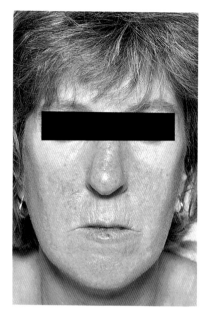

Figure 6.17 Facial appearance in systemic sclerosis. Note 'beaked nose' with pinched cheeks and small mouth.

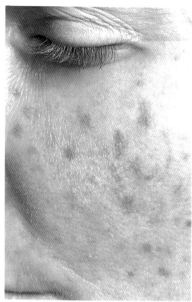

Figure 6.18 Macular telangiectasia of facial skin in systemic sclerosis.

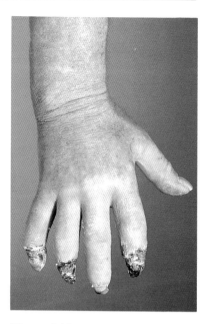

Figure 6.19 Ischaemic necrosis of tips of fingers in systemic sclerosis.

> Systemic sclerosis is a multisystem autoimmune disorder in which fibroblasts are stimulated to produce new collagen and vascular endotheluim is damaged. Stiff skin (Scleroderma) is a common manifestation. Arthritis, glomerulonephritis and gut involvement are also common.

PATHOLOGY AND LABORATORY FINDINGS
Biopsy of affected skin shows excess new collagen which has an eosinophilic and almost homogeneous appearance. Anti-nuclear antibodies occur in up to 30% of patients. Diagnosis is usually made from the constellation of clinical signs and confirmatory laboratory findings due to the typical involvement of other organ systems.

TREATMENT
There is no satisfactory way of reliably altering the course of this disorder. Nonetheless some improvement can be obtained by skilful management of the Raynaud's phenomenon. Some improvement is occasionally produced with penicillamine and immunosuppressive treatment with steroids and azathioprine or cyclosporine. Retinoid drugs and colchicine have also been used.

Morphoea

Morphea is localized scleroderma.

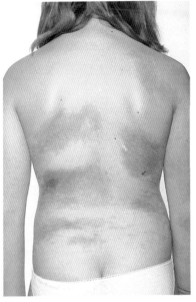

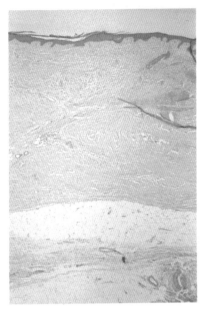

Figure 6.20 Plaques of morphoea.

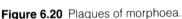

Figure 6.21 Pathology of morphoea. The dermal connective tissue is thickened and has a more homogeneous appearance than usual.

CLINICAL FEATURES

One or several thickened sclerotic plaques develop over the trunk or limbs. They range in size from 2–3 to 10 cm in diameter. A mauve colour at first, they become brownish later (Figure 6.20). They mostly occur in young adults but occasionally develop in children where their presence can lead to serious deformity as when it occurs on the scalp, producing an *en coup de sabre* appearance. Morphea generally gradually remits after a period of two to three years.

PATHOLOGY

There is marked replacement of the subcutaneous fat with new collagen which has a pale homogenized appearance (Figure 6.21).

TREATMENT

Luckily the condition rarely causes symptoms as there is no effective treatment.

Variants

Generalized morphoea

This is a rare type of scleroderma which is confined to the skin but develops over wide expanses of skin, causing considerable limitation of movement and even impeding breathing.

Lichen sclerosus et atrophicus

There is disagreement as to whether this is really a form of morphoea or not. Many would agree that there are sufficient similarities for it to be included here.

CLINICAL FEATURES

Small irritating whitish areas occur on the genitalia (Figure 6.22) or around the anus, or less commonly elsewhere over the skin. In men the condition occurs on the glans penis or prepuce. It is then known as **balanitis xerotica obliterans** and may cause discomfort and paraphimosis. There is a characteristic pathological picture in which there is intense oedema in a subepidermal band (Figure 6.23).

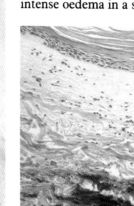

Figure 6.22 Lichen sclerosus et atrophicus of vulval skin. Note the whitish patches.

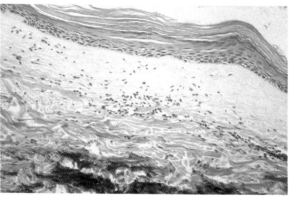

Figure 6.23 Pathology of lichen sclerosus et atrophicus showing the typical subepidermal oedematous zone.

TREATMENT

Good results have been obtained with high potency topical corticosteroids (e.g. clobetasol 17-propionate). Circumcision is recommended for the condition in men.

Dermatomyositis

Both muscle and skin are affected in this disabling disorder. Polymyositis is the identical disorder without skin involvement.

CLINICAL FEATURES

Skin

In dermatomyositis dull red to mauve areas develop over the face, backs of the hands, elbows, knees and elsewhere.

Dull red to mauve areas develop over the face, backs of the hands, elbows, knees and elsewhere. A particularly characteristic sign is the presence of erythema on the upper lids and around the eyes where the erythema is traditionally likened to the colour of the heliotrope flower (Figure 6.24). On the backs of the hands the erythema typically affects the paronychial folds and the skin over the metacarpals (Figure 6.25).

78

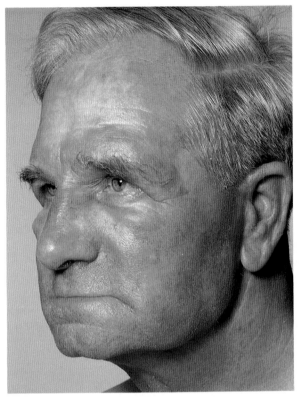

Figure 6.24 Mauve discolouration of facial skin in dermatomyositis with particular involvement of periocular area.

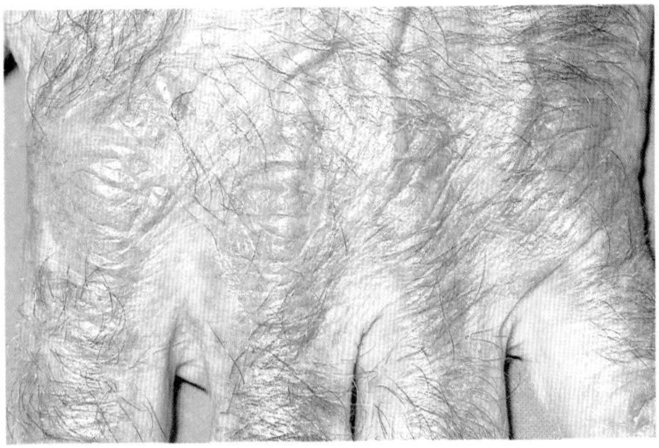

Figure 6.25 Streaky mauve-red appearance over back of metacarpals and fingers in dermatomyositis.

Sometimes small areas of necrosis appear, due to an accompanying vasculitis. Calcium is deposited in long-standing skin lesions.

Muscle

There is a proximal myositis which causes pain and tenderness as well as profound weakness. If progressive, pharyngeal and respiratory muscles are affected and the condition becomes life-threatening. However, the disease generally spontaneously remits in most patients.

> There is also a proximal myositis which causes pain and tenderness as well as profound weakness.

LABORATORY FINDINGS

Muscle enzymes such as phosphocreatinekinase, aldolase and lactic dehydrogenase are increased in the blood, sometimes to extraordinarily high levels. Urine creatine is also a good indicator of disease activity. Muscle damage can also be assessed by muscle biopsy and electromyography.

TREATMENT

Oral steroids are the mainstay of treatment and are given in sufficient dosage to prevent further progress of the disease. Azathioprine and other immunosuppressive drugs are sometimes prescribed.

The vasculitis group of diseases

There are several disorders where the major focus of the disorder seems to be on the vasculature. Anywhere can be affected in these diseases but the major focus of attack seems to be on the kidneys, the respiratory system, the joints and the skin. The central nervous system and the gut are also involved on occasion.

> In the vasculitis group of disorders, the major focus of the disorder seems to be on the vasculature.

Allergic vasculitis (Henoch Schönlein purpura)

Although any age group can be affected, children and young adults seem especially prone to the disorder.

CLINICAL FEATURES

Generally allergic vasculitis (AV) starts suddenly with fever, painful joints and a rash. The rash is both urticarial and papular, and particularly marked on extensor surfaces. It is also quite definitely purpuric in that it can't be 'blanched' by pressure with a microscope slide (Figure 6.26). The lesions come in recurrent crops over the first few days.

> Generally allergic vasculitis (AV) starts suddenly with fever, painful joints and a purpuric urticariol and papular rash.

Joint pain with some swelling is quite commonly noted. Cramping abdominal pain and malaena occasionally develop as a result of submucosal haemorrhagic oedema. Acute glomerulonephritis occurs ranging from microscopic haematuria when mildly affected, to oliguria with renal failure in a very few severely affected patients. The disorder remits spontaneously in most patients but may recur in some.

> Arthritis, glomerulonephritis and gut involvement are also common.

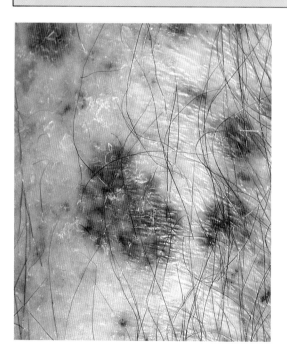

Figure 6.26 Purpuric papules of Henoch Schönlein purpura.

PATHOLOGY AND PATHOGENESIS
The cause is unknown but hypersensitivity to streptococcal antigens may play a role in some patients. Immune complexes formed are believed to be deposited in endothelium initiating the reaction. Histologically, collections of polymorphonuclear leukocytes and fragments of their nuclei are found around small blood vessels in the dermis (leukocytoclasis) alongside oedema and some bleeding. The endothelium is swollen and may show degenerative change (Figure 6.27). This picture, known as leukocytoclastic angiitis, is not specific to this disease.

TREATMENT
Rest and monitoring for renal involvement is all that is required for most patients. Severely affected patients will need systemic steroids.

Polyarteritis nodosa
Polyarteritis nodosa is a serious rare inflammatory disorder of large and medium-sized arteries. Inflammation affects the vessel wall, which dilates aneurysmally. This results in rupture in some instances and ischaemic changes in others. The clinical features will depend on which vessels are affected. Central nervous system, cardiovascular, gastrointestinal and renal problems may all arise in this potentially fatal disease. In the skin a livedo reticularis pattern may be seen, and persistent ulcers have been recorded. Steroids and immunosuppressive agents have been used in treatment.

Nodular vasculitis
This is an uncommon inflammatory disorder of the cutaneous vasculature of the legs seen in women predominantly.

CLINICAL FEATURES
Painful red and purpuric papules and nodules develop on the calves and

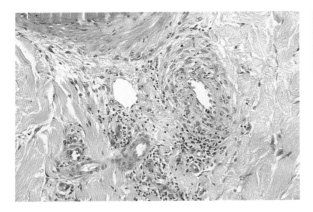

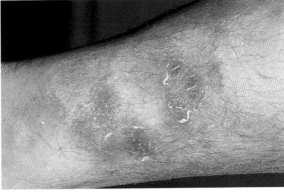

Figure 6.27 Pathology of allergic vasculitis. Polymorphonuclear cells and fragments of polymorph nuclei are seen around small damaged blood vessels (leukocytoclastic angiitis).

Figure 6.28 Papules and nodules on lower leg of woman with nodular vasculitis. These were painful and some were purpuric.

elsewhere on the legs in recurrent crops (Figure 6.28). Some may ulcerate but generally they disappear without sequel. The condition may last for many years.

PATHOLOGY AND PATHOGENESIS
Nothing is known of the cause. Histologically there is a leukocytoclastic angiitis.

TREATMENT
Steroids, immunosuppressive agents and anti-inflammatory drugs have been tried with little success.

Other types of cutaneous vasculitis

The development of crops of purple purpuric papules with darker and occasionally crusted central areas and sometimes pustules is seen in the course of subacute bacterial endocarditis, gonococcaemia and meningococcaemia (Figure 6.29). Drugs such as the thiazides may also cause a vasculitis. Renal involvement sometimes accompanies the skin lesions. Clearly the importance of such lesions is that they are recognized for what they are – signs of an underlying systemic disorder – so that this can be rapidly diagnosed and treated.

> Cutaneous vasculitis may cause crops of purple purpuric papules with crusted central areas and pustules in the course of subacute bacterial endocarditis, gonococcaemia and meningococcaemia.

Capillaritis

There is a group of benign, persistent, mildly inflammatory skin disorders where the focus of the abnormality appears to be in the papillary dermis and the immediately subepidermal capillary vasculature. As a group, the term persistent pigmented purpuric eruption seems appropriate, because not only are they persistent but, because of the damage to capillaries, there is leakage of blood and both purpura and pigmentation from haemosiderin staining. Clinically the lesions mostly occur on the lower legs and vary from a macular spattered appearance ('Schamberg's disease') (Figure 6.30) to an itchy papular

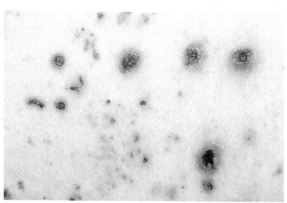

Figure 6.29 Purpuric and necrotic papules in cutaneous vasculitis.

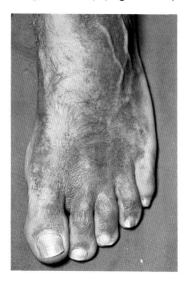

Figure 6.30
Pigmented and purpuric eruptions due to Schamberg's disease.

eruption (lichenoid purpuric eruption) or a macular golden eruption (lichen aureus) (Figure 6.31). These disorders generally cause little disability and remit spontaneously after a variable period. Generally no treatment is required.

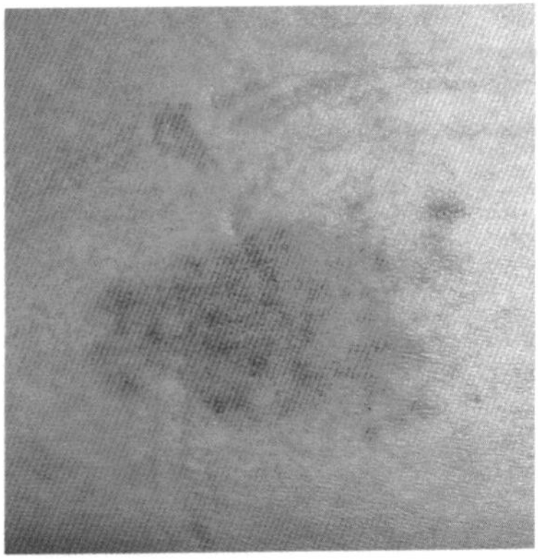

Blistering diseases

Many inflammatory skin disorders can produce blistering at some stage in their natural history. In the primary blistering diseases blistering is the major feature of the disease and a direct result of the initial pathological process. The different blistering diseases are given in Table 6.5. They are conventionally divided into 'subepidermal' and 'intraepidermal' blistering disorders.

Figure 6.31 Golden patch due to purpura in 'lichen aureus'.

Subepidermal blistering diseases

Bullous pemphigoid (senile pemphigoid)
Bullous pemphigoid (BP) is an uncommon, acute blistering disease occurring mainly in the over-60s.

CLINICAL FEATURES
Large tense, often blood-stained blisters develop over a few days anywhere on the skin surface (Figure 6.32). Mostly they do not affect the buccal mucosa. New crops of blisters continue to appear for many months without adequate treatment, and the disease is painful and disabling. In a very small proportion of patients the disorder is a sign of an underlying malignancy.

In bullous pemphigoid large tense, often blood-stained subepidermal blisters develop over a few days.

Table 6.5 The 'primary' blistering disorders

Subepidermal blistering disorders	
Senile pemphigoid	Acute, widespread, severe
Cicatricial pemphigoid	Chronic, limited in extent, mucosa-affected scarring
Erythema multiforme	Acute, mucosae as well, variously caused
Dermatitis herpetiformis	Itchy, persistent, associated with gluten enteropathy
Epidermolysis bullosa	Genetically and phenotypically diverse, varies from mild to lethal

Intraepidermal		
Pemphigus:	Vulgaris Vegetans	} Suprabasal epidermal split
	Erythematosus Foliaceous	} Subcorneal epidermal split

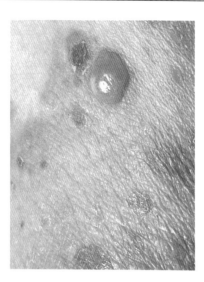

Figure 6.32 Tense blisters due to bullous pemphigoid

Figure 6.33 There is a fluorescent band at the dermoepidermal junction in this fluorescence photomicrograph due to deposition of immunoglobulin (IgG). A biopsy from the skin around the site of blistering was frozen and the cryostat section treated with fluorescein tagged anti-immunoglobulin antibodies.

Figure 6.34 Pathology of bullous pemphigoid showing subepidermal blister.

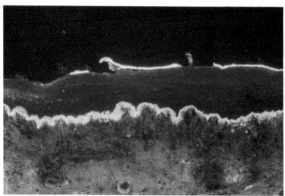

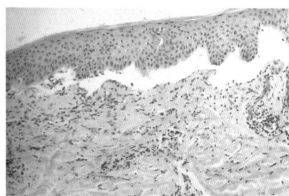

There is a circulating antibody directed to the epidermal basement membrane zone in 85–90% of patients which can be detected using the immunofluorescence method. Antibodies of the IgG type and the complement component C3 are also deposited in the subepidermal zone around the lesions in the majority of patients and can also be detected using the direct immunofluorescence technique.

LABORATORY FINDINGS

There is a circulating antibody directed to the epidermal basement membrane zone in 85–90% of patients which can be detected using the immunofluorescence method. The titre of this antibody is to some extent a reflection of the activity of the disease. Antibodies of the IgG type and the complement component C3 are also deposited in the subepidermal zone around the lesions in the majority of patients and can also be detected using the direct immunofluorescence technique (Figure 6.33). Biopsy of new blisters reveals that there is subepidermal fluid with polymorphs and eosinophils in the infiltrate subepidermally (Figure 6.34).

TREATMENT

Patients with widespread blistering may need to be nursed in hospital and treated as though they had severe burns. High doses of corticosteroids (60 mg per day of prednisone or even more) are needed to control the disease. Immunosuppressive treatment with azathioprine or methotrexate is usually started simultaneously. The blisters themselves should be treated with 'wet dressings'.

Variants of bullous pemphigoid

There are other rare blistering diseases in which the blister forms subepidermally. These include (1) benign mucous membrane pemphigoid, in which lesions occur chronically in the mouth and in the conjunctivae as well as on the skin, and (2) 'bullous disease of childhood' where bullous lesions occur in infancy, particularly in the buttock and perigenital area. In the latter disorder, and in some blistering conditions in adults, IgA is deposited instead of IgG.

Dermatitis herpetiformis

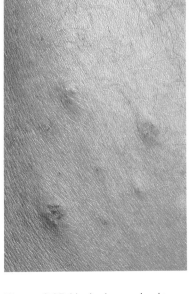

This is a chronic remittent itchy blistering disorder in which there is gluten hypersensitivity.

> Itchy vesicles and urticarial papules on exterior surfaces due to subepidermal inflammation and blister formation occur in dermatitis herpetiformis.

CLINICAL FEATURES
Vesicles, papulovesicles and urticarial papules appear in crops over the knees, elbows, scalp, buttocks and around the axillae (Figure 6.35). They are intensely irritant. Most patients with dermatitis herpetiformis (DH) have a mild gastrointestinal absorptive defect which does not lead to clinical disease in many. It has been found that this is due to gluten hypersensitivity (gluten enteropathy) as in patients with coeliac disease. Some diseases with a pronounced immunopathogenetic component are more common in patients with DH. These include thyrotoxicosis, rheumatoid arthritis, myasthenia gravis and ulcerative colitis. The disorder is persistent but fluctuates in intensity.

Figure 6.35 Vesiculopapules in dermatitis herpetiformis.

LABORATORY FINDINGS
Small bowel mucosal biopsy reveals partial villous atrophy in 70–80% of patients with DH. Minor abnormalities of small bowel absorptive function are also common. Biopsy of new lesions demonstrates that the

> Small bowel mucosal biopsy reveals partial villous atrophy in 70–80% of patients with DH.

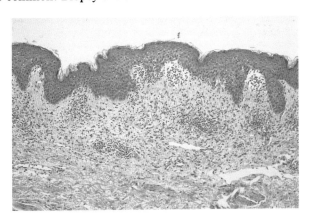

Figure 6.36 Pathology of dermatitis herpetiformis. There are collections of polymorphs in the tips of the dermal papillae where the subepidermal blistering begins.

Direct immunofluorescent examination reveals the presence of IgA in the papillary tips in the skin around the lesions in all patients.

vesicle forms subepidermally and develops from collections of inflammatory cells in the papillary tips (the papillary tip abscess) (Figure 6.36). Direct immunofluorescent examination reveals the presence of IgA in the papillary tips in the skin around the lesions in all patients.

TREATMENT

The skin lesions can be suppressed with the drug dapsone (50–200 mg per day) in most patients. Dapsone unfortunately has many toxic side effects including mild haemolysis, methaemoglobinaemia, sulphaemoglobinaemia and rashes such as fixed drug eruption. Most patients tolerate the drug quite well. However, a severe haemolytic crisis can occur in patients with glucose 6-phosphate dehydrogenase deficiency given dapsone. A gluten-free diet will improve the gastrointestinal lesion and improves the skin disorder in many patients after some months.

Epidermolysis bullosa

This is not a single disorder but a group of similar congenitally determined blistering diseases. The blistering is caused by various congenital structural and metabolic defects and unlike the blisters described thus far, does not have a marked immunopathological component.

Epidermolysis bullosa simplex

The blistering in these rare disorders appears subepidermal but is actually through the basal layer of the epidermis. It is usually limited to hands and feet and the sites of trauma (Figure 6.37). They are dominantly inherited. The blisters may just be confined to the soles of the feet and not prove troublesome till adolescence. As with most genodermatoses these conditions persist throughout life. There is no effective treatment other than to avoid trauma and to keep the blistered areas clean and dry.

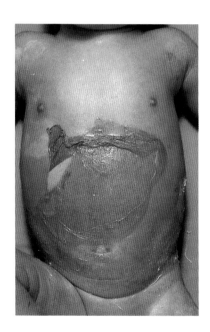

Figure 6.37 Blisters on the trunk due to epidermolysis bullosa simplex.

Blistering develops subepidermally in the inherited blistering disorders known as epidermolysis bullosa. In dystrophic forms there is great scarring and disability.

Dystrophic epidermolysis bullosa

Disorders in this rare group of conditions cause severe scarring and indeed some forms are not compatible with life. They are also subepidermal, but the split is lower down than epidermolysis bullosa simplex, and within the upper dermis. They are mostly recessive but there are some dominant types too. Blistering and scarring cause marked tissue loss over the hands and feet with eventually webbing of the fingers and toes and maybe loss of these structures. There is also marked scarring of the mucosae which affects the pharynx and oesophagus too so that severe dysphagia is a problem. Squamous cell carcinoma develops on the most severely affected sites in some patients. This is a terrifyingly destructive and disabling group of disorders for which there is at present no adequate treatment.

Other subepidermal blistering disorders

Erythema multiforme may cause extensive subepidermal blistering (pages 69–70). *Herpes gestationis* also causes subepidermal blisters (page 259). *Porphyria cutanea tarda* also gives rise to subepidermal blistering (page 262).

Pemphigus

Pemphigus causes blistering because of a loosening of desmosomal links between epidermal cells caused by immunological attack. There are several types. They are all rare, but *pemphigus vulgaris* (PV) is the least rare. In PV the split occurs within the epidermis just above the basal layer (suprabasal). The lesions are thin-walled delicate blisters that usually rapidly rupture and erode (Figure 6.38). They occur anywhere on the skin surface and very frequently occur within the mouth and throat where they cause much discomfort and disability. The disease may cause widespread blistering and erosion and is persistent, although fluctuating in intensity. Before adequate treatment it was usually fatal.

> Pemphigus causes intraepidermol blistering because of a loosening of desmosomal links between epidermal cells caused by immunological attack.

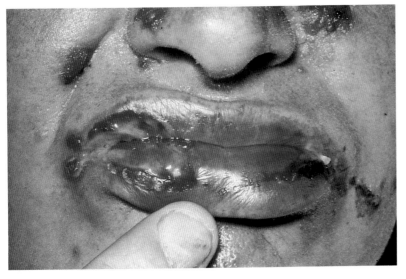

Figure 6.38 Eroded area on lips and face due to pemphigus vulgaris.

LABORATORY FINDINGS

In more than 90% of patients there is a detectable circulating antibody directed to the area between epidermal cells. The titre of the antibody reflects the severity of the disease. The presence of the antibody and its titre are determined by indirect immunofluorescence methods. Biopsy reveals the intraepidermal split with rounded up epidermal cells

> In more than 90% of patients there is a detectable circulating antibody directed to the area between epidermal cells.

> Direct immunofluorescence examination of the perilesional uninvolved skin will show the presence of antibody of the IgG class and the complement component C3 between epidermal cells.

(known as acantholysis). Direct immunofluorescence examination of the perilesional uninvolved skin will show the presence of antibody of the IgG class and the complement component C3 between epidermal cells.

TREATMENT

The patients should be treated as though they had burns, and if severely affected they need inpatient care. Doses of systemic steroids are required to control the blistering (doses of up to 100 mg prednisone are sometimes given). Immunosuppressive therapy with azathioprine or methotrexate should be started simultaneously. Treatment with cyclosporin and with gold as for rheumatoid arthritis has also been used.

Variants

Pemphigus vegetans

There is a more inflammatory component to this very rare intraepidermal blistering condition in which the lesions are usually limited in extent.

Pemphigus foliaceaous

Here the dissolution of desmosomal links occurs higher up within the epidermis just below the stratum corneum. Erosions occur around the upper trunk and head and neck mainly, and the disorder is not quite so serious as in pemphigus vulgaris. However, there is a very serious South American type which occurs endemically in this region that may be caused or precipitated by a virus spread by an insect vector.

Pemphigus erythematodes

This is another rare, superficial type of pemphigus in which the lesions have some resemblances to discoid lupus erythematosus. This occurs around the face and scalp particularly.

Drug eruptions

Most drugs have side effects as well as pharmacological effects, and skin disorders are a frequent form of drug side effect. These can mimic many of the spontaneously occurring skin disorders as well as producing quite specific changes. Drug-induced skin disorder can develop after the initial dose or need a short period of time during which sensitization takes place. Other problems, such as pigmentations or hair anomalies, may take some months before appearing. Often a rash occurs after taking the drug for some time without apparent reason.

It is important that drug reactions are suspected when the nature and cause of a skin disorder is in doubt as 'drugs' in one shape or form are taken by a substantial proportion of the population. Drug eruptions don't only stem from orthodox prescribed drugs but are also caused by cough medicines, analgesics, laxatives or other 'over-the-counter' symptomatic remedies and enquiry must also be made about this possibility. Drug rashes may also be caused by medication absorbed through the skin or any of the mucosae, or even inhaled.

The diagnosis of a drug eruption is difficult to confirm as there are few laboratory tests available. Currently the only useful specific laboratory tests are those dependent on there being specific immunoglobulin IgE directed to the particular drug – penicillin is the only drug of importance that can be detected in this way (radio allergo adsorbent test, RAST). Lymphocyte transformation tests and migration inhibition tests of cell-mediated hypersensitivity fail because the 'allergen' is some metabolite of the drug or a tissue component altered by the drug, or because of some pharmacokinetic consideration.

Skin biopsy may assist in eliminating other causes for an eruption. Intracutaneous prick or scratch tests may be helpful on rare occasions as with penicillin hypersensitivity. Patch tests are rarely helpful as these tests are designed to detect contact allergens. The most useful diagnostic test is the 'challenge' in which the suspected agent is administered to determine whether the condition recurs or is aggravated. Clearly this is not possible in the case of potentially severe or life-threatening conditions. Even when this is not the case it should only be performed with the patient's consent and if important information may be obtained which is relevant to the care of the patient. The smallest possible dose should be given and the patient should be carefully observed subsequently.

Types of drug eruption

Severe life-threatening eruptions

Angioedema/anaphylactic shock
These are sudden in onset and IgE-mediated reactions of the immediate hypersensitivity type. They are provoked by serum-containing products and by penicillin and its derivatives when given parenterally. The patient becomes pale and collapses with severe hypotension and maybe bronchospasm. Treatment is required urgently with oxygen, intravenous hydrocortisone and adrenalin.

Erythema multiforme (Stevens Johnson syndrome)
For a clinical description see page 69. Sulphonamides, hydantoinates, carbamazepine, some nonsteroidal anti-inflammatory agents and maybe penicillin can cause this disorder.

Toxic epidermal necrolysis
This drug reaction, which has a mortality approaching 50%, occurs predominantly in middle-aged and elderly women. The drugs incriminated include sulphonamides, indomethacin, the hydantoinates and gold salts. There is erythroderma with extensive desquamation and in places blistering and erosion. The mucosae are also severely affected.

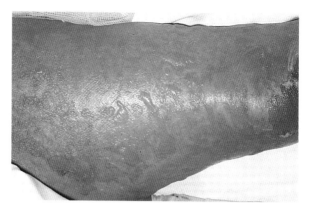

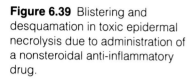

Figure 6.39 Blistering and desquamation in toxic epidermal necrolysis due to administration of a nonsteroidal anti-inflammatory drug.

The patients rapidly become dehydrated and are very sick. They need to be nursed as though they had extensive burns (Figure 6.39). They need intensive support treatment with parenteral fluids, antibiotics and systemic steroids.

Exanthematic eruptions

This is probably the commonest group of drug eruptions. Red/pink macules develop over the trunk and limbs. When intense, the rash is said to be *morbilliform* or measles-like. Ampicillin, the psychotropic drugs and the nonsteroidal anti-inflammatory agents cause this type of rash.

A lichenoid rash (with some resemblance to lichen planus, see pages 142–146) may be caused by gold salts, mepacrine and carbamezepine.

Vascular eruption or purpuric lesions develop over the legs and less frequently the arms and trunk. The thiazide diuretics and the hydantoinates are especially linked with this type of rash.

Urticarial rashes may be produced by penicillin, aspirin, tartrazine (and other dyes) and opioid drugs.

Photosensitivity rashes

In this group of drug-induced conditions the rash is confined to the light exposed areas and is wavelength-dependent, i.e. only reacts to particular wavelengths in the solar ultraviolet spectrum. The rash itself is red and papular or plaque-like (Figure 6.40). Some drugs seem able to provoke a phototoxic eruption which is seen in many patients to whom the drug is given and is dose dependent, and others cause a photoallergic rash in which a photoallergen has formed and which only affects a few individuals. Tetracyclines and sulphonamides may cause a phototoxic response. The phenothiazines may cause either a phototoxic or a photoallergic reaction.

Blistering rashes

Erythema multiforme and toxic epidermal necrolysis have already been discussed. Naproxen and frusemide may cause a 'pseudoporphyria-like' rash (Figure 6.41) in the light exposed sites. Nalidixic acid may also cause blistering. Captopril and penicillamine may cause a pemphigus or a pemphigoid-like eruption.

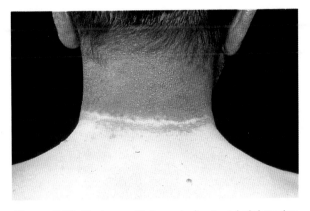

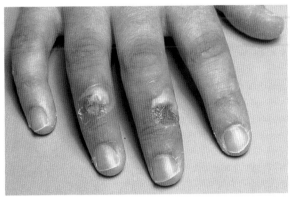

Figure 6.40 Photosensitivity rash due to administration of a tetracycline drug.

Figure 6.41 'Pseudophorphyria' with erosions on the backs of the fingers due to frusemide.

Fixed drug eruptions

This not uncommon drug reaction causes inflammatory patches to appear within hours at the same sites on every occasion the drug is administered. The areas become inflamed, and may even blister before subsiding when the drug is stopped, leaving pigmentation (Figure 6.42). Numerous drugs, including dapsone, the sulphonamides, tetracycline and mefenamic acid may be responsible.

Lupus erythematosus-like rashes

These may be caused by penicillamine, hydralazine, hydantoinates and procaineamide amongst others. The drugs may precipitate or initiate lupus erythematosus.

As pointed out elsewhere, drugs can have many other effects on the skin, including changes in pigmentation and hair distribution.*

TREATMENT

Treatment of all drug eruptions consists of identifying the causative drug and then stopping it. Care must be taken to see that the offending agent or one with cross-reacting chemical groups isn't given again. When the drug is stopped the rash remits in most cases and all that is required is symptomatic treatment.

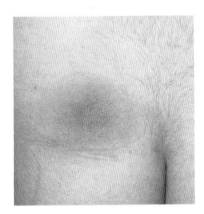

Figure 6.42 Round dusky erythematous patch on buttock due to 'fixed drug eruption' caused by mefenamic acid.

* For further information the reader is referred to *A Guide to Drug Eruptions*.

CHAPTER

7

Skin disorders in AIDS, immunodeficiency and venereal disease

Acquired immune deficiency syndrome (AIDS) is caused by a lympho-tropic retrovirus, now known as the human immunodeficiency virus (HIV). The virus is acquired either by sexual intercourse (homo- or heterosexual) or from the accidental introduction of material contaminated by the HIV into the systemic circulation. Currently it is most common in homosexuals, drug addicts and the recipients of contaminated blood in the form of transfusions or concentrates. However, the disease is now starting to spread in the heterosexual population. In Africa, spread is predominantly by heterosexual contact. The virus incapacitates the T-helper lymphocytes and thus prevents proper functioning of the cell-mediated immune response. It uses the T4 antigen as its receptor and employs the T-cell's genomic apparatus to replicate, destroying the cell as it does so. It can also infect reticuloendothelial cells (including Langerhans cells) and B-cell lymphocytes.

> The human immunodeficiency virus is spread by sexual contact or by contaminated blood being introduced into the blood or tissues of the victim causing AIDS after a long latent interval.

After gaining access, the virus usually stays latent for long periods but may cause a systemic illness a relatively short time after infection and before or at the time of seroconversion. This is characterized by pyrexia, malaise and a rash which have been described as resembling infectious mononucleosis.

For the most part there are no symptoms even after an antibody response develops for several years until the virus is 'activated' by unknown events or an intercurrent infection such as herpes simplex. Skin disorders are prominent in AIDS and patients often present with a skin complaint.

> AIDS has gradually spread and has reached Pandemic proportions.

Infections

When the disease is activated the patient becomes subject to a wide variety of opportunist infections as well as an increased incidence of, and severe manifestations of, usually mild and commonplace infections.

The AIDS patient is subject to a wide variety of opportunist infections as well as an increased incidence of, and severe manifestations of, usually mild and commonplace infections.

Fungus infections

Dermatophyte infections, including nail infection, are extensive and difficult to clear. *Candidiasis* is often a major problem, especially in the mouth and in the oropharyx. Systemic spread of candida infection is unfortunately not uncommon and often a terminal event. *Pityrosporon ovale* causes extensive eruptions of *pityriasis versicolor*. It may also be responsible for a troublesome and persistent truncal *folliculitis* in some patients (Figure 7.1) and the common problem of persistent and severe *seborrhoeic dermatitis* seen in others (see below). Various 'deep fungus' infections are common, particularly in hot and humid parts of the world.

Viral infections

Viral warts may become very extensive and troublesome. Mollusca contagiosa lesions may be both larger than usual and present in very large numbers (Figure 7.2). *Herpes simplex* infection may be a particular problem, with extensive and persistent skin involvement resulting in scarring. *Herpes zoster* is similarly a troublesome infection in AIDS and may be the initial manifestation. It may look unlike

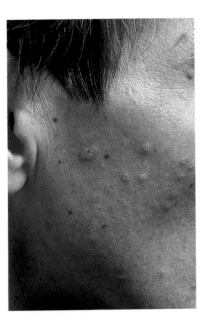

Figure 7.1 Folliculitis due to *Pityrosporon ovale* infection in a patient with HIV infection.

Figure 7.2 Mollusca contagiosa – multiple lesions in a patient with advanced AIDS.

'ordinary' herpes zoster and cause considerable pain and tissue destruction as well as spreading outside the dermatomes in which it began.

Bacterial infections

Tuberculosis and *syphilis* are both major problems for individuals with AIDS. Both disorders progress more rapidly and are responsible for more florid manifestations in AIDS patients than in the normal population. Infections with mycobacterial species that do not generally infect human beings may also be seen. *Epithelioid angiomatosis* is an odd widespread infection with a bacterial micro-organism that is probably caused by a similar micro-organism to the bacillus causing 'cat scratch' disease. It causes Kaposi's sarcoma-like lesions (see below) and a widespread eruption of red papules.

Skin cancers

Depressed delayed hypersensitivity also results in failure of 'immune surveillance' and the development and rapid progression of many forms of skin cancer. However, other mechanisms, including other viral infections, may also be at work in the development of the disorder known as Kaposi's sarcoma (KS). Interestingly the condition does not seem to accompany AIDS contracted from blood transfusion. Mauve, red, purple or brown macules, nodules or plaques which may ulcerate involve the skin at any site and may spread to involve the viscera. It is a frequent cause of death in patients with AIDS.

> AIDS patients are also subject to pruritus, dry skin and seborrhoeic dermatitis; homosexual patients with AIDS are prone to rapidly progressive Kaposis' Sarcoma.

Other skin manifestations

Pruritus

There are several disorders that give rise to generalized itching in AIDS. The papular folliculitis rash that is mentioned above as due to *Pityrosporon ovale* is often distressingly pruritic. The skin of patients with AIDS may become dry and ichthyotic looking, so that AIDS may be counted as one of the causes of 'acquired ichthyosis' and this is also a cause of persistent irritation.

Scabies

Scabies seems to spread very quickly and cause extensive and severe involvement in patients with AIDS and causes severe itching.

Seborrhoeic dermatitis

Another cause of itching in AIDS is *seborrhoeic dermatitis*. This is peculiarly common and often extensive in patients with AIDS –

presumably this is due to massive overgrowth of *Pityrosporon ovale* and whatever other micro-organisms are involved. The manifestations are similar to ordinary seborrhoeic dermatitis although more florid and extensive (Figure 7.3).

Psoriasis

Pre-existing psoriasis may develop an 'explosive phase', or psoriasis may develop de novo as an aggressive, rapidly spreading eruption. It is not clear why psoriasis is aggravated in this manner in HIV infection. It is no more common in the HIV positive population than in normal controls.

Treatment of skin manifestations of AIDS

Treatment with zidovudine (azidothymidine, AZT) (500–1500 mg per day in 4–5 divided doses) is indicated to slow the progress of the HIV infection. It causes nausea, malaise, headache, rash and many other side effects. Ganciclovir and Foscarnet are indicated for cytomegalovirus complications. Acyclovir is used for herpes simplex and herpes zoster. Various antibiotics and other antimicrobials are used as indicated for the bacterial infections. Fluconazole, itraconazole and keto-conazole are particularly useful for the serious and life-threatening Candida infections. Recombinant interferon-alpha 2β and other interferons have been used with some success in Kaposi's sarcoma.

Drug-induced immunodeficiency

Patients who have organ transplants of kidneys, heart or liver are maintained on corticosteroids and either azathioprine or cyclosporin for the rest of their lives. Patients with autoimmune disorders such as systemic lupus erythematosus, systemic sclerosis or dermatomyositis, rheumatoid arthritis or chronic renal disease, and those with psoriasis, atopic dermatitis and other eczematous diseases, amongst others, are also treated with these immunosuppressive drugs for varying lengths of time. The cutaneous side effects from the immunosuppression are not usually as prominent as in AIDS patients but depend on the extent and length of the immunosuppression.

Patients with renal allografts appear to have most problems, maybe because they are treated continuously for longer periods than most of the other groups. They are prone to the development of numerous warty lesions on the hands and face – after about eight years of immunosuppression some 25% were found to have warty patches in one British study (Figure 7.4). These are either viral warts or solar keratoses, or lesions which are somewhere in between! It may be that many of the viral warts directly transform into preneoplastic lesions.

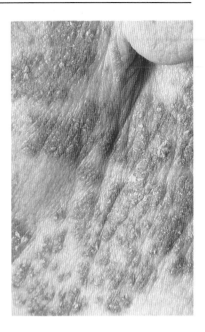

Figure 7.3 Extensive florid seborrhoeic dermatitis in a patient with HIV infection.

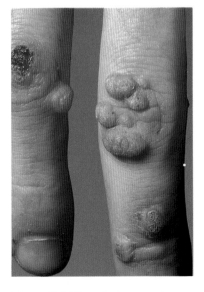

Figure 7.4 Warty lesions on the hands in patient after eight years on azathioprine and prednisolone following renal allograft, which are either viral warts or solar keratoses or somewhere in between.

Certainly Bowen's disease and squamous cell carcinoma of the exposed areas are not uncommon but the exact role and contributions of solar ultraviolet radiation, human papilloma virus infection and the drugs themselves are uncertain.

It should be noted that photochemotherapy with ultraviolet radiation of the 'A' type (320–400 nm, the long wave part of the spectrum) (PUVA) treatment (page 318) causes depression in delayed hypersensitivity but it is not certain what role this has in the subsequent development of skin cancer in patients with psoriasis treated with PUVA some years previously.

Other causes of acquired immundeficiency

Lymphoreticular diseases such as Hodgkin's disease can result in depressed delayed hypersensitivity. The same is true for the leukaemias. Carcinomatosis also causes depressed immune defences. Sarcoidosis also results in depressed delayed hypersensitivity. There are depressed immune defences of the skin in atopic dermatitis (page 107) but these have not been adequately characterized and do not seem to result in anything other than skin infections (viral warts, mollusca contagiosa, herpes simplex and staphylococcal infection in particular). Hypovitaminosis A, chronic malnutrition and chronic alcoholism also result in depressed immune defences.

> Causes of immunodeficiency include treatment with immunosuppressive drugs, PUVA therapy, alcoholism, malnutrition and some congenital disorders.

Congenital immunodeficiencies

There are various congenital causes of depressed immunity resulting in either depressed immediate hypersensitivity or depressed cell-mediated immunity or a combination of both of these. Infantile agammaglobulinaemia is inherited as an X-linked recessive disorder. There are no plasma cells in the marrow and the patients are susceptible to severe pyoderma and numerous warts. In severe combined immunodeficiency there is depression of circulating lymphocytes and levels of all immunoglobulins. Patients are susceptible to all infections and usually die between the ages of 1 and 2 years. It is inherited as either a sex-linked recessive or an autosomal recessive characteristic. Ataxia telangiectasia (autosomal recessive) is characterized by cerebellar degeneration, telangiectasia on exposed skin developing progressively, lymphopaenia and depressed levels of IgA. There are also syndromes with defective neutrophil function such as the autosomal recessively inherited Job syndrome resulting in staphylococcal abscesses. In some congenital disorders the underlying problem has not been well characterized as, for example, epidermodysplasia verruciformis, in which plane warts due to particular antigenic types of the wart virus are widespread over the limbs and trunk.

Dermatological aspects of venereal disease

Several skin infections, while not exclusively 'venereal', are nonetheless spread by venereal contact. Such disorders include genital warts, molluscum contagiosum, scabies and pubic lice.

Reiter's syndrome

This disorder occurs as a sequel to nonspecific urethritis in men and less commonly bowel infection, and probably results from infection with a mycoplasma organism in most cases. There is usually an accompanying arthritis and spondylitis and occasionally a conjunctivitis. Psoriasiform skin lesions develop on the soles and toes. These are often severe, aggressive and pustular (**keratoderma blenorrhagica**). The psoriasiform lesions may be extremely persistent and very disabling. Inflamed red scaling patches may also develop on the glans penis (**circinate balanitis**). There is a curious preponderance of patients with the HLA B27 haplotype.

Gonorrhoea

This venereal disease which predominantly affects urethral epithelium is caused by the delicate intracellular Gram-positive diplococcus – the gonoccoccus. The skin is only affected during gonococcaemia, when small purpuric and pustular vasculitic lesions suddenly appear in the course of a pyrexal illness (Figure 7.5).

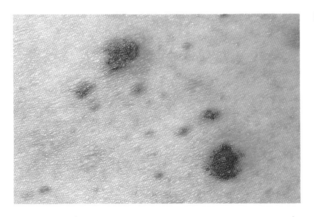

Figure 7.5 Vasculitis.

Chancroid (soft sore)

This venereal infection is caused by the Gram-negative bacillus *Haemophilus ducreyi*. One to five days postinfection a soft sloughy ulcer appears on the penis or vulva. Other sites in the perineal and genital areas may be affected, and sometimes extragenital sites are affected. Inguinal adenitis occurs in 50% of patients. The chancroid lesion must be carefully distinguished from the chancre of syphilis, herpetic ulceration, granuloma inguinale and the results of trauma, by clinical bacteriological and serological methods. The treatment of choice is erythromycin (500 mg 6-hourly for 14 days).

Syphilis

Syphilis has been of enormous historical importance and has once again become of major importance with the emergence of AIDS. This is both because the syphilitic chancre serves as a portal of entry for the HIV virus and because the manifestations of syphilis are much more dramatic in AIDS patients.

The disease is caused by the delicate spirochaetal micro-organism *Treponema pallidum* that is transmitted by contact between mucosal surfaces as in sexual intercourse.

> The primary chancre of syphilis occurs at the site of inoculation after 9–90 days and is then followed by a generalized secondary stage with rash and fever and eventually by a localized destructive (gummatous) tertiary stage 5–50 years later.

CLINICAL FEATURES

Characteristically the incubation period is 9 to 90 days and the first sign is the appearance of the chancre at the site of inoculation, usually on the glans penis, prepuce or less often on the shaft in men and on the vulva in women. In homosexuals the chancre appears around or in the anus. Chancres less often appear on the lips and buccal mucosa or around the inguinal regions or buttocks. The chancre is of variable size (0.5–3 cm in diameter) and has a sloughy and markedly indurated base.

Figure 7.6 Palmar rash in secondary syphilis.

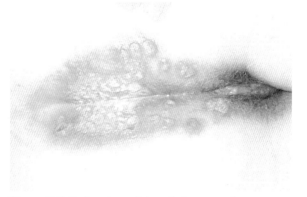

Figure 7.7 Perianal condylomata in secondary syphilis.

Untreated, it heals after three to eight weeks. This primary stage of the disease is followed by a brief quiescent phase of from two months to up to three years before the secondary stage occurs. In secondary syphilis there are signs of systemic upset with mild fever, headache, mild arthralgia, generalized lymphodenopathy and skin manifestations. These latter include an early widespread macular rash, including on the palms (Figure 7.5) and a later papular or lichenoid eruption. Thickened warty areas (condyloma lata) appear perianally and in other moist flexural sites (Figure 7.7). Ulcers appear on the oral mucosa (snail trail ulcers).

After resolution of the secondary stage there is a latent period without signs or symptoms lasting for 5 to 50 years. The tertiary stage takes protean forms and includes cardiovascular disease with aneurysm formation, central nervous disorder either as tabes dorsalis or general paralysis of the insane, and ulcerative or gummatous lesions that may occur on the skin or on mucosal surfaces.

DIAGNOSIS

Diagnosis is made by identification of the spirochaete from wet preparations of the chancre or moist secondary stage lesions and by serological tests detecting either lipoidal substance liberated by tissues or by the presence of antibodies to the micro-organism.

The serological tests are very important. The older Wasserman reaction (WR) was a complement fixation test and has been replaced by the venereal disease reference laboratory (VDRL) test which is a 'flocculation test', which although not specific is quite sensitive and becomes positive early in the disease. It also responds to effective treatment by becoming negative some six months after therapy. The WR and the VDRL tests (and other similar tests) depend on lipoidal antigens. The *Treponema pallidum* haemagglutination assay is currently the most used specific test depending on antibodies to the micro-organism.

TREATMENT

The treatment of syphilis is by parenteral penicillin over a 10-day period. One intramuscular injection of procaine penicillin 600 000 IU daily for 10 consecutive days is adequate. A proportion of patients develop a fever and maybe a rash after starting treatment (Jarisch Herxheimer reaction) – more serious reactions can also occur.

CHAPTER
8

The eczematous dermatoses

This group of disorders is characterized by the presence of a particular type of inflammation of the skin in which the main focus of damage is in the epidermis. The epidermal cells become separated by oedema fluid (spongiosis) (Figure 8.1). Other signs of inflammation, including the accumulation of inflammatory cells and vasodilatation, are seen in the upper dermis immediately beneath the epidermis.

This type of response is provoked by a wide variety of stimuli including direct injury from toxic chemicals and mechanical trauma and immunological reactions although the cause of some eczematous disorders has not yet been discovered.

Traditionally, eczematous disorders are divided into endogenous (or constitutional) types in which the cause of the problem stems from the patient's inherent constitution rather than the environment, and exogenous types which result from an external influence of some kind. In fact the division is not that simple as endogenous eczema is often precipitated or aggravated by external factors and exogenous eczema occurs more readily in patients who have had endogenous eczema.

The clinical picture of the eczematous diseases is quite varied, depending on the nature of the provoking stimulus and the acuity of the process. The common types of eczema are set out in Table 8.1. The terms eczema and dermatitis are synonymous.

Figure 8.1 Pathology of eczematous reaction showing spongiosis in one segment of the epidermis.

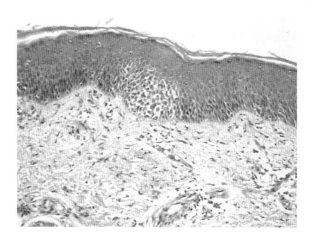

Table 8.1 Common types of eczema

Type	Synonyms	Frequency/age group	Remarks
Atopic dermatitis	Neurodermatitis Besnier's prurigo Infantile eczema	Very common, mostly occurs in infants and the very young	Cause unknown but appears to be immunologically mediated
Seborrhoeic dermatitis	Infectious eczematoid dermatitis	Very common, all age groups	Probably has a microbial cause with overgrowth of normal skin flora being responsible
Discoid eczema	Nummular eczema	Uncommon — mainly in middle-aged individuals	Cause unknown
Lichen simplex chronicus	Circumscribed neurodermatitis	Quite common, mainly in young and middle-aged adults	Initial cause appears to be a localized itch causing an 'itch–scratch cycle'
Eczema craquelée	Ateatotic eczema	Uncommon, restricted to the elderly	Low humidity and vigorous washing seem responsible
Venous eczema	Stasis dermatitis Gravitational eczema	Common in the age group that has gravitational syndrome	Multiple causes, a common variety is allergic contact dermatitis to medicaments used
Allergic contact dermatitis		Common in all adult age groups save the very old	Delayed hypersensitivity response to a specific agent
Primary irritant contact dermatitis	Occupational dermatitis 'Housewives' eczema'	Very common in all adult age groups save the very elderly	Both mechanical and chemical trauma responsible
Photosensitivity eczema		Not uncommon — mainly in adults	Both phototoxic and photoallergic types occur

> Eczema is an inflammatory skin response to many injurious agents characterized by epidermal oedema.

Atopic dermatitis

DEFINITION
This is a very common, extremely itchy disorder of unknown cause that characteristically but not invariably affects the face and flexures of infants, children, adolescents and young adults.

> Persistent pruritus with secondary effects from scratching are characteristic of atopic dermatitis.

101

CLINICAL FEATURES

Signs and symptoms
The major issue as far as this disease is concerned is itching. When the disorder is in an 'active phase' the patient is constantly itchy and restless but subject to irregular episodes of intense and quite disabling intensification of the pruritus. The itchiness is made worse by changes in temperature, by rough clothing (such as woollens) and by sundry other minor environmental alterations. This symptom greatly disturbs sleep and when young children are affected the whole family becomes affected. Scratching results from the severe pruritus in all save infants under the age of two months. In addition to scratching, patients with atopic dermatitis often rub the affected itching parts – they frequently rub their eyes with the index finger knuckles (Figure 8.2). The incessant scratching and rubbing results in considerable injury to the skin, the most obvious of which is the simple linear scratch mark or excoriation (Figure 8.3). More significant than the excoriation is the chronic thickening of the skin that results from the perpetual scratching. This is also characterized by accentuation of the skin markings at the site involved. The thickening and accentuation of skin markings is

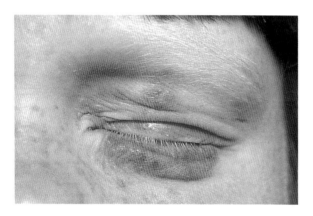

Figure 8.2 Inflammation and thickening of skin of eyelids due to continual rubbing in atopic dermatitis.

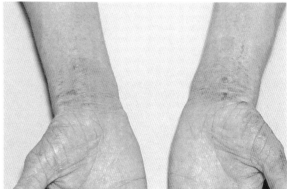

Figure 8.3 Scratch marks (excoriations) and eczematous patches on wrists in atopic dermatitis.

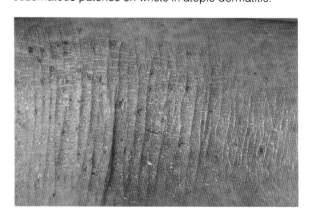

Figure 8.4 Accentuation of skin marking in lichenification in a patient with atopic dermatitis.

known as lichenification (Figure 8.4) and is due to massive epidermal hypertrophy as well as oedema and inflammatory cell infiltrate in the upper dermis (Figure 8.5).

In many patients there is a widespread fine scaling of the skin surface described as 'dryness' or xeroderma, but which is not really a form of ichthyosis (page 249) as sometimes described incorrectly, but the results of the eczematous process itself. Another feature sometimes incorrectly ascribed to ichthyosis is the presence of increased prominence of the skin markings on the palms (Figure 8.6) – the so-called hyperlinear palms. Luckily these give rise to no particular disability and the true cause is unknown. In the most severely affected patients there is in addition a background pinkness of the skin as well as cracking and fissuring at some sites because of the inelasticity of the abnormal stratum corneum.

The skin of the cheeks is often quite pale in contrast to the rest of the skin and this feature, taken together with crease lines just below the eyes (known as Denny Morgan folds) probably the result of continual rubbing, makes the facial appearance quite characteristic (Figure 8.7).

When the skin of the back of an atopic dermatitis patient is firmly stroked with a blunt object such as a key, a white line results in some

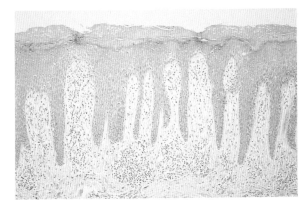

Figure 8.5 Pathology of lichenification showing epidermal thickening and inflammation.

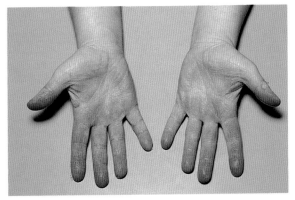

Figure 8.6 Increased markings on palms typical of atopic dermatitis.

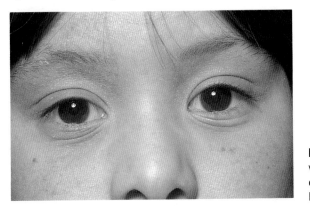

Figure 8.7 The face of a patient with atopic dermatitis showing an extra 'fold' beneath the eyes – the Denny Morgan fold.

70% of patients (Figure 8.8) – 'white dermographism'. This is the reverse of the normal triple response and tends to disappear when the condition improves. The cause of this paradoxical blanching is unknown but is presumably similar to a blanching observed after intracutaneous injection of methacholine or carbamyl choline into the skin of atopic dermatitis patients.

Sites affected

The sites mostly affected are the flexures, particularly the antecubital and popliteal fossae, the face and neck, the wrists and ankles, but truncal skin and indeed anywhere on the skin surface can be involved (Figures 8.9 and 8.10). Because of the continual rubbing the nails tend to be smooth and shiny and the eyelashes and eyebrows may be obviously deficient for the same reason.

Clinical variants

In patients with black skin there is a marked follicular component to the disorder in which there are numerous follicular papules in affected areas (Figure 8.11). In lichenified areas in black-skinned patients there may be irregular pigmentation with hyperpigmentation at some sites and loss of pigment at other sites.

Some individuals lose their childhood eczema only to develop chronic palmar eczema in later years. This is believed also to be a manifestation of atopic disease.

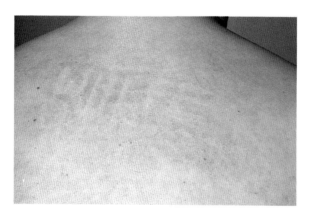

Figure 8.8 White dermographism in a patient with atopic dermatitis.

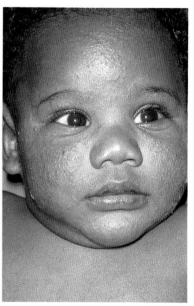

Figure 8.9 Atopic dermatitis affecting the face.

Associated disorders

Patients with atopic dermatitis quite often also suffer from asthma. Approximately 30% of atopic dermatitis patients will also have had asthma before their skin disorder has healed. There is no particular synchronization and the worsening or remission of one has no particular implication as far as the state of the other is concerned. Patients with atopic dermatitis also have an increased prevalence of hay fever and once again the activity of one seems to bear no particular relationship with the activity of the other.

Atopic dermatitis, asthma and hay fever seem to share pathogenetic mechanisms in which aberrant immune processes play an important part. These three 'atopic' disorders cluster in families and the tendency to one or the other or all is inherited in an as yet uncharacterized way.

> Atopic dermatitis, asthma and hay fever seem to share pathogenetic mechanisms in which aberrant immune processes play an important role.

Other disorders that are said to occur more frequently in 'atopic' patients include chronic urticaria (pages 66–69) and migraine. Alopecia areata (pages 274–276) occurs more often in atopic dermatitis patients than normal control subjects and is more intractable when it does.

In addition to these associations, the skin of patients with atopic dermatitis is more vulnerable to both chemical and mechanical trauma and has an unfortunate tendency to develop irritant dermatitis.

Complications

Patients with atopic dermatitis are frequently troubled by skin infections. The appearance of pustules and the development of impetiginized areas (page 38) represent pyococcal infection and are the most

> Patients with atopic dermatitis are frequently troubled by skin infections. The appearance of pustules and the development of impetiginized areas are common.

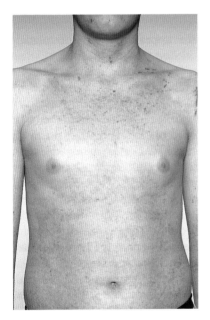

Figure 8.10 Atopic dermatitis involving much of the front of the trunk.

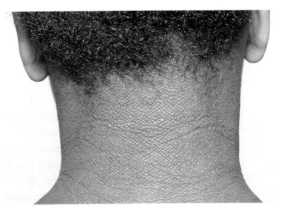

Figure 8.11 Follicular papules in a patient with black skin, due to atopic dermatitis.

infection and pituitary–adrenal axis suppression, probably outweighs the short-term benefits.

Cyclosporin is a fungal metabolite with immunosuppressive effects that is also useful for some patients with severe psoriasis (page 140). It is a cyclic peptide that has been found useful to suppress the rejection response in patients with renal or cardiac transplants. It has been found to have a dramatic effect in patients with severe generalized atopic dermatitis when given at a dose of 3–5 mg/kg/body weight per day. Unfortunately, as with most effective drugs, there are toxic side effects which in the case of cyclosporin include nephrotoxicity and hypertension.

None of these systemic drugs or PUVA should be given without consultation of a specialist with experience in the benefits and side effects of the various treatments.

> Patients with severe atopic dermatitis may need PUVA systemic cyclosporin or steroids. Many benefit from appropriate antibacterial treatments.

Antimicrobial agents

As already mentioned, patients with atopic dermatitis are particularly prone to skin infection. Infection with staphylococci and maybe other bacteria cause pustules, impetiginized lesions and cellulitis in these patients and may also be responsible for flare-ups of the dermatitis. This is the reason that appropriate antibacterial measures by themselves seem to be beneficial for the eczema sufferer.

For those patients having recurrent infected lesions, bacterial swabs must always be taken before starting treatment with either topical or systemic antibacterial agents. It is sometimes useful to recommend an antimicrobial bath additive such as a povidone iodine or a hexachlorophane preparation. The infected area can be soaked or bathed in 1 in 8000 potassium permanganate solution or aluminium subacetate solution. Topical antibiotics are not recommended save perhaps topical tetracycline because of the problems of encouraging the emergence of resistant strains.

If there is evidence of significant infection in several sites which may be aggravating the atopic state then systemic antibiotics should be given. The particular agents used will depend on local practice and current policy but provision to deal with a penicillin-resistant Staphylococcus should be made and for this reason either flucloxacillin or a quinolone is often prescribed.

Seborrhoeic dermatitis

DEFINITION

A common eczematous disorder that characteristically occurs in 'hairy areas', both in the flexures and on the central parts of the trunk, and is now believed to be at least in part due to overgrowth of the normal skin flora in the regions affected.

Overgrowth of normal skin flora causes itchy, red scaling and crusted areas in flexures, over central areas of the face and on scalp in seborrhoeic dermatitis.

CLINICAL FEATURES

Signs and symptoms

Reddened itching patches appear at the affected sites which may become either scaly or exudative and crusted. Scaling is a common feature when the condition develops insidiously (Figure 8.14) and scaling lesions are the most frequently seen. Often mild scaling occurs without erythema as it does, for example, on the scalp as 'dandruff'. When severe, the eyebrows may also be affected. Other facial areas may become involved such as the nasolabial folds, the paranasal sites and the retroauricular folds. Scaling and erythema of the eyelid margins (marginal blepharitis) may also occur. Another type of lesion seen in seborrhoeic dermatitis is a form of folliculitis. This seborrhoeic folliculitis is marked by the presence of sheets of small papules and papulopustules which if closely examined seem to derive from the hair follicle in the region. At least in some of these patients the usually commensal yeast-like micro-organism *Pityrosporon ovale* seems to have taken on an aggressive role and to have been responsible for the inflammatory lesions seen.

The condition may also erupt suddenly and cause exudative lesions in the flexures. This is especially prone to occur in the summer months in overweight individuals. In the elderly, seborrhoeic dermatitis sometimes rapidly spreads, becoming generalized. This 'erythrodermic' picture is disabling but luckily quite uncommon.

The disorder causes considerable itchiness, as do all the eczematous disorders. It also gives rise to soreness and much discomfort when it is exudative and affects the major flexures.

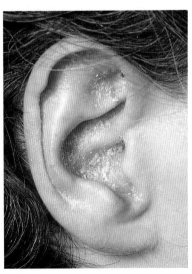

Figure 8.14 Scaling in seborrhoeic dermatitis.

111

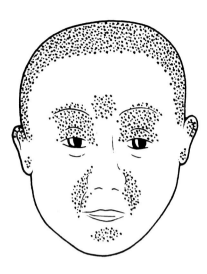

Figure 8.15 Sites of involvement in facial seborrhoeic dermatitis.

Sites affected

The facial sites affected are highlighted in Figure 8.15. Scaling patches occurring on the central chest (Figure 8.16) and over the upper back are less common now than they once were in middle-aged and elderly men. Itchy erythematous areas occurring in the groins, especially in the overweight and especially in middle-aged and elderly men, are extremely common (Figure 8.17). When acute and severe the condition becomes exudative and other flexural sites such as the axillae and the umbilicus also become involved (sometimes known as infectious eczematoid dermatitis).

DIFFERENTIAL DIAGNOSIS

In the groin area it is important to distinguish flexural psoriasis (pages 125–126) and ringworm infection (tinea cruris, page 34). Ringworm rashes are usually asymetrical and don't reach up right into the groin apices. There is usually a raised advancing edge to ringworm and a tendency to clear centrally. Mycological testing is so simple and useful

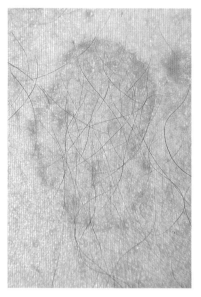

Figure 8.16 Scaling patch on chest in seborrhoeic dermatitis.

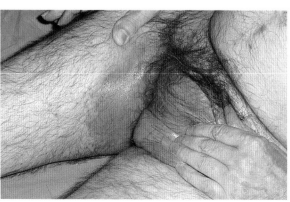

Figure 8.17 Infectious eczematous dermatitis affecting the groin in an elderly man.

Table 8.2 Differential diagnosis of rashes in the groin

	Clinical features	Tests
Ringworm	Often not symmetrical, very itchy, rapidly spreading	Microscopy and culture of scales
Seborrhoeic dermatitis Intertrigo	Tends to be symmetrical and to involve apices of groins as well, other areas may be affected	None available
Clothing dermatitis	May resemble seborrhoeic dermatitis, likely to affect other areas	Patch testing
Chronic benign familial pemphigus	Exudative, fissured appearance, often a family history	Biopsy

and the results of misdiagnosis so embarrassing that all should become proficient at skin scraping and recognition of fungal mycelium (page 32). Rarely, Hailey–Hailey disease (chronic benign familial pemphigus) presents with persistent exudative lesions that may resemble seborrhoeic dermatitis (see Table 8.2).

> Seborrhoeic dermatitis has become notorious recently as a sign of AIDS, and presumably this is a result of the underlying immunosuppression.

NATURAL HISTORY AND EPIDEMIOLOGY

The condition is extremely common at all ages and in both sexes. Severe and widespread seborrhoeic dermatitis is a particular problem for elderly men but the milder forms are probably no more common in the elderly than in younger age groups. A rash diagnosed as seborrhoeic dermatitis in infancy is now thought by some to be a form of atopic dermatitis. 'Cradle cap' occurring in the newborn is probably not related to proper seborrhoeic dermatitis but represents a minor and transient abnormality of desquamation from the scalp.

As far as is known, there is no racial predilection for the disorder and it appears to affect all social groups and occupations. The disorder has become notorious recently as a sign of AIDS, and presumably this is a result of the underlying immunosuppression (page 94).

Left untreated, the condition waxes and wanes over many years. Indeed some individuals seem curiously prone to develop lesions of seborrhoeic dermatitis and are rarely free of one type of seborrhoeic dermatitis or another over long periods.

113

In treatment of seborrhoeic dermatitis, removal of the precipitating microbial cause and suppression of the eczematous response with topical preparations containing both 1% hydrocortisone and a miconazole or clotrimazole may be all that is required.

TREATMENT

The major aims in treatment of seborrhoeic dermatitis are the removal of the precipitating microbial cause and the suppression of the eczematous response. For this purpose topical preparations containing both 1% hydrocortisone and an imidazole such as miconazole or clotrimazole may be all that is required for patients with limited disease. A recently introduced preparation containing lithium succinate has also been useful. Occasionally, if these agents are unsuitable or unsuccessful, a traditional empirical approach may be tried using sulphur and salicylic acid preparations. These agents are antimicrobial and keratolytic, and although inelegant, appear quite effective when all else fails!

When there are exudative intertriginous areas in the major body folds then bed rest is indicated to avoid further friction between opposing skin surfaces and to minimize continued irritation from clothing. Bland lotions or weak nonirritating antibacterial solutions should be used to bathe the affected areas frequently or as wet dressings that *must* be kept moist. Broad-spectrum systemic antibiotics should also be employed: ampicillin or a tetracycline are suitable. This treatment usually succeeds in improving the situation within a few days, after which topical corticosteroid–imidazole preparations can be used.

Discoid eczema (syn. nummular eczema)

DEFINITION

Discoid eczema is a quite common eczematous disorder of unknown cause distinguished by the appearance of reddened scaling rounded areas on the arms and legs.

CLINICAL FEATURES

Signs and symptoms

Slightly raised, pink-red scaly discs, varying in diameter from 1 to 4 cm, appear on the arms and legs and less frequently on the trunk (Figure 8.18). The disorder is usually quite itchy but not usually as itchy as many other eczematous disorders. It is not usually acute and exudative, but can be. The skin on the arms and legs often shows dryness as well.

NATURAL HISTORY AND EPIDEMIOLOGY

Discoid eczema is one of the less common eczematous conditions but is by no means rare. It is most common in the middle aged and elderly. The condition is not as persistent as many types of eczema and is not usually troublesome after a few months.

DIFFERENTIAL DIAGNOSIS

The condition has to be distinguished from psoriasis, in which the margins are more distinct, from ringworm, which usually spreads peripherally and has a raised margin, and from Bowen's disease, which

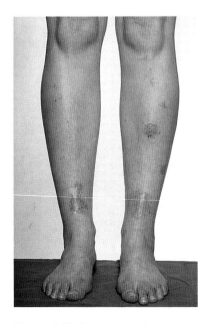

Figure 8.18 Patches of discoid eczema on legs.

Table 8.3   Differential diagnosis of round, red scaling patches

Psoriasis	Well-defined, thickened, scaly plaques, usually multiple
Discoid eczema	Only a moderately well-defined edge. Slightly scaly pink patches, limited in number
Ringworm	May be annular with central clearing. Microscopy and culture of scales will reveal
Bowen's disease	Often slightly irregular in shape. Infiltration is varied. Edge is well defined. Biopsy settles

is mostly restricted to the light exposed areas and is usually one or two solitary red scaling patches (see Table 8.3).

PATHOLOGY AND PATHOGENESIS
The changes of eczema are present in histological sections but nothing is known of the cause of this disorder.

TREATMENT
Weak and moderately strong corticosteroid preparations (e.g. 1% hydrocortisone, clobetasone or desoximethasone are all suitable) applied once or twice daily usually suppress the disorder. Tar preparations (e.g. Clinitar® cream) or tar-corticosteroid preparations (e.g. Tarcortin) are also helpful. Emollients and emollient cleansers are also helpful as adjuncts.

Eczema craquelée (syn. asteatotic eczema)

DEFINITION
Eczema craquelée is an uncommon eczematous disorder that occurs on the extensor aspects of the limbs of elderly subjects and is characterized by a 'crazed' and fissured appearance.

CLINICAL FEATURES

Signs and symptoms
The most common affected sites are the shins, but the sides of the thighs and extensor aspects of the upper arms and forearms, as well as the back, are all sometimes involved. Involved skin is pink, roughened and superficially fissured, giving a crazed appearance (Figure 8.19). The areas affected are more sore than itchy. The condition has a very characteristic appearance and it is uncommon for it to be mistaken for any other disorder.

Figure 8.19 Eczema craquelée – note dry, 'crazed' scaling appearance.

NATURAL HISTORY AND EPIDEMIOLOGY
The disorder is restricted to the elderly and is mainly seen in the newly hospitalized or institutionalized individual when there is low ambient relative humidity and after unaccustomed vigorous bathing. The condition persists if untreated but rapidly remits with treatment.

PATHOLOGY AND PATHOGENESIS
The disorder seems to be an unusual response of already vulnerable skin to minor mechanical and chemical trauma.

TREATMENT
The main element to the treatment is rehydration of the skin surface using emollients and emollient cleansers and at the same time stopping vigorous washing and drying. Use of 1% hydrocortisone ointment may also speed up resolution.

Lichen simplex chronicus (syn. circumscribed neurodermatitis)

DEFINITION
This is a disorder localized to one or, less frequently, two or more sites that is intensely pruritic and is characterized by thickening and exaggeration of skin markings on the surface.

CLINICAL FEATURES

Signs and symptoms
Some areas seem predisposed to the development of lichen simplex chronicus (LSC) including the medial aspect of the ankle, the back of the scalp, the extensor aspects of the forearms around the wrists, and

the genitalia. The condition is extremely itchy and patients complain bitterly about the intense local irritation that they experience.

The lesions are characteristically raised irregular red plaques with a well-defined margin which have exaggerated skin markings (lichenification) over the scaling surface (Figure 8.20). If the itching is persistent and intense and the resultant scratching vigorous, the affected sites may become very thickened, raised and excoriated. The resultant lesion is known as a prurigo nodule and unlike LSC many such nodules may occur over the skin in an uncommon disorder known as prurigo nodularis (Figure 8.21).

NATURAL HISTORY AND EPIDEMIOLOGY

This not uncommon condition is mainly seen in tense and anxious middle-aged subjects of either sex and all races. It may be more common in the Indian subcontinent. It is a very stubborn and persistent disorder which may stay unchanged for many years. Prurigo nodularis is similarly stubborn and persistent.

DIFFERENTIAL DIAGNOSIS

Hypertrophic lichen planus (page 144) may be difficult to distinguish although this disorder tends to be more mauve and be less regularly lichenified than LSC. Biopsy may be needed to distinguish these disorders with certainty. Lichen simplex chronicus may also resemble a patch of psoriasis (page 124) although the distinct lichenification of LSC should distinguish it.

PATHOLOGY AND PATHOGENESIS

Histologically there may be striking hypertrophy of the epidermis (Figure 8.22) which in extreme cases may resemble epitheliomatous change (pseudoepitheliomatous hyperplasia). There is also hyperkeratosis and a variable amount of inflammation in the subepidermal zone. There is a marked increase in the rate of epidermal cell production accounting for the hypertrophy and it is believed that the persistent

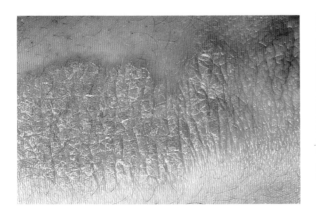

Figure 8.20 Thickened scaling erythematous patch of lichen simplex chronicus.

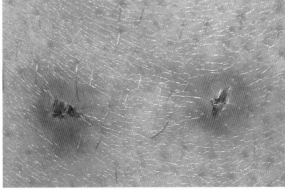

Figure 8.21 Prurigo papules – note excoriations.

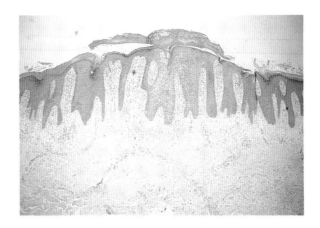

Figure 8.22 Pathology of lichen simplex chronicus. Note marked psoriasiform epidermal thickening.

trauma of scratching and rubbing is responsible for this. The major question as to what provokes the pruritus in the first place remains unanswered.

TREATMENT
The condition tends to persist regardless of the treatment prescribed. High potency topical corticosteroids, intralesional corticosteroids or preparations of coal tar are sometimes helpful.

Contact dermatitis

This term is used to describe an eczematous rash developing as a result of contacting injurious materials. These materials may injure by a direct toxic action on the skin or may induce an immunological reaction of delayed hypersensitivity type. The former is known as a primary irritant contact dermatitis. The latter is allergic contact hypersensitivity. They may be difficult to distinguish clinically. Both types of contact dermatitis are common and extremely important as they cause a great deal of loss of work and disability.

Primary irritant dermatitis

DEFINITION
Primary irritant dermatitis is an eczematous rash that results from direct contact with toxic 'irritating' materials.

> Primary irritant dermatitis is an eczematous rash that results from direct contact with toxic 'irritating' materials.

CLINICAL FEATURES
Scaly red and fissured areas appear on the irritated skin (Figure 8.23). The hands are the most frequently affected. The palmar skin and the palmar surfaces of the fingers are often affected but the areas between the fingers and elsewhere on the hands may also be involved. The condition may become exudative and very inflamed if the substances contacted are very toxic.

> Scaly red and fissured areas appear on the irritated skin. The hands are the most frequently affected.

    This form of contact dermatitis causes considerable soreness and

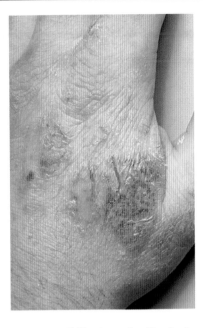

Figure 8.23 Primary irritant dermatitis affecting hand.

irritates. The fissures make movement very difficult and effectively disable the victims.

DIFFERENTIAL DIAGNOSIS

The condition must be distinguished from allergic contact dermatitis by a carefully taken history and patch testing (see below). Psoriasis of the palms may resemble contact dermatitis but is usually accompanied by signs of psoriasis elsewhere and distinguished by having an easily discernible margin.

Ringworm usually affects one palm only and is marked by diffuse erythema and silvery scaling. If there is any doubt, scales should be examined for fungal mycelium under the microscope.

NATURAL HISTORY AND EPIDEMIOLOGY

An 'irritant' substance will injure anyone's skin if there is sufficient contact. However, some individuals are more prone to develop primary irritant contact dermatitis – especially atopic subjects and those with fair skins who sunburn easily.

The disorder is particularly often seen in manual workers (occupational dermatitis) and housewives (housewife's eczema). Builders, mechanics, hairdressers, cooks and laundry workers are some of the groups who are frequently affected. The condition causes considerable economic loss from the loss of work caused. Contact with alkalis, organic solvents, detergent substances, cement and particulate waste is often responsible.

> Some individuals are more prone to develop primary irritant contact dermatitis – especially atopic subjects and those with fair skins who sunburn easily.

PATHOLOGY AND PATHOGENESIS

The condition can be thought of as a kind of 'epidermal failure' in which after prolonged minor injury from one or several substances the epidermis responds by developing an eczematous reaction.

MANAGEMENT

Identification of potential hazards and prevention is important. Use of the least irritating substances, prevention of skin contact, the use of protective gloves, proper skin care by removal of irritants and the use of emollients and worker education are all important in prevention.

When present the cause must be identified and further contact prevented. When the condition is severe, rest from manual work is required. Emollients are an important part of treatment to make affected skin more supple and to minimize fissuring. Weak and moderately potent corticosteroids should accelerate healing. Some patients who suffer repeated attacks may need to be transferred to work which is less damaging to the skin.

Allergic contact dermatitis

> Allergic contact dermatitis is an eczematous rash that develops after contact with an agent to which delayed (cellular) hypersensitivity has developed at the sites of skin contact with the 'allergen'.

DEFINITION

Allergic contact dermatitis is an eczematous rash that develops after contact with an agent to which delayed (cellular) hypersensitivity has developed.

CLINICAL FEATURES

The rash develops at the sites of skin contact with the 'allergen' but occasionally spreads outside these limits for unknown reasons. The vigour and speed of the reaction vary enormously depending on the particular individual. When very acute, the reaction develops within a few hours of contacting the responsible substance – such a speedy response is seen, for example, in the condition of 'poison ivy' which is common in the USA. Itching is noticed at first and then the area involved becomes red, swollen and vesicular. Later the area becomes scaling and fissured.

An enormous number of substances are potentially capable of causing 'sensitization' so that allergic contact dermatitis develops after contact with these materials. Nickel dermatitis is one of the commonest examples of allergic contact dermatitis – some 5% of women in the UK are said to be nickel sensitive. They cannot wear stainless steel jewellery because of the nickel in the steel (Figure 8.24). Similarly they develop a rash beneath steel 'studs', clips and buckles in contact with the skin. Patients who are nickel sensitive may also react to 'dichromate' and other chromate salts.

Other examples of allergy of this type include allergy to chemicals in rubber, for example, mercaptobenzthiazole (MBT) and thiouram, and to formalin. These allergies may cause dermatitis when wearing particular clothes, as indeed may sensitivities to dyes.

Allergies to lanolin (in sheepwool fat and used in many ointments and creams) and to perfumes, can cause dermatitis after the wearing of cosmetics. Lanolin is also one of many substances that also include ethylene diamine, Vioform, neomycin and local anaesthetics that cause a dermatitis after using a cream or an ointment (dermatitis medicamentosa) (Figure 8.25).

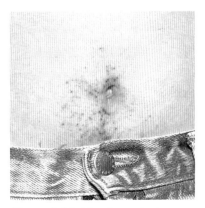

Figure 8.24 Allergic contact dermatitis to nickel in a stainless steel stud.

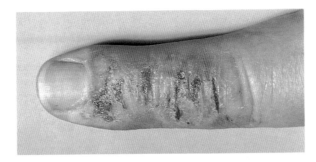

Figure 8.25 Allergic contact dermatitis to Cetavlon PC in an antiseptic cream.

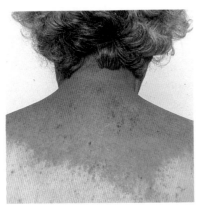

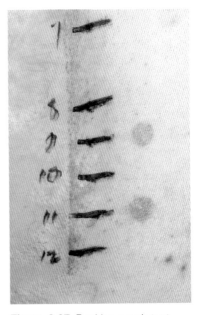

Figure 8.26 Allergic contact dermatitis to paraphenylene diamine in hair dye.

Dyes (such as the black hair dye paraphenylene diamine) can also be the cause of allergic contact dermatitis (Figure 8.26). Plants such as garlic and flowers such as primulas and chrysanthemums often sensitize as well.

Some materials are notorious for causing sensitivity and are not often used topically because of this, for example, penicillin, sulphonamides.

NATURAL HISTORY AND EPIDEMIOLOGY

Allergic contact dermatitis is not as prevalent as primary irritant dermatitis but is nonetheless quite common. It is rare in children and less common in the elderly. It is seen in all racial groups although is less common in black-skinned individuals. The sensitivity, once established, is theoretically permanent, though in practice some patients seem to lose their sensitivities.

DIAGNOSIS OF ALLERGIC CONTACT HYPERSENSITIVITY

Accurate history taking is important to learn of possible contactants. Similarly, careful examination identifying all involved areas and the possible contactants of these sites is very important. The definitive technique for diagnosing allergic contact hypersensitivity is the patch test. In this test possible allergens are placed in occlusive contact with the skin for 48 hour periods and the area inspected 48 hours after removal of the patch. A positive test is revealed by the development of an eczematous patch with erythema, swelling and vesicles at the site of application (Figure 8.27). In practice, low concentrations of allergen are applied to avoid false positive primary irritant reactions.

Figure 8.27 Positive patch test reactions 24 hours after removal of a 'patch test battery' that had been in occlusive contact for 48 hours.

> The definitive technique for diagnosing allergic contact hypersensitivity is the patch test. Possible allergens are placed in occlusive contact with the skin for 48 hour periods and the area inspected 48 hours after removal of the patch.

121

Table 8.4 Common antigens used in patch testing and concentrations in which they are used

Antigen	%
Nickel sulphate	5
Balsam of Peru	25
Colophony	10
Chlorocresol	1
PPD base	1
MBT	2
Formalin	1
Potassium dichromate	0.5
Wool alcohols	30
Epoxy resin (Araldite)	1
Chloroxylenol	1
Neomycin	20
Cobalt chloride	1
Dowicil 200	1
Parabens	15
Thiuram-mix	1
Mercapto-mix	2
Perfume-mix	8
Kanthon CG	0.67
Primin	0.01
Ethylene diamine	1
Benzocaine	5

MBT = mercaptobenzthiazole. PPD = paraphenylene diamine

In most cases a battery of the commonest allergens in appropriate concentrations is applied. Such a battery is set out in Table 8.4

> The antigen crosses the stratum corneum and is picked up by epidermol Langerhans cell who 'process' it and pass it to T-lymphocytes. These lymphocytes develop a specific memory for the antigen and then divide. Those cells are then involved in subsequent exposures.

PATHOLOGY AND PATHOGENESIS

The sensitizing chemical (antigen) crosses the stratum corneum barrier and is picked up by the Langerhans cells in the epidermis (Figure 8.28). The antigen is then 'processed' by the Langerhans cell and then passed on to T-lymphocytes in the peripheral lymph nodes. Here some of the T-lymphocytes develop a specific 'memory' for the particular antigen and the population of these expands. This process of sensitization takes some 10–14 days in humans. After this period, when the particular antigen contacts the skin the primed T-lymphocytes with the 'memory' for this chemical species rush to the contacted site and liberate cytokines and mediators that injure the epidermis and cause the eczematous reaction. The pathology of allergic contact hypersensitivity is quite similar to that seen in other types of eczema.

TREATMENT

It is vital to identify the sensitizing material and prevent further contact. The eczema will subside rapidly in most cases after removal from the antigen. Use of weak or moderately potent topical corticosteroids and emollients will speed the resolution of the eczematous patches.

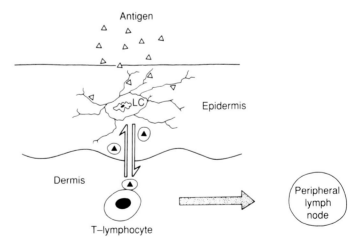

Figure 8.28 Diagram to show processes in allergic contact dermatitis. △ = antigen. ▲ = antigen processed by Langerhans cell. LC = Langerhans cell. Antigen is processed by T-Langerhans cells in the epidermis and then presented to T-lymphocytes.

Venous eczema (*syn*. gravitational eczema; stasis dermatitis)

DEFINITION

This is an eczematous disorder occurring predominantly on the lower legs in individuals with chronic venous hypertension.

CLINICAL FEATURES

Itchy pink scaling areas which become exudative and fissured intermittently develop on a background of the changes of chronic venous hypertension (Figure 8.29). The affected areas are often around venous ulcers but the margins of the eczematous process are poorly defined. Occasionally the process spreads to the contralateral leg and even to the thighs and arms.

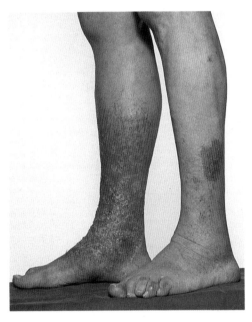

Figure 8.29 Gravitational eczema.

PATHOGENESIS

In most cases the eczema is due to an allergic contact hypersensitivity to one of the substances used to treat the venous ulcer. Such substances include lanolin, neomycin, Vioform, ethylene diamine and rubber additives. No allergic hypersensitivity is found in some patients, and it has been suggested that such patients develop a sensitivity to the breakdown products of their own tissues (autosensitization).

TREATMENT

Care must be taken to ensure that any contact hypersensitivity is identified and the patient advised not to use any substance to which he or she is sensitive. The simplest of topical applications should be used – white soft paraffin is suitable as an emollient and 1% hydrocortisone ointment is suitable as an anti-inflammatory agent.

Psoriasis and lichen planus

Psoriasis

Psoriasis is one of the most important skin disorders because of its frequency, persistence and/or recurrent nature and tendency to disable in a proportion of those it affects. The clinical features, combined with some understanding of the genetic background and cascade of events involved in the production of the skin lesions have served to focus the attention of researchers on to the disorder. One issue that has not yet been answered satisfactorily is whether psoriasis is one disease or several. Certainly there are several variants that differ sufficiently to question as to whether they represent separate diseases or not. 'Psoriasis-like' (psoriasiform) tissue reactions also occur as a reaction to a range of stimuli, suggesting that the tissue alterations in psoriasis may only represent one important type of tissue response to injury.

DEFINITION

Psoriasis is a common, genetically determined, inflammatory skin disorder of unknown cause which in its most usual form is character-ized by well-demarcated raised red scaling patches that preferentially localize to the extensor surfaces.

> Psoriasis is a genetically determined inflammatory disorder of unknown origin affecting 1–2% population causing well defined red scaling patches on extensor surfaces.

CLINICAL FEATURES

The lesions

The typical lesion is distinctive. It has a very well demarcated margin and is raised above the skin surface (plaque). The affected skin is a variable shade of red and the surface is often thrown up into large silvery scales (Figure 9.1). Plaques vary enormously in size and shape. They often start out discoid but end up polycyclic (Figure 9.2) as several lesions coalesce.

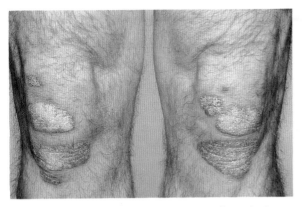

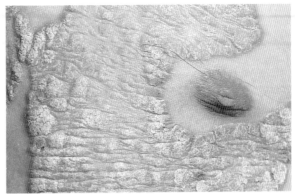

Figure 9.1 Typical red scaling plaques of psoriasis on knees.

Figure 9.2 Polycyclic plaque of psoriasis.

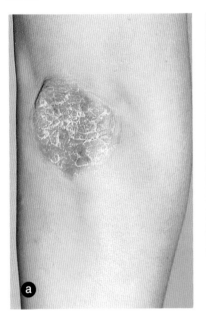

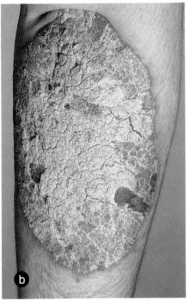

Figure 9.3 (a) Psoriatic patch on elbow – a site of predilection. (b) Thick plaque of psoriasis with heaped up adherent scale.

Sites affected

In its most usual form psoriasis affects the extensor aspects of the trunk and limbs preferentially. The knees, elbows and scalp are especially frequently affected (Figure 9.3). In fact virtually anywhere on the skin surface can be affected, although the mucosae seem spared.

The nails are often affected and may show the so-called thimble pitting, separation of the nail plate from the nail bed (onycholysis), subungual debris, brownish-black discolourations and deformities of the nail plate (Figure 9.4). Rarely the nails are affected in the absence of any changes on the skin surface.

Although the extensor surfaces are predominantly affected in the majority of patients, the reverse sometimes occurs, so that flexural lesions are more prominent. This is most often seen in the major body folds in the elderly, especially in those who are overweight. The groins and genitalia, the axillae, the inframammary folds in women and the skin of abdominal folds and the umbilicus in either sex are affected by sore red patches whose surfaces are not as scaly as in ordinary psoriasis as the moistness of the flexural areas decreases the scaling and produces a moist and glazed appearance (Figure 9.5).

The face is not usually severely affected in psoriasis although the scalp margin, the paranasal folds and the retroauricular folds are quite often involved (Figure 9.6).

Psoriasis sometimes appears at the site of a minor injury such as a scratch, a burn or a graze (Figure 9.7). This curious reaction is known as the isomorphic response or the Koebner phenomenon. It mostly occurs when the psoriasis is in a particularly active and spreading phase. The development of a skin disorder at the site of injury is characteristic of, but not specific to, psoriasis as it is also seen in other

Figure 9.4 (a) A minor degree of involvement of nail plate with pitting and onycholysis. (b) Severe nail involvement with deformity of nail plates and discolouration. (c) Typical psoriatic nail with onycholysis and some discolouration.

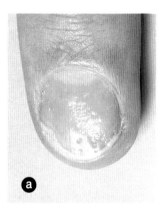
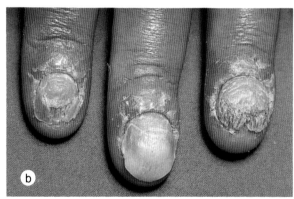
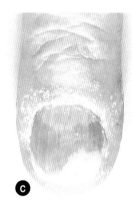

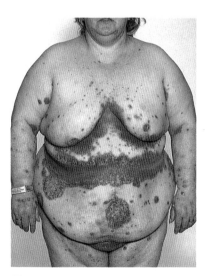
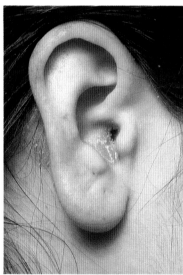
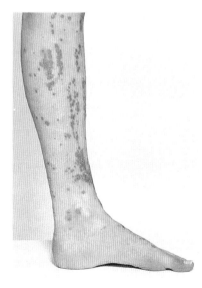

Figure 9.5 Flexural psoriasis affecting body folds in obese patient.

Figure 9.6 Psoriasis of retroauricular folds.

Figure 9.7 Psoriasis appearing at sites of injury (scratch marks). This is known as the isomorphic response (Koebner phenomenon).

disorders, including lichen planus (page 74) and discoid lupus erythematosus (page 142). Its cause is unknown.

NATURAL HISTORY AND EPIDEMIOLOGY

Surveys in the UK, the USA and Scandinavia have all reported that psoriasis is found in between 1 and 3% of the population at the time of the survey. It has been claimed that the disorder is less common in African and Asian groups but detailed figures aren't available. It does appear less of a problem in the Japanese and some other Asian populations but it has been suggested that it is becoming more frequently seen in these groups with the trend to westernization. Whatever the exact frequency and whatever the particular population under discussion, the nature of the disease makes it a skin disorder of major importance.

Interestingly, the disease has been found to be of greater frequency in men than in women in some studies. There are two main peaks of incidence. The commonest age at which the disorder first appears is in the second half of the second decade of life. Recently it has been recognized that psoriasis also appears quite often for the first time in the seventh decade. In general, the younger the age of onset the worse the outlook as far as frequency, severity and persistence of the disease is concerned.

Psoriasis is a life-long disorder subject to unpredictable remissions and relapses. Single episodes are uncommon and in the most frequent variety an episode in the teenage years is followed by a series of attacks, each lasting weeks or months, in the succeeding years. Less frequently the disorder is persistent but fluctuates in intensity.

> Psoriasis is a life-long disorder subject to unpredictable remissions and relapses.

GENETICS

Psoriasis is often familial, but does not appear to be inherited in any regular dominant, sex-linked or recessive way. With one parent affected there is approximately a 30% chance of a child being affected. With both parents suffering from psoriasis the chances rise to 60% that a child will develop psoriasis. In a recent survey in Sweden it was found that 6.4% of relatives of families in which there was a patient with psoriasis were affected, compared to 1.94% of controls. Nonidentical twins have an approximately 20% chance of both being affected, and the 'concordance' rate for identical twins seems to be of the order of 70%. These figures do not suggest a regular Mendelian form of inheritance but are consistent with either a 'polygenic' form of inheritance or perhaps an autosomal dominant with so-called incomplete penetrance.

It has been found that certain leukocyte antigens (HLA) occur more frequently in patients with psoriasis than in the general population. The HLA characteristics of an individual are carried on chromosome 6, are inherited in a regular Mendelian way and are of vital importance in the body's immune response. There are A, B and C (class I) and D (class II) types of antigen (or loci) with several alleles for each locus. One at each locus is received from each parent.

Several diseases have been found to have associations with particular HLA groupings but the associations are 'statistical' and not absolute. Psoriasis is one such disease and is linked with several HLA types. The specific HLA groups associated are HLA-B13, HLA-B17 and HLA-B37. In addition there is an association with the class II antigen DR7. It is said that an individual with one of these groups has a five or six times increased chance of having the disease compared to the population without these groupings. These groupings are said to be associated particularly with psoriasis of early onset. Another HLA group, CW6, apparently has an even greater association with psoriasis (13 times increased risk in Caucasians and 25 times in Japanese!).

DIFFERENTIAL DIAGNOSIS

Any red, scaling disorder can be mistaken for psoriasis and vice versa (see Table 9.1). On the scalp the most frequently seen disorder to be mistaken is seborrhoeic dermatitis (page 111) although this usually affects the scalp diffusely rather than in distinct plaques. Lichen simplex chronicus (page 116) of the scalp typically presents with a red scaling patch on the occiput which can look very psoriasis-like. The intense itching and lichenified surface should serve to distinguish the two disorders.

Multiple patches of ringworm may appear very like psoriasis (Figure 9.8) but the lesions are often more ring-like than psoriasis and can be distinguished by microscopical examination of potassium hydroxide (KOH)-treated skin scraping (page 32). Mycosis fungoides – a T-cell lymphoma of skin – often evolves through a phase in which there are many red psoriasiform lesions on the trunk. They differ from psoriasis

Table 9.1   Differential diagnosis of red scaling rashes

	Discriminants
Psoriasis	Nail changes, family history, multiple patches on extensor surfaces
Discoid eczema	Round scaly patches on arms and legs
Lichen simplex chronicus	Itchy, lichenified, persistent
Bowen's disease	Plaques tend to be smaller and more limited in number, biopsy decides
Superficial basal cell carcinoma	Thin, slightly raised edge, biopsy decides
Mycosis fungoides	Multiple psoriasiform patches, but irregularly thickened, biopsy helps
Ringworm	Often annular, spreads peripherally, microscopy and culture of scale important

by being more irregular in shape and being persistent and at differing stages of development.

On the legs, raised round red scaling 'psoriasiform' patches often turn out to be Bowen's disease in the elderly, but could also be psoriasis or discoid eczema. Lichen simplex chronicus around the ankles may also be difficult to distinguish.

Psoriasis of the palms (Figure 9.9) and/or soles can be very difficult to distinguish from eczema affecting these sites. Even after several investigations, including biopsy, the clinician may remain undecided as to the correct diagnosis.

Superficial basal cell carcinoma lesions are sometimes several centimetres in diameter and quite psoriasiform in appearance but have a fine raised 'hair-like' margin. There are also disorders characterized by the development of pink scaling patches of unknown cause that have (inappropriately) been termed the 'parapsoriasis' diseases. They probably have no proper relationship to psoriasis other than a superficial morphological similarity in some instances.

The psoriasiform appearance is common to a number of dermatoses and biopsy and other investigations are often required to reach a definitive diagnosis.

> Psoriasis must be distinguished from other red/scaling disorders including eczematous conditions, ring worm, neoplastic disorders of epidermis and mycosis fungoides.

CLINICAL VARIANTS

Guttate psoriasis
This disorder is mainly seen in children aged 7–14 years. Often it develops some two to four weeks after an episode of tonsillitis or pharyngitis, mostly due to beta-haemolytic streptococci. It behaves like

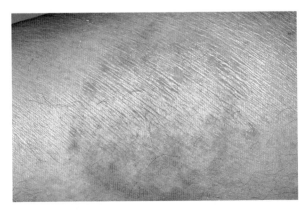

Figure 9.8 'Psoriasiform' plaque in leg due to ringworm.

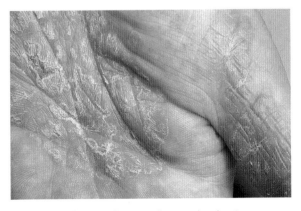

Figure 9.9 Red scaling patch on palm due to psoriasis. Such a presentation can be very difficult to distinguish from eczema.

an exanthem as the characteristically 'drop' sized lesions (Figure 9.10). All appear at the same time and usually don't last longer than eight to ten weeks.

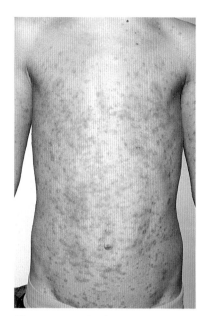

Figure 9.10 Multiple small patches of 'guttate' psoriasis seen after a streptococcal tonsillitis.

Napkin psoriasis

Infantile napkin dermatitis (page 232) sometimes takes on a very psoriasis-like appearance and typical psoriatic lesions develop on the scalp and trunk. Generally this clears with appropriate treatment without recurrence of psoriatic lesions during childhood, so that the true relationship with psoriasis is unknown.

Erythrodermic psoriasis

Patients with severe and widespread plaque-type psoriasis sometimes progress to generalized skin involvement. When this happens the typical plaque-like appearance disappears and the skin is universally red and scaly and the condition is known as erythrodermic psoriasis. Such patients are seriously ill (Chapter 21). They suffer from a number of complaints.

1. Heat loss, and they are in danger of hypothermia because of the increased blood supply to the skin.
2. Water loss, leading to dehydration because of the disturbed barrier function of the abnormal stratum corneum.
3. They also have a hyperdynamic circulation because effectively there is a vascular shunt in the skin. When the patient's myocardium is already compromised because of other factors there is a danger of high output failure.
4. Erythrodermic patients also lose protein, electrolytes and metabolites via the shed scale and exudate and may develop deficiency states.
5. They also become depressed because of the malaise, pruritus and discomfort they experience.

Erythrodermic patients may be improved or put into remission by treatment but their outlook is none too good because such patients are prone to develop further attacks of generalized disease.

> Patients with generalized psoriasis suffer from heat loss, dehydration loss of other nutrients and hyperdynamic solution.

Pustular psoriasis

Most dermatologists consider this as a manifestation of psoriasis, although there are some who believe it is a separate disorder. It seems probable to the writer that pustular psoriasis is indeed part of the disorder we know as psoriasis, with exaggeration of one particular component of the disease (see Pathology below). There are two main types:

1. *Palmoplantar pustulosis*
   Patients with palmoplantar pustulosis (PPP) develop yellowish-

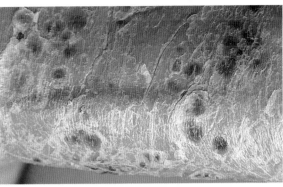

Figure 9.12 Pustular psoriasis of the sole of the foot with several older brown scaling lesions that were pustules.

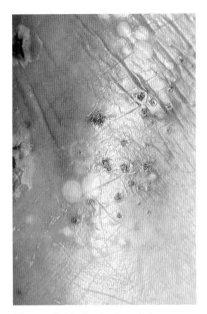

Figure 9.11 Typical pustular psoriasis affecting the sole of the foot.

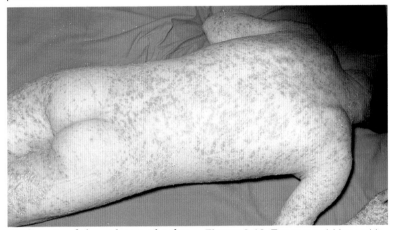

white, sterile pustules on the central parts of the palms and soles (Figure 9.11). Older lesions take on a brownish appearance and later are shed in a scale at the surface (Figure 9.12). The affected area can become generally inflamed, scaly and fissured, and although relatively small areas of skin are affected the condition can be very disabling.

Figure 9.13 Ten-year-old boy with severe generalized pustular psoriasis.

The disorder tends to be resistant to treatment (see below) and is subject to relapses and remission over many years.

Palmoplantar pustulosis is characterized by yellowish pustules on palms and soles.

2. *Generalized pustular psoriasis*
This is also known eponymously as Von Zumbusch disease, and is one of the most serious disorders dealt with by dermatologists. In its classical form attacks occur suddenly and are characterized by severe systemic upset, a swinging pyrexia, arthralgia and a high polymorphonuclear leukocytosis accompanying the skin disorder.

The skin first becomes erythrodermic and then develops sheets of sterile pustules over the trunk and limbs (Figure 9.13).

In generalized pustular psoriasis the skin suddenly becomes erythrodermic and then develops sheets of sterile pustules over the trunk and limbs. Pyrexia, leukocytosis and severe malaise accompany the condition.

Sometimes the pustules become confluent so that 'lakes of pus' develop just beneath the skin surface. In other areas there is a curious type of superficial peeling without pustules forming.

These patients are very unwell and require hospitalization. Mostly they can be brought into remission by modern treatments (see below) but are subject to recurrent attacks. The disorder sometimes affects infants and small children.

> 'Seronegative' rheumatoid type polyarthropathy occurs in 5–6% psoriasis. There is also a destructive arthropathy affecting distal interphalangeal joints known as psoriatic arthropathy.

Other forms of pustular psoriasis
Occasionally pustules may develop after strong corticosteroids have been used and then abruptly withdrawn. The same is true for systemic steroids and it is generally acknowledged that pustular psoriasis may occur as a consequence of the use of corticosteroids in psoriasis.

Other rare variants of pustular psoriasis include:

1. Acrodermatitis continua (also known as dermatitis repens) in which there is a recalcitrant pustular erosive disorder on the fingers and toes around the nails and occasionally elsewhere.

2. Pustular bacterid, in which sterile pustules suddenly appear on the palms and soles after an infection.

Subcorneal pustular dermatosis is another quite rare disorder which is probably a variant of pustular psoriasis and in which there is a generalized eruption of sterile superficial pustules.

Arthropathic psoriasis
There is a higher prevalence of a rheumatoid-like arthritis with symmetrical involvement of the small joints of the hands and feet, wrists and ankles in patients with psoriasis (5–6%) compared to a matched control population (1–2%). This 'rheumatoid arthritis-like' disorder differs in one important respect from ordinary rheumatoid arthritis – there is no circulating rheumatoid factor.

In addition to the above pattern of polyarthritis, there is a distinctive and destructive form of joint disease that seems specific to psoriasis. In this 'psoriatic arthropathy' the distal interphalangeal joints, the posterior zygohypophysial, the temporomandibular and the sacroiliac joints are particularly picked out by the inflammation. The disorder is also more destructive than in rheumatoid disease, so that bony erosion and destruction take place leading to 'collapse' of affected digits (Figure 9.14) justifying the term often used for this dreadful disease – arthritis mutilans.

Although remissions may occur and treatment may temporarily improve these inflammatory joint complications of psoriasis they tend to run a progressive course subject to remissions and relapses.

PATHOLOGY AND PATHOGENESIS

The histopathological appearance of psoriasis is distinctive but not specific. The main features may be subdivided into (1) the epidermal thickening, (2) the inflammatory component, and (3) the vascular component, but of course all are closely interlinked.

The epidermal thickening

The epidermis shows marked exaggeration of the rete pattern and elongation of the epidermal downgrowths with bulbous club-like enlargement of their ends (Figure 9.15). The average thickness is increased from about three to four cells in the normal skin to approximately 12–15 cells in the psoriatic lesion. Many mitotic figures can be seen and the rate of epidermal cell production seems to be greatly enhanced. When epidermal cells are labelled in DNA synthesis by exposing them to a radiolabelled precursor of DNA *in vitro* or *in vivo* and an autoradiographic technique to demonstrate the labelled cells, there is an obvious increase of cells in division in psoriasis compared to normal (Figure 9.16). The turnover time of psoriatic epidermis and stratum corneum is consequently very much shortened. Normally it

> There is an obvious increase of cells in division in psoriasis compared to normal. The turnover time of psoriatic epidermis and stratum corneum is consequently very much shortened.

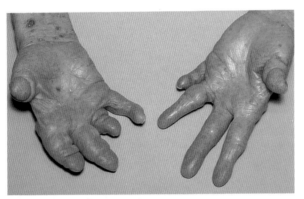

Figure 9.14 The results of psoriatic arthropathy (arthritis mutilans).

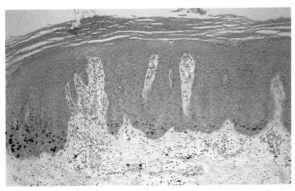

Figure 9.15 Regular epidermal thickening in psoriasis with parakeratosis. There are cells at the base of the epidermis that are darkly labelled by the process of autoradiography after incubation in radiolabelled thymidine indicating that they are in the DNA synthesis of cell division.

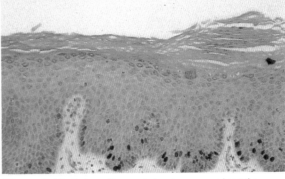

Figure 9.16 Autoradiograph to show prominently darkly labelled cells in DNA synthesis after incubation with radiolabelled thymidine.

Normally it takes some 28 days for a newly born cell to ascend from the basal layer and travel through the epidermis and the stratum corneum and reach the surface and desquamate off. In psoriasis it takes some 4 days.

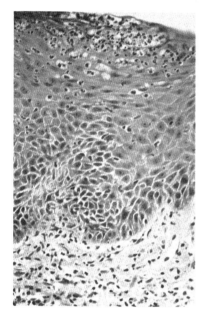

Figure 9.17 This photomicrograph shows many inflammatory cells in the thickened epidermis in psoriasis.

takes some 28 days for newly born cells to ascend from the basal layer and travel through the epidermis and the stratum corneum and reach the surface and desquamate off. In psoriasis it takes some four days!

Surmounting the thickened epidermis is a stratum corneum in which the epidermal nuclei have not disappeared during differentiation ('parakeratosis').

The inflammatory component

Interspersed between the 'parakeratotic' horn cells are collections of desiccated polymorphonuclear leukocytes known as Munro microabscesses. The epidermis is oedematous and itself infiltrated by inflammatory cells. The dermis immediately below the epidermis also contains many inflammatory cells, mostly lymphocytes. In pustular psoriasis the epidermal component is much less in evidence and there are collections of inflammatory cells within the epidermis (Figure 9.17). It has been suggested that chemotactic influences attract the inflammatory cells into the epidermis and stratum corneum and both complement components and eicosanoids – particularly leukotriene B4 – have been identified in psoriatic stratum corneum.

The vascular component

The papillary capillaries are greatly dilated and tortuous to a degree not seen in other inflammatory skin disorders. Ultrastructurally it can be seen that there are larger gaps than usual between the endothelial cells. These abnormal capillaries are the last of the features to go during resolution and it has been claimed that abnormal capillaries can be detected in the apparently normal uninvolved skin of psoriatic subjects.

The pathology of psoriasis is characterized by epidermal hypertrophy collections of polymorphs in the parakeratotic stratum corneum and dilated tortuous papillary capillaries.

AETIOLOGY

The cause of psoriasis is unknown, despite the enormous research effort that has been made in the past two to three decades. Various hypotheses have been popular at different times. One very obvious abnormality in psoriasis is the hyperplastic epidermis with increased mitotic activity, and one line of intense investigation has been directed at determining whether there is a defect in the control of epidermal cell production in this disease. As there is incomplete information concerning normal regulation of epidermal cell division, the question has been difficult to answer, but anyway attention has moved away from this possibility and focused more on the inflammation and possible immunopathogenesis. Several subtle immunological defects have been described but of more interest is that the disorder often responds to immunosuppressive agents such as cyclosporin and methotrexate.

Various potentially heritable biochemical abnormalities have been suggested and/or described which could explain both the increased epidermal proliferation and the inflammatory component. At different times, alterations in the skin content or activity of cyclic nucleotides, polyamines, eicosanoids, cytokines and growth factors have been described, but in most cases these changes are secondary to other less well characterized events.

Infection has been recurrently considered as a possible cause and in recent years the involvement of retroviruses has been suggested. In this respect it is worth noting that in acquired immune deficiency syndrome (AIDS) patients a very severe and aggressive form of psoriasis may develop.

Evidence for any one particular mechanism as the cause of psoriasis is extremely slim and clearly more research effort is needed.

TREATMENT

1. Patients with limited plaque-type psoriasis. Many patients with two or three plaques affecting the knees, elbows or elsewhere require very little treatment. Some don't bother as their lesions do not progress and cause no disability. In other patients simple treatment with an emollient such as white soft paraffin, by itself or with the addition of a mild keratolytic such as 2% salicylic acid, is sufficient when used once or twice daily.

2. When there are more lesions and the disorder is producing symptoms, more active treatments are required. The simplest and often quite effective are the traditional tar-containing preparations. Their mode of action is uncertain but it seems probable that they have several suppressive and cytotoxic effects which summate to give an anti-inflammatory activity. Tar ointment and tar and salicylic acid ointment BP are simple and effective but are not popular as they soil and stain as well as having a distinctive tarry smell. Proprietary tar-containing preparations such as Clinitar® cream and Alphosyl® cream are better looking and smelling. Used once or twice per day these agents are effective and safe. Tar-containing shampoos are also prescribed for the treatment of psoriasis of the scalp. They should be used three or four times per week in conjunction with a topical application for the scaling areas of scalp skin. 'Tar baths' are also employed as part of the treatment for patients with multiple psoriatic lesions. In this form of treatment tar liquid (liquor picis detergens BP) is added to the bath water (50 ml per bath). Topical application of tar in one form or another has often been used to photosensitize patients for subsequent treatment with ultraviolet irradiation (see below). This is mainly applicable to inpatient treatment.

3. Dithranol (Anthralin) is a potent reducing agent (1.8-dihydroxy-9-(1-hydroxy)-anthaphenine). It is one of the most effective remedies available, clearing up to 80% of patients in a six-week period. Unfortunately its use has some disadvantages including being an irritant and causing redness and soreness, making it unsuitable for some patients with sensitive skin and causing a

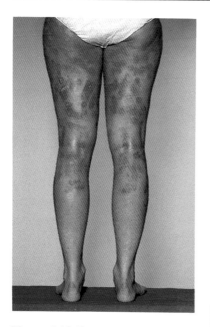

Figure 9.18 Brownish-purple staining on skin due to dithranol.

brownish or purplish stain on the skin treated, as well as on clothes and bedding (Figure 9.18). It is generally used in ascending concentrations, starting at 0.1 or 0.05%. A traditional method of applying dithranol has been in a stiff zinc oxide paste vehicle (Lassar's paste) so that the preparation did not flow onto and irritate uninvolved skin. This treatment requires some skill and is best used on an inpatient basis. To make dithranol treatment suitable for outpatients the tendency has been to use either dithranol in white soft paraffin or one of the proprietary preparations such as Dithrocream® which is available in different strengths. Apart from the irritation and staining dithranol has no serious side effects.

A recently introduced topical treatment is with an analogue of vitamin D3 known as calcipotriol (Dovonex®). This agent appears quite effective and without serious toxicities. It is likely that other vitamin D3-like agents will be available in the next few years.

> Limited plaque type psoriasis usually responds to topical preparations containing tars or dithranol and emollients. Flexural psoriasis may be helped by weak topical corticosteroids.

There is only a very limited role for topical corticosteroids in the treatment of psoriasis. They are useful for patients with flexural lesions for which irritant tar and dithranol preparations are not suitable. For the same reason weak topical corticosteroids are also suitable for lesions on the genitalia and the face. Potent topical corticosteroids should NOT be used because frequent use is likely to lead to side effects (pages 310–311) and because eventual withdrawal may lead to severe rebound and even the appearance of pustular lesions. Potent topical steroids (such as fluocinolone acetonide or betamethasone dipropionate) may be suitable for use on the scalp and they are sometimes justifiable for use on the palms and soles if other treatment is not helping. Nonetheless, potent (and very potent) topical corticosteroids, sometimes with plastic film occlusive bandaging, are used as a first-line treatment in some countries. This treatment damps down the lesions and is 'cleaner' than many of the traditional topical treatments but the added benefits are not worth the potentially serious side effects in this writer's view.

4. Patients with very widespread, erythrodermic and pustular psoriasis require other forms of management. As pointed out above, these individuals are often quite seriously ill and may need inpatient treatment to ensure that they don't become hypothermic, dehydrated or nutritionally deficient and to ensure that they are receiving appropriate regular treatment. For the most part, topical treatment is impractical and inadequate, although the use of emollients may be soothing and may give some slight help. Mostly systemic treatments are needed.

Patients with widespread recalcitrant psoriasis, erythrodermic
psoriasis or generalized pustular psoriasis may require
methotrexate, retinoids or the new immunosuppressive,
cyclosporin.

5. The antimetabolite methotrexate is a competitive antagonist of
    tetrahydrofolate reductase, blocking the formation of thymidine
    and thus DNA. It is thought that this antiproliferative activity
    may be important both as far as the epidermal abnormality is
    concerned and with regard to lymphocyte proliferation and its
    action as an immunosuppressive agent. Whichever way it works it
    is a highly effective treatment for patients with severe psoriasis.
    Unfortunately it is also quite toxic, producing hepatotoxicity in
    most patients who stay on the drug for long periods. The drug
    also suppresses haematopoiesis and may cause gastrointestinal
    upset.
        It is given in doses of 5–25 mg/week orally or intramuscularly.
    To minimize the possibility of serious side effects patients must
    be monitored frequently (preferably monthly) by blood counts
    and blood biochemistry. It is recommended that a liver biopsy is
    performed both before treatment begins and after a cumulated
    dose of 1.5 g methotrexate. If serious liver toxicity is found this
    treatment should stop.
        Methotrexate is also a teratogen and fertile women should use
    contraceptive measures. Although this drug can be dramatically
    successful it must be used with caution. It is mainly suitable for
    those who would otherwise be disabled by the disease, and seems
    particularly suitable for some elderly patients with severe psoria-
    sis.

The retinoids
Retinoids are analogues of retinol (vitamin A) and have been found to
exert important actions on cell division and maturation. The orally
administered retinoid etretinate, and its newer water-soluble derivative
acitretin, has been found to be of particular value in psoriasis. This
drug when given in doses of 0.5–1.0 mg/kg/day benefits patients to
some extent with all types of severe psoriasis after three to four weeks,
but is of most help when used in combination with ultraviolet treatment
(see below) or dithranol. Its major drawback is that it is teratogenic and
can only be given to fertile women if they use contraception. Other
significant toxicities include a hyperlipidaemia producing effect and a
possibility of hyperostosis and extraosseous calcification. In addition it
does have some hepatotoxicity in a few patients (Table 9.2). These
'significant' toxicities are luckily not common but minor mucosal side
effects occur in all patients. These include drying of the lips and the
buccal, nasal, conjunctival and anogenital mucosae. Minor generalized
pruritus and slight hair loss also occur. For this reason these drugs need
to be prescribed and their effects monitored by an experienced
dermatologist. Despite the large number of potential problems they are

Table 9.2   Toxic side effects of etretinate

Toxic side effect	Comment
Major	
Teratogenicity	Contraception necessary for fertile women
Hyperlipidaemic effect	Causes a rise of serum lipids in about 30% of patients; care is needed in chronic use
Hepatotoxicity	Hepatotoxicity is possible but uncommon
Bone toxicity	Disseminated interstitial skeletal hyperostosis and other changes in chronic use
Minor	
Drying and cracking of lips	Seen in most patients
Drying of eyes and nose	Seen in about 25% of patients
Increased rate of hair loss	Seen in about 25% of patients
Pruritus, peeling palms and soles	Seen in about 25% of patients
Myalgia and arthralgia	Seen in about 10% of patients

Table 9.3   Skin disorders helped by ultraviolet radiation

Disease	Comment
Psoriasis	PUVA and UVB are often used
Atopic dermatitis	A few patients benefit
Acne	Only occasionally used
Mycosis fungoides	Often used as initial treatment
Pityriasis lichenoides chronica	Good treatment for rare disease

PUVA = photochemotherapy with ultraviolet radiation of the 'A' type (320–400 nm, long wave part of the spectrum)
UVB = ultraviolet radiation in the 280–320 nm range (the medium wave part of the spectrum)

extremely useful drugs, controlling the psoriasis and being well tolerated by many patients with severe disease.

Treatment with ultraviolet radiation
Ultraviolet radiation (UVR) (pages 20–29) has long been known to have therapeutic effects in a number of skin disorders, including psoriasis (Table 9.3). A form of UVR treatment known as PUVA is mainly used. PUVA is an acronym for Photochemotherapy with Ultra Violet radiation of the A (long wave) type. The UVA is supplied by special fluorescent lamps that emit at wavelengths of 300–400 nm housed in cabinets or special frames over beds.

A photosensitizing psoralen drug is given 2 hours before. The particular psoralen used is mainly 8-methoxy psoralen, but 5-methoxy psoralen and trimethoxy psoralen are sometimes used. The dose of the most frequently used psoralen, 8-methoxy psoralen, is 0.6 mg/kg. The treatment starts off three times per week with exposure gradually increasing till there is a sustained therapeutic effect. Usually improvement starts in the second or third week and after clearance further treatments are given if further lesions appear.

> UVR treatment (either UVB or PUVA) may be useful treatment for patients with generalized recalcitrant plaque type psoriasis.

The dose of UVA is calculated from the output of the lamps and the time of exposure and is calculated in joules. The dose required for clearance is approximately 50–100 joules per cm^2 and care is taken to keep the dose as low as possible and certainly below a total cumulated dose of 1500 joules per cm^2 to reduce the possibility of long-term side effects.

There are several long-term side effects (Table 9.4).

1.   Increased incidence of squamous cell carcinoma of the skin (pages 213–216) (up to 10 or 12 times that in a control group of psoriatics after 10 years) occurs and perhaps an increased incidence of basal cell carcinoma and melanoma as well.

Table 9.4   Side effects of PUVA treatment

Side effect	Comment
Major (long term)	
Skin cancer	Considerable increase in incidence of squamous cell carcinoma and maybe other types of skin cancer
Cataract	UVA screening spectacles must be used during and 24 hours after exposure
'Photoaging'	Damage to the dermis results in the appearance of aging and altered elastic properties
Minor (short term)	
Nausea	Probably due to the psoralen
Burning	In some sensitive people, or if the dose of UVR is too great
Pruritus and xeroderma	Emollients are helpful

UVA = ultraviolet radiation in the 320–400 nm range (the long wave part of the spectrum). UVR = ultraviolet radiation. PUVA = photochemotherapy with UVA.

2. Increased solar elastotic degenerative change with the appearance of aging and alteration of skin elasticity.

3. Cataracts can develop and all patients who receive PUVA must wear effective UVA protective goggles or sun glasses during exposure and for 24 hours afterwards.

In the short term, nausea is often experienced and if too long an exposure is given, burning can occur. Patients who are 'sensitive to the sun' or who coincidently have a disorder that can be aggravated by UVA exposure, such as lupus erythematosus or porphyria cutanea tarda should not be treated by PUVA.

Photochemotherapy with UVA is quite popular with patients because no 'messy ointments' are used and they develop a deep sun tan.

An alternative approach to PUVA which may reduce the total dosage of UVA is called bath PUVA in which the patient bathes in a solution of a psoralen. At the time of writing this is becoming more popular and is likely to supplant oral PUVA treatment for a substantial proportion of patients. Another form of PUVA is used in conjunction with retinoids (RePUVA) in which the total dose of UVA necessary is much reduced, as is the dose of etretinate.

Medium wave UVR (UVB, 280–320nm), once popular, has recently become popular again and certainly is capable of clearing psoriasis especially in combination with tars (page 135) or dithranol (page 135).

Cyclosporin

Cyclosporin is an immunosuppressive agent used in organ transplantation. It appears to work by inhibiting the synthesis of cytokines by T-lymphocytes. It is also dramatically effective in psoriasis when given in doses of 3–5 mg/kg/day. Because of its toxic side effects, which include renal damage with gradually increasing nitrogen retention, it can cause (and aggravate pre-existing) hypertension. Its place in the treatment of severe psoriasis is assured but the long-term usefulness of the drug is currently being explored.

Pityriasis rubra pilaris

DEFINITION

Pityriasis rubra pilaris (PRP) is an uncommon skin disorder of unknown cause which often has a superficial resemblance to psoriasis as it is characterized by redness and scaling but has a distinctive histological appearance and a distinctive component of follicular involvement.

CLINICAL FEATURES

The commonest type of PRP occurs in the late middle-aged or elderly and is often of sudden onset. Usually the disease begins on the face and scalp with pinkness and scaling and spreads within a few days or a week or two to involve the rest of the body. There is a characteristic orange type of hue to the redness (Figure 9.19) and on the thickened palms this is a characteristic yellowish discolouration (Figure 9.20). Scattered

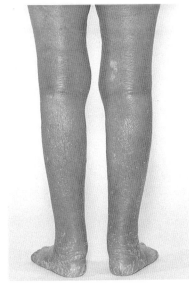

Figure 9.19 Pityriasis rubra pilaris. Note the orangey hue to the erythema. This is a characteristic feature.

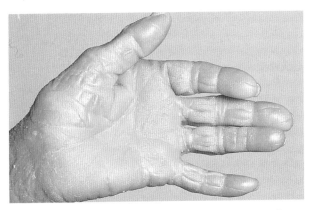

Figure 9.20 Palmar thickening due to hyperkeratosis in pityriasis rubra pilaris.

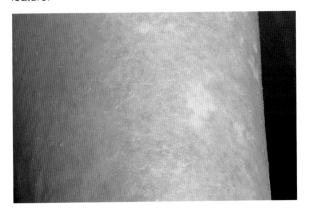

Figure 9.21 An 'island of white spared skin' in pityriasis rubra pilaris.

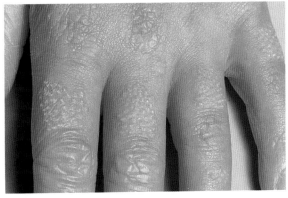

Figure 9.22 Follicular distribution of eruption in pityriasis rubra pilaris.

amongst the red scaling eruption are islands of spared white skin (Figure 9.21) and on the hands, thighs and sometimes elsewhere there is a typical follicular accentuation due to the presence of hyperkeratotic spines (Figure 9.22).

There is also an infantile type which, although similar in many ways to the adult form, tends to be much more stubborn and resistant to treatment.

EPIDEMIOLOGY AND NATURAL HISTORY

Although uncommon, PRP is by no means rare, and most large departments deal with two or three patients per year. The adult form

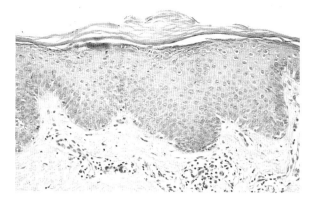

Figure 9.23 Pathology of pityriasis rubra pilaris with epidermal thickening but without the marked accentuation of the rete/papillary pattern as seen in psoriasis.

tends to improve spontaneously after 18 months to two years but the infantile variety may persist for many years.

PATHOLOGY AND PATHOGENESIS

The histological appearance is distinctive in that although there is considerable epidermal thickening the accentuation of the dermal papillae and the undulations of the dermoepidermal junction are much less marked than in psoriasis (Figure 9.23). In addition the follicular canals tend to be filled with compacted horny spines. The inflammatory component of psoriasis is missing in PRP which is why it has often been classified as a disorder of keratinization.

TREATMENT

Many patients respond well to oral retinoids by mouth (page 316) given in the same manner as for psoriasis. Treatment by methotrexate has also been advocated.

Lichen planus

DEFINITION

Lichen planus (LP) is an inflammatory disorder of skin of unknown origin but with a prominent immunopathogenetic component. It is characterized by an eruption of variable extent of typical mauve or pink flat-topped itchy papules.

> Lichen planus (LP) is an inflammatory disorder of skin of unknown origin but with a prominent immunopathogenetic component. It is characterized by an eruption of variable extent of typical mauve or pink flat-topped itchy papules.

CLINICAL FEATURES

The typical lesion of LP is a mauve or pink, flat-topped polygonal papule which often has a whitish lacework pattern on its surface (Wickham's striae) (Figure 9.24). The papules are often aggregated in some sites, for example, the front of the wrist, but may also occur scattered sparsely over the skin of the limbs and trunk. Lichen planus is mostly a mild disorder with only a few lesions developing but many lesions may occur, making life quite uncomfortable for affected patients. In a few the eruption may be dense and generalized (Figure 9.25).

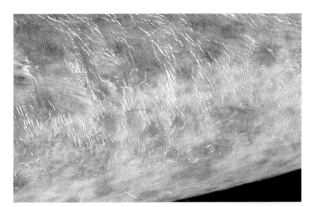

Figure 9.24 Red-mauve papules of lichen planus. Some of these have a faint white network pattern on the surface (Wickham's striae).

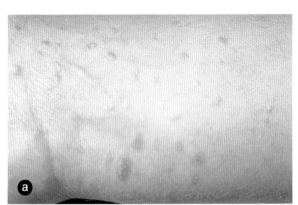

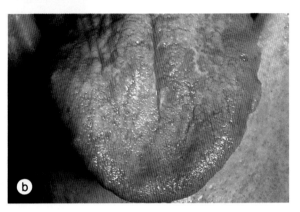

Figure 9.25 Many papules of lichen planus affecting (a) the wrist, (b) the tongue.

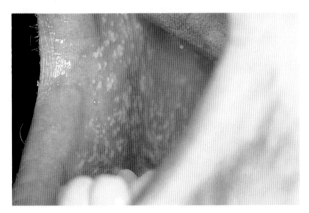

Figure 9.26 White lacework pattern on the buccal mucosa due to lichen planus.

The mucosae are often affected and lesions occur in the mouth in some 30% of patients. A white lacework pattern on the buccal mucosa is the most frequently observed type of lesion (Figure 9.26) but the tongue and elsewhere in the mouth may also be involved with either a white lacework, whitish macules or punctuate lesions. The male genitalia are also sometimes affected (Figure 9.27). Lesions on the oesophageal and vaginal mucosae have rarely been reported. The nails are affected in 5–10% of patients. When they are, longitudinal ridges develop (Figure 9.28). Less frequently a destructive process develops in

143

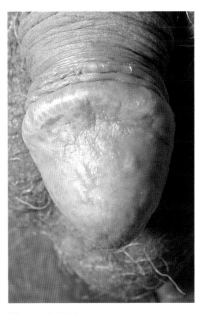

Figure 9.27 Lichen planus papules affecting the glans penis.

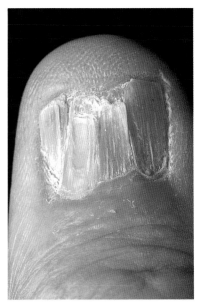

Figure 9.28 Longitudinal ridging of the nails in lichen planus.

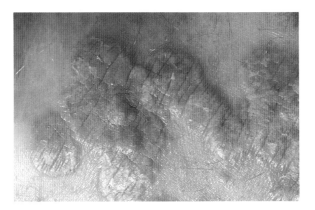

Figure 9.29 Thickened patch of hypertrophic lichen planus.

which the nail plate is lost and the nail forming tissue – the nail matrix – is damaged.

The scalp is sometimes affected and then localized patches of hair loss and scalp scarring occur.

Affected areas are usually very itchy although for some reason excoriations are not often seen in affected skin. As lesions heal they flatten and often leave a pigmented patch at the site of the lesion which persists for some weeks.

Clinical variants

The commonest variant is the hypertrophic lesion. ***Hypertrophic lichen planus*** lesions are thickened mauvish papules or nodules of irregular shape which often have a warty or scaling surface (Figure 9.29). Solitary hypertrophic lesions may appear in the course of a 'routine' attack of lichen planus or develop as solitary lesions in which case they are usually on the lower legs.

Atrophic lichen planus is really quite uncommon. Flat or very slightly raised pink macules develop in this variant.

Annular lichen planus describes the situation in which lichen planus lesions have fused to give a ring-type configuration. This odd variant sometimes occurs on the male genitalia and lower abdomen but rarely occurs elsewhere.

Lichen nitidus is a rare variant of lichen planus in which numerous tiny pink flat-topped papules develop.

Bullous lichen planus is a very rare variant in which blistering occurs on some lesions.

Lichen plano-pilaris is the name for lichen planus which predominantly involves the hair follicles. Affected sites lose their terminal hair and develop horny spines which project from the affected hair follicles.

Very uncommonly an attack of lichen planus may be both very severe and of very sudden onset so that large areas of the skin surface may be affected, causing an erythroderma.

> Patients with Lichen planus have a higher incidence of autoimmune disorders than a control population.

ASSOCIATIONS

Lichen planus appears to be in the general category of autoimmune diseases and patients affected by it have a higher frequency of other autoimmune disorders than a comparable unaffected population. Myasthenia gravis and vitiligo seem particularly associated.

NATURAL HISTORY AND EPIDEMIOLOGY

The disease seems not uncommon in Europe, accounting perhaps for some 2–4% of new patients in skin clinics, but is quite uncommon in the USA. It appears to be a more frequent problem in parts of Asia, but accurate figures are not available. It is rare in children but occurs in most other age groups. It seems rare in families and there does not appear to be a major genetic component to the disease.

For the most part lichen planus is quite benign, most patients being free of lesions after a year. Occasionally repeated attacks may occur. Hypertrophic lesions tend to last for many years.

PATHOLOGY AND AETIOPATHOGENESIS

The characteristic histopathological changes are seen in Figure 9.30.

1. A band of lymphocytes and histiocytes immediately subepidermally. Amongst the inflammatory cell infiltrate are clumps of melanin pigment as a result of damage to the epidermis.
2. Damage to the basal epidermal cells with a 'sawtooth' profile, vacuolar degenerative change and scattered eosinophilic cytoid bodies representing dead epidermal cells.

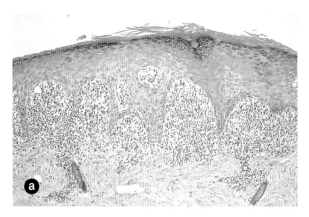

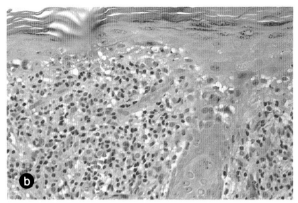

Figure 9.30 (a) Pathology of lichen planus showing typical changes with a band of lymphocytes and histiocytes in the subepidermal region (lichenoid band) and epidermal thickening with hypergranulosis but 'sawtooth' pattern of erosion in the basal epidermal region. (b) Detail of pathology of lichen planus showing basal epidermal region with erosion, cytoid bodies and a dense lymphocytic infiltrate.

> Variable epidermal thickening with increase in thickness of the granular cell layer and a subepidermal band of lymphocytes are typical pathological features.

> The basic alteration is thought of as an immunological attack on the basal layer while the presence of inflammatory cells and the other epidermal alterations are believed to be secondary events.

3. Variable epidermal thickening with increase in thickness of the granular cell layer.

Immunofluorescence studies show a dense band of fibrin at the dermoepidermal junction and clumps of IgM deposit.

The basic process is thought of as an immunological attack on the basal layer while the presence of inflammatory cells and the other epidermal alterations are believed to be secondary events. Very little is known about the initiating event but it is interesting to note:

1. Very similar 'lichenoid' rashes are produced in the course of some drug eruptions.
2. In the course of the graft versus host reaction after marrow transplantation a lichen planus-like reaction occurs, suggesting that the grafted lymphocytes are behaving 'autoaggressively'.
3. As pointed out on page 145 there are associations with other autoimmune diseases.

TREATMENT

As mentioned above, the disease mostly remits spontaneously so that in most patients very little treatment is required. Weak topical corticosteroids may be helpful in relieving the pruritus and reducing the prominence of the eruption. When patients are severely affected with a generalized eruption, systemic corticosteroids are sometimes helpful in giving relief. The oral retinoid drug etretinate (page 137) has also been found successful for some patients.

10

Acne, rosacea and similar disorders

The disorders described in this chapter are common, inflammatory, tend to be characterized clinically by papules and occur on the face pre-eminently. These features do not imply a common aetiopathogenesis.

Acne

Acne is one of the commonest of skin disorders – if not the commonest. It has been estimated that 70% of the population have some clinically evident acne at some stage during adolescence!

> It has been estimated that 70% of the population have some clinically evident acne at some stage during adolescence.

DEFINITION
Acne (acne vulgaris) is a disorder of hair-bearing skin in which hair follicles develop obstructing horny plugs (comedones) as a result of which inflammation later develops around the obstructed follicles, causing tissue destruction and scar formation.

> Increased sebum secretion and formation of horny plugs (comedones) in follicular lumens are the earliest abnormalities in acne.

CLINICAL FEATURES

The lesions
The earliest feature of the disorder is an increased rate of sebum secretion making the skin look greasy (seborrhoea). Blackheads or comedones usually accompany the greasiness. They are often seen at the sides of the nose and over the forehead but can occur anywhere over the sites usually affected by acne (Figure 10.1). Comedones are follicular plugs composed of follicular debris and compacted sebum. They have pigmented tips from the melanin pigment deposited by the follicular epithelium at this level (Figure 10.2). It is not true that the blackened tip to the comedo is the result of oxidation of fatty material as was once believed, just as there is no truth to the ancient myth that

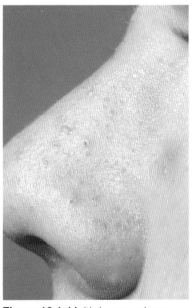

Figure 10.1 Multiple comedones and seborrhoea in acne.

the whole comedone represents a tiny worm! Visible comedones can be expressed out by pressure on the surrounding tissues but they reform within a few days. Accompanying the visible comedones are numerous invisible comedones many of which do not have pigmented tips.

Inflamed reddened papules develop from blocked follicles. These are often quite tender to the touch and may be set quite deep within the skin (Figure 10.3). Sometimes they develop pus-containing vesicles at their tips (pustules) but these may also arise independently. In a few patients some of the papules become quite large and very unsightly and are then spoken of as nodules.

In severely affected patients the nodules liquify centrally so that fluctuant cysts are formed. In reality the lesions are pseudocysts as they have no epithelial lining. This type of acne, which is luckily quite uncommon, is known as cystic or nodulocystic acne and can be very disabling and disfiguring.

When the large nodules and cysts eventually subside they leave in their wake firm fibrotic nodular scars which sometimes become hypertrophic or even keloidal (Figure 10.4). The scars are often quite irregular and tend to form 'bridges' (Figure 10.5). Even the smaller inflamed papules can cause scars and these tend to be pock like or are triangular indentations ('ice pick scars').

There is a very rare and severe type of cystic acne known as acne fulminans in which the acne lesions quite suddenly become very inflamed. At the same time the affected individual is unwell and develops fever and arthralgia. Laboratory investigation reveals a polymorphonuclear leukocytosis and odd osteolytic lesions in the bony

Inflamed reddened papules develop from blocked follicles.

Some of the papules become large nodules.

In some, nodules liquify centrally so that fluctuant cysts are formed. In reality the lesions are pseudocysts as they have no epithelial lining.

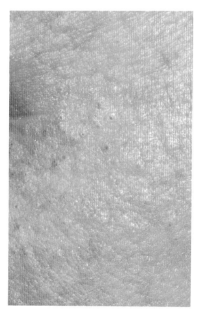

Figure 10.2 Multiple comedones in acne. Note the blackened tips from melanin.

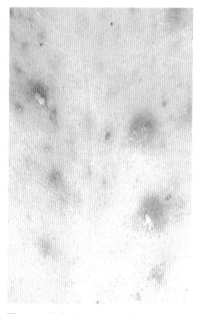

Figure 10.3 Acne papules.

148

skeleton. The cause of this disorder is not clear although it has been suggested that it is due to the presence of a vasculitis somehow precipitated as a result of the underlying acne.

> Nodules and cysts subside giving rise to scarring.

Sites affected
Any hair-bearing skin can develop acne but certain areas are much more prone than others (Figure 10.6). These acne prone areas tend to have hair follicles with terminal hairs and larger sebaceous glands (sebaceous follicles). The face and particularly the skin of the cheeks, lower jaw, chin, nose and forehead are usually affected. The scalp is not involved but the back of the neck often develops lesions. The front of the chest, the shoulders and the upper back are all 'favoured areas' for the development of lesions. They are usually affected together with the face but are occasionally involved in isolation.

> Any hair-bearing skin can develop acne.

In patients with severe acne and many lesions on the above sites it is quite common for other areas to be affected as well. The outer aspects of the upper arms, the buttocks and the front and sides of the thighs are such areas – although it is rare for these to be affected as extensively as the face, back or chest.

Clinical course
For most of those affected the disorder is annoying and may be troublesome but not of enormous significance because it is limited in

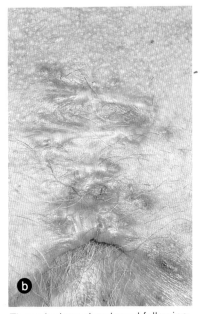

Figure 10.4 (a) Nodular scars in acne. These lesions developed following the resolution of inflamed acne papules. (b) Hypertrophic scarring in bridging pattern.

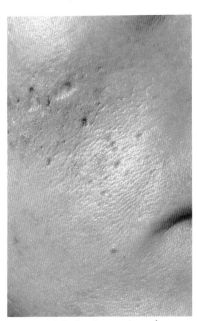

Figure 10.5 Pock scarring of acne.

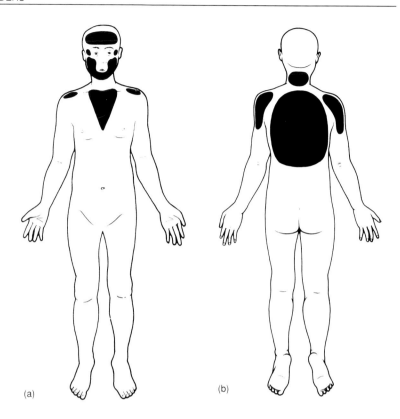

Figure 10.6 (a) Diagram to show common sites of involvement due to acne on the front of the trunk and face. (b) Diagram to show common sites of involvement due to acne on the back of the trunk and face.

(a)

(b)

extent and only lasts a few months or at the most a year or two. For the unfortunate few the condition is a disaster as it is disfiguring and disabling and persistent, with wave after wave of new lesions. Although the natural tendency is for resolution it is difficult to know in any individual patient when the condition will improve. The majority of individuals have lost their acne spots by the age of 25 years but some, particularly young women, tend to have the occasional lesion for very much longer. In some women there is a pronounced premenstrual flare of their acne some 7–10 days before the menses begin.

Many patients will say spontaneously that their acne improves in the summer time and there can be little doubt that sun exposure seems to improve many patients. Although the sun improves acne the heat does not, and indeed can make it worse. Soldiers with acne in hot, humid climates, for example, are sometimes quite disabled by a sudden marked aggravation of their acne and in some cases have to be evacuated home or sent to a cooler station because of this.

EPIDEMIOLOGY

As mentioned at the start, acne is an extremely common disease with some 70% of the population developing some clinically evident acne at some point during adolescence and early adult life. Luckily the proportion in whom the condition is more than trivial and persists is not great and perhaps only 10–20% request medical attention for the problem. This proportion will vary in different parts of the world depending on the incidence in the particular ethnic group, the degree of affluence and sophistication of medical services and the predominant medical problems of the area.

The variations in incidence in different ethnic groups have not been well characterized although it does appear that Eskimos and Japanese suffer from less acne than do Western Caucasians.

The age of onset is that of puberty or a little after although many patients do not appear troubled untill the age of 16 or 17 years. Men appear to be affected earlier and more severely than women.

Acne lesions sometimes appear on the cheeks and chin of infants a few weeks or months of age and even a little later than that (Figure 10.7). This infantile acne is usually trivial and short lived but can occasionally be troublesome.

The disorder is usually thought of as a disorder of adolescence but as pointed out above, exceptions do occur. Not only does it sometimes occur in the very young it can rarely also occur for the first time in late middle age and the elderly (Figure 10.8).

> Not only does acne occasionally occur in the very young it can rarely also occur for the first time in late middle age and the elderly.

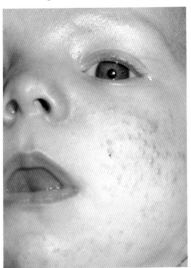

Figure 10.7 Infantile acne.

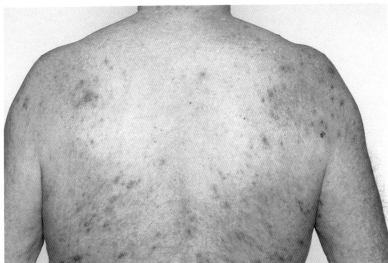

Figure 10.8 Extensive acne affecting the back in a man of 65 years.

SPECIAL TYPES OF ACNE

Acne from drugs and chemical agents

Androgens provide the normal 'drive' to the sebaceous glands and because of the increased secretion of these hormones they are responsible for the increased sebum secretion at puberty. When given therapeutically for any reason they can also cause an eruption of acne spots.

Glucocorticoids, such as prednisolone, when given to suppress the signs of rheumatoid arthritis, an autoimmune disease or some other chronic inflammation, can also induce troublesome acne spots (Figure 10.9). Why this should be has never been adequately explained. Glucocorticoids do not seem to increase the rate of sebum secretion and

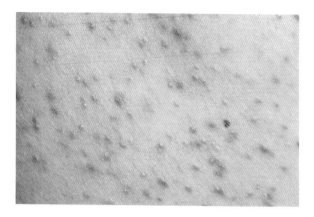

Figure 10.9 Steroid acne. The lesions tend to be more uniform in appearance than in 'ordinary' acne.

the acne that results is curiously monomorphic in that sheets of acne lesions appear (unlike ordinary acne) all at the same stage of development. Interestingly, corticosteroid creams can uncommonly also cause acne spots at the site of application.

Other systemically administered drugs such as phenytoin and isoniazid have also been incriminated as causing an acne type of eruption but the evidence for this effect from these agents has never been very strong.

Oil acne

Engineers, mechanics and factory workers who come into contact with lubricating and cutting oils develop an acne-like eruption at the sites of contact. The eruption consists of small papules, pustules and comedones and is often observed on the fronts of the thighs and forearms of affected workers as this is where oil-soaked overalls contact the skin. A quite similar 'acneiform folliculitis' sometimes arises at the sites of application of tar-containing ointments during the treatment of skin diseases (Figure 10.10).

Some cosmetics seem to aggravate or even cause acne in some

> Engineers, mechanics and factory workers who come into contact with lubricating and cutting oils develop an acne-like eruption at the sites of contact.

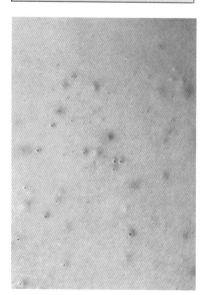

Figure 10.10 Comedones and inflamed follicular papules from tar application.

Figure 10.11 Acne due to cosmetics.

patients. This is because they sometimes contain comedo-inducing (comedogenic) agents (such as cocoa butter and derivatives, and some mineral oils) that can induce acne. This cosmetic or 'pomade' acne is less of a problem now that cosmetic manufacturers are aware of the problem but nonetheless it still does occur on occasions and can be difficult to detect (Figure 10.11).

Chloracne

Chloracne is an extremely severe form of industrial acne which occurs in individuals who have been exposed to complex chlorinated organic naphthalenic compounds and dioxin. Epidemics have occurred after industrial accidents such as occurred in Serveso in Italy, in which the population around the chemical plant concerned were affected. The compounds responsible are extremely potent and lesions may continue to develop for some months after the original exposure. Typically numerous large cystic-type lesions occur in this form of industrial acne.

Excoriated acne

This disorder is most often seen in young women. Small acne spots around the chin, forehead and on the jaw line are picked, squeezed and otherwise altered by manual interference. The resulting papules are crusted and often more inflamed than routine acne spots. When questioned as to why the individual concerned should do this there is either flat denial or the explanation that they were trying 'to get rid of the spots'. Often the patients involved have very little true acne and the main cosmetic problem is the results of the labour of their fingers.

PATHOLOGY, AETIOLOGY AND PATHOGENESIS

Histologically the essential features are those of a folliculitis but it is sometimes difficult to make out just what is going on in a biopsy of an acne lesion as there is so much inflammation present. Of course, the exact histological picture will depend on what lesion has been sampled and at what stage it was when the biopsy was taken. Usually it is possible to make out a ruptured follicle or at least fragments of follicular epithelium. In the earliest stages a follicular plug of horn (comedone) can be identified. In later stages fragments of horn appear to have provoked a violent mixed inflammatory reaction which may consist of masses of polymorphs (the signs of an acne 'cyst' developing) and in places a granulomatous reaction with many giant cells and histiocytes (Figure 10.12). In older lesions, fibrous tissue is deposited, indicating scar formation.

What provokes this inflammatory reaction? It would seem important to try to find out as most of the clinical manifestations of acne are due to the inflammation. It is worthwhile summarizing what has been discovered by a programme of careful clinical research by many researchers over the past three decades. In the first place patients with acne have a higher rate of sebum secretion (SER) compared to matched control subjects and furthermore there is some correlation between the extent of the increase in the SER and the severity of the acne.

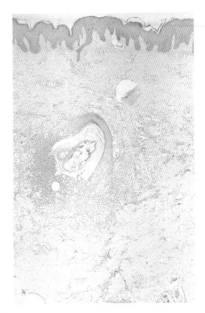

Figure 10.12 Pathology of inflamed acne papules showing ruptured follicle and a dense inflammatory cell infiltrate composed predominantly of polymorphs.

> Histologically the essential features in acne are those of a folliculitis.

> Patients with acne have a higher rate of sebum secretion (SER) compared to matched control subjects. There is some correlation between the increase in the SER with the severity of the acne.

> Acne first appears at puberty at which time there is a sudden increase in the level of circulating androgens. Experimental work suggests that sebaceous glands are 'androgen driven' and that few other influences, endocrine or otherwise, are as important as the level of androgen secretion. Follicular obstruction seems also to play an important role.

> The normal flora – particularly the proprionibacteria which are microaerophilic and lipophilic, so that they are ideally suited to living in the depths of the hair follicle in an oily milieu, increase in numbers during puberty when their food supply, in the form of sebum, increases. One possibility is that the normal follicular flora are responsible for hydrolysing the lipid esters of sebum, liberating potentially irritating fatty acids.

> It is clear that increased sebum secretion, follicular obstruction and the proliferation of follicular bacteria and the consequent hydrolysis of the lipids of sebum are all aspects of the pathogenesis of acne.

Acne first appears at puberty at which time there is a sudden increase in the level of circulating androgens. Eunuchs don't get acne, and the administration of testosterone provokes the appearance of acne lesions. Experimental work suggests that sebaceous glands are 'androgen driven' and that few other influences, endocrine or otherwise, are as important as the level of androgen secretion. Follicular obstruction seems also to play an important role. Comedones are early lesions clinically, and microscopically it is commonplace to find horny plugs in the follicular canals. Furthermore, interesting changes have been described in the follicular epithelium in the follicular canal, suggesting that there is abnormal keratinization in the mouth of the hair follicle.

Pathogenic bacteria are not found in acne lesions and are not thought to be involved in the pathogenesis of the disease. It is possible, nonetheless, that the normal flora has a role to play. The flora consists of Gram-positive cocci – the micrococci (also known as staphylococci epidermidis), and Gram-positive bacteria – *Proprionibacterium acnes*. In addition there are also yeast-like micro-organisms known as *Pityrosporum ovale*. The proprionibacteria are microaerophilic and lipophilic so that they are ideally suited to living in the depths of the hair follicle in an oily milieu, and it is not surprising that they increase in numbers during puberty when their food supply, in the form of sebum, increases. One frequently discussed possibility is that the normal follicular flora are responsible for hydrolysing the lipid esters of sebum, liberating potentially irritating fatty acids. The constituents of sebum and of skin surface lipid (after bacterial hydrolysis) are given in Table 10.1.

From the above it is clear that increased sebum secretion, follicular obstruction and the proliferation of follicular bacteria and the consequent hydrolysis of the lipids of sebum are all aspects of the pathogenesis of acne. But the question inevitably arises, how can these events be linked? There is as yet no entirely satisfactory answer but an acceptable hypothesis is set out in Figure 10.13. From this it can be seen that it is

Table 10.1 Main constituents of sebum and skin surface lipid

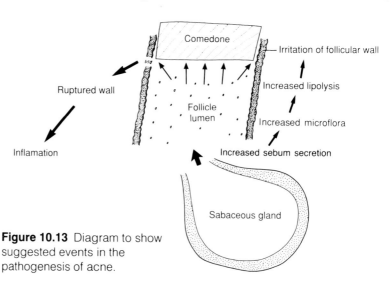

Figure 10.13 Diagram to show suggested events in the pathogenesis of acne.

154

suggested that the papules and cysts, which are the most important lesions from the patients' point of view, are caused by follicular rupture.

Treatment

There is no acne patient who cannot be substantially helped by appropriate treatment. It must also be borne in mind that before the patient presents at the physician's office he or she has almost certainly been advised by his or her mother, father, aunt, grandmother and local 'healer', whether such advice is requested or not. Often the young sufferer is blamed in one way or another for having the disorder and accused of doing too much of one thing or not enough of the other. Consequently many forms of familial or folk treatments seem to be more in the nature of punishments than anything else. Dietetic and social restrictions are typical restrictive measures imposed on the unfortunate acne patient. Exhortation to more abrasive and frequent washing is another tactic adopted by well meaning but misguided family and friends.

Luckily most acne patients survive this onslaught and improve spontaneously after a few months. A proportion do not improve and find their way to the pharmacist where many excellent treatments can be purchased. Some of these contain benzoyl peroxide or other antimicrobial compounds, or sulphur or salicylic acid, and are quite similar to those available on prescription (see below). Many with milder degrees of acne will be helped by these medications. It is only those with resistant, recalcitrant and more severe types of acne that reach the physician. It will vary in different countries but perhaps only 10% of those with clinical acne in the UK see their practitioner.

Basic principles

Treatment may be aimed at:

1. reducing the bacterial population of the hair follicles to cut down the hydrolysis of lipids;
2. encouraging the shedding of the follicular horny plugs to free the obstruction (comedolytic agents);
3. reducing the rate of sebum production, either directly by acting on the sebaceous glands or indirectly by inhibiting the effects of androgens on the sebaceous glands (anti-androgens);
4. reducing the damaging effects of acne inflammation on the skin with anti-inflammatory agents (Table 10.2 and Figure 10.14).

General measures

Patients with acne are often depressed and may need sympathetic counselling and support. In particular the inevitability of their improvement needs to be stressed. As mentioned above there is no evidence that particular foodstuffs have any deleterious effect or that washing vigorously will help remove lesions. These and other myths should be dispelled along with a straightforward explanation of the nature of the disorder, its natural history and treatment.

Treatment may be aimed at (a) reducing the bacterial population of the hair follicles to cut down the hydrolysis of lipids, (b) encouraging the shedding of the follicular horny plugs to free the obstruction (comedolytic agents), (c) reduction in the rate of sebum production, either directly by acting on the sebaceous glands or indirectly by inhibiting the effects of androgens on the sebaceous glands (anti-androgens), (d) anti-inflammatory agents to reduce the damaging effects of acne inflammation on the skin.

Table 10.2   Main treatments for acne

Topical	Oral
Antimicrobial	*Amtimicrobial*
Benzoyl peroxide	Tetracycline
Tetracycline	Minocin
Erythromycin	Erythromycin
Clindamycin	
Azelaic acid	
Comedolytic	*Sebum suppressive*
Tretinoin	Isotretinoin
Isotretinoin	Cyproterone and ethinylestranol
Salicylic acid	Spironolactone

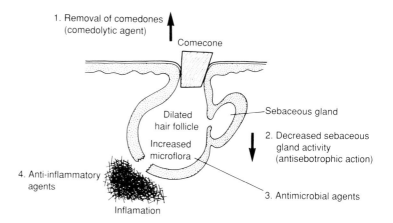

Figure 10.14 Diagram to demonstrate the main therapeutic pathways in acne.

TOPICAL TREATMENTS

There are many topical preparations available and it is best to become familiar with a few rather than try to understand the benefits and shortcomings of them all. Currently the most popular form of topical preparation is either a gel, a cream or an alcohol-based lotion.

Comedolytic preparations

Tretinoin-containing preparations are most popular in the USA but are also used extensively elsewhere. They are not bacteriocidal but are nonetheless effective. Recently the *cis* isomer of tretinoin – isotretinoin – has also been used successfully for the treatment of acne.

Side effects from the use of tretinoin preparations include some pinkness and slight scaling of the skin surface especially in fair, sensitive-skinned individuals. For the most part this 'dryness' of the treated area is tolerable and anyway decreases after continual usage. In fact most of the topical preparations for acne have some irritative and drying effects. Tretinoin may also produce increased sensitivity to the sun because the use of the compound causes thinning of the stratum corneum. Concern has been expressed about the percutaneous penetration of tretinoin and its possible teratogenicity. However, experiments indicate that only very small amounts are absorbed which do not even match the endogenously produced tretinoin from the metabolism of vitamin A.

Sulphur (as elemental sulphur 2–10%) has been used traditionally as a treatment for acne. It seems to be helpful for some patients but has dropped out of fashion. Its efficacy probably depends both on its antimicrobial action and its comedolytic activity. Other 'traditional' and now not frequently used agents for acne include resorcinol and salicylic acid. The latter agent is both antimicrobial and keratolytic and has wide usage in dermatological treatments.

Other agents employed to remove blackheads include abrasive preparations. These contain particles of such substances as aluminium oxide or polyethylene beads which literally abrade the skin surface and 'liberate' the comedones.

Topical antimicrobial compounds

Preparations containing benzoyl peroxide (2–10%) are designed to assist patients with superficial acne who have many comedones, and are widely used and quite effective. Benzoyl peroxide is also bacteriocidal, it releases oxygen, proving lethal to the microaerophilic *Proprionibacterium acnes*.

A variety of other nonantibiotic antimicrobial agents have been employed in 'face washes', lotions and creams. Hexachlorophane, chlorhexidine and miconazole are some of the other antibacterial compounds employed. One that has only been developed in recent years is an interesting fatty acid known as azelaic acid. Used in 20% concentrations it has proved very effective in trials with very little in the way of side effects.

> Topical treatments for acne include cornedolytics (eg tretinoin) and antibacteral agents including antibiotics e.g. erythromycin.

Topical antibiotics

Topical chloramphenical has been used in the treatment of acne for many years but it is only in the past decade that preparations containing other antibiotics have been shown to be effective and have become popular medicaments. Tetracycline (2%), erythromycin (1–2%) and clindamycin (2%) seem to be as effective as 5% benzoyl peroxide (50% improvement in the numbers of acne spots over a 12 week period) but are less irritating to the skin. Luckily these substances have a low tendency to sensitize and are not often responsible for allergic contact dermatitis (page 120) although they may cause a minor degree of direct primary irritation.

Some concern has been expressed over the possibility of systemic toxic side effects from the percutaneous absorption of antibiotics but although the possibility should be borne in mind, examples of this problem are extremely rare. Of considerably more concern is the emergence of antibiotic resistance in the cutaneous microflora which can then be transferred to more pathogenic microbial species. As yet few clinical sequelae have resulted but there seems to be a good chance that more will occur if the use of these agents is not controlled.

SYSTEMIC TREATMENTS

Antibiotics

Tetracyclines

Systemic tetracyclines have been the sheet anchor for treatment of moderate and severe acne for many years. Patients with many papular lesions involving several sites are suitable for systemic tetracyclines. It is usual to start treatment with a dose of 250 mg t.i.d. or 6-hourly, and then when a response has been attained to reduce the dose to that required to keep the patient free of new lesions. The improvement usually begins four to eight weeks after starting treatment and continues over the next two to three months. Some 70% of patients can be expected to improve on this regimen. Treatment may have to be maintained for several months, or exceptionally even up to two years, dependent on whether new lesions develop after stopping the drug. With tetracycline and oxytetracycline the drug should be given 30 minutes before a meal to prevent interference with absorption. The newer minocycline or doxycycline are given in smaller doses (50 or 100 mg) once or twice per day and their absorption does not seem affected by food.

Side effects with the tetracyclines are few and not usually serious. Gastrointestinal discomfort and diarrhoea occasionally occur and may necessitate stopping the drug in some instances. Photosensitivity may occur with any of the tetracyclines but was mainly a problem with older, now no longer used, analogues. Fixed drug eruption (page 91) may occur with this group of drugs and rarely other acute drug rashes develop (page 89). Minocycline can cause a dark brown pigmentation of the skin of acne scars or acral areas or the exposed part of the skin after long-continued use in a small number of patients.

Tetracyclines must not be given to pregnant women as they are teratogenic, and must not be given to infants as they cause a bone and tooth dystrophy in which these structures become deformed and discoloured and fluoresce.

Erythromycin

This is also an effective antibiotic for acne. Its efficacy is similar to the tetracyclines but luckily patients who do not respond to these latter drugs may respond to erythromycin. The starting dosage is 250 mg 6-hourly for the first few weeks with reduction after a response has begun. Subsequent management is as for the tetracyclines. Side effects with erythromycin are not uncommon but are minor and usually restricted to nausea.

Systemic tetracyclines or erythromycin are effective in some 70% patients with moderately severe acne when given over several weeks. Their mode of action is unknown.

Other antibiotics and antimicrobials

Clindamycin, the quinolines and the sulphonamides are other drugs that have been used systemically for acne. None is more effective than the tetracyclines but they may be suitable for patients who are either intolerant or who no longer respond to the tetracyclines or erythromycin. Side effects are more common and sometimes of a serious nature (e.g. blood dyscrasias). There is some evidence (admittedly anecdotal) that patients respond to systemic antibiotics more readily if topical treatments are prescribed at the same time.

Isotretinoin (13-*cis*-retinoic acid)

The large majority of patients with acne will respond to topical or some combination of topical and systemic drugs. However, some severely affected patients may not, and for them there is another drug that can offer relief. This agent is a member of the retinoid group of drugs and is known as isotretinoin (it is the same *cis*-isomer of tretinoin used topically). Its action is primarily to reduce sebum secretion by shrinking the sebaceous glands but it may also have effects on the keratinization of the mouth of the hair follicle and an anti-inflammatory action as well.

It is given in a dose of 0.5–1.0 mg/kg/body weight/day usually for a four-month period. The response to this regimen is often dramatic, with inhibition of new lesions and resolution of the old in more than 80% of patients. Patients with many large cystic lesions affecting the trunk as well as the head and neck region take longer to respond and may need more than one four-month course.

Unfortunately toxic side effects are many and frequent. They range from the trivial, of which the most frequent is drying and cracking of the lips (Figure 10.15), to the very serious which include teratogenicity, hepatotoxicity, bone toxicity and a blood lipid elevating effect. The teratogenic effects are amongst the most worrisome as of course the

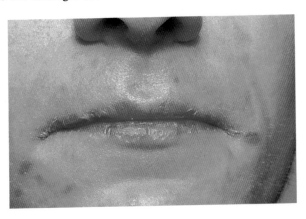

Figure 10.15 Cracking of the lips due to administration of isotretinoin.

acne age group is almost identical with the reproductive age group. The effects on the foetus include facial, cardiac, renal and neural defects and are most likely to arise if the drug is taken during the first trimester. Some 30–50% of pregnancies during which the drug was taken have been affected. Because of this it is strongly recommended that if it is planned to prescribe isotretinoin for a women who can conceive that effective contraceptive measures must also be planned and used during and for up to one month after stopping the drug.

Hepatotoxicity is rare although a small rise in liver enzymes is not uncommon. A rise in triglycerides and cholesterol such that the ratio of very low density lipoproteins to high density lipoproteins is increased regularly occurs, such that overall there is a 30% rise in lipid levels. This is not likely to be a problem for patients with acne but may be for patients with psoriasis and disorders of keratinization who are sometimes also treated with retinoid drugs because they are older and take the drugs for longer periods (pages 315–316). The same is true for the bone toxicity. A variety of bone anomalies have been described including disseminated interstitial skeletal hyperostosis and osteoporosis but they are not likely to be a problem for acne subjects. *Because of the toxicities of this important drug it can only be prescribed from hospitals in the UK*.

Antiandrogens

Administration of antiandrogens inhibits androgenic activity and reduces sebum secretion. Reducing the rate of sebum secretion will lessen the tendency to form comedones and reduce the number of inflammatory lesions as well. Although many antiandrogens have been tried, most have proved unsatisfactory for one reason or another. Currently only one antiandrogen preparation is available – Dianette. This is a mixture of an antiandrogen, cyproterone acetate (2 mg), and an oestrogen, ethinyl oestradiol (35 µg). It is a central antiandrogen blocking the pituitary drive to androgen secretion. It also suppresses ovulation and acts as an oral contraceptive. It is not suitable for men because of its feminizing properties. It improves acne after some six to eight weeks of use but is not as effective as isotretinoin. It is associated with a number of minor side effects, essentially those associated with taking oral contraceptives.

Spironolactone, the potassium-sparing diuretic, has also been found to have antiandrogenic effects and has occasionally been used as a treatment for acne.

Systemic isotretinoin should be reserved for the most severely affected acne patients. Given over a 4 month period it has an 80% success rate but many toxic side effects including teratogenicity. The drug greatly reduces serum secretion.

Rosacea

Rosacea used to be known as acne rosacea but as the only relationships between the two disorders seem to be that both are characterized by inflammatory lesions occurring on the face and that both respond to antibiotics there seems no sense in retaining the 'acne' prefix.

DEFINITION

Rosacea is a chronic inflammatory disorder of the skin of the face characterized by persistent erythema and telangiectasia punctuated by acute episodes of swelling and papules.

CLINICAL FEATURES

Sites affected

The cheeks, forehead, nose and chin are the most frequently affected areas, making a typical cruciate pattern of skin involvement (Figure 10.16). The flexures and periocular areas are conspicuously spared. Uncommonly the neck and the bald area of the scalp in men are also affected. Sometimes only one or two areas are affected and this makes diagnosis quite difficult. In rare instances extrafacial lesions occur, the limbs being particularly subject to these very unusual manifestations of what is otherwise quite a common disease.

The lesions

The most characteristic physical sign is that of persistent erythema (Figure 10.17) which is often accompanied by marked telangiectasia (Figure 10.18). The disorder may not progress beyond this

> Rosacea is a chronic inflammatory disorder of the skin of the face characterized by persistent erythema and telangiectasia of the cheeks, chin and forehead punctuated by acute episodes of swelling and papules.

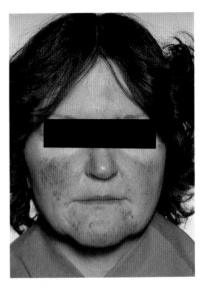

Figure 10.16 Typical rosacea with involvement of the cheeks, forehead and chin.

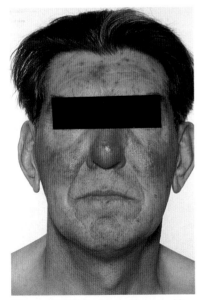

Figure 10.17 Typical rosacea with erythema of the cheeks and forehead.

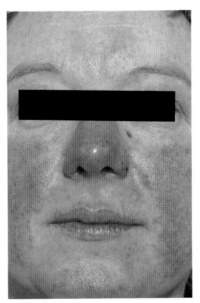

Figure 10.18 Erythema and telangiectasia in rosacea.

Patients flush and blush more frequently, more deeply and for longer periods than do non rosaceous controls.

'erythemato-telangiectatic' state but even if it does not, the bright red facies it causes is sufficient to cause considerable social discomfort and often marked depression. Such patients also complain of frequent flushing and blushing at the most trivial stimuli. They certainly appear to flush and blush more frequently, more deeply and for longer periods than do nonrosaceous controls.

Superimposed on this noninflammatory and persistent background of erythema are episodes of swelling and papules which develop for no very obvious reason (Figure 10.19). The papules are a dull red, dome shaped and nontender in contrast to acne, where they tend to be irregular and tender. Pustules also occur but are less frequent than in acne, and blackheads, cysts and scars do not.

DIFFERENTIAL DIAGNOSIS
Any red rash of the face may be confused with rosacea, and the diagnosis may not be straightforward at first. The major skin disorders and systemic diseases with which rosacea may be confused are set out in Table 10.3.

Papular rashes of the face seem to cause most problems. Acne occurs in a younger age group and is usually distinguished by the greasy skin, comedones and scars as well as lesions outside the face. However, in some patients the presence of persistent erythema can make distinction quite difficult. Perioral dermatitis (page 168) should not be difficult to differentiate as this disease is mainly distributed around the mouth and there is no background of erythema. Rarely discoid lupus erythematosus (page 74) presents with papular lesions which may be difficult to distinguish, and in systemic lupus erythematosus there may be a symmetrical eruption on the face which may superficially resemble

Figure 10.19 (a,b) Papules of facial skin in rosacea.

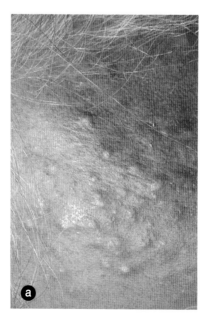
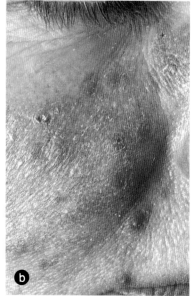

Table 10.3 Differential diagnosis of rosacea

Disorder	Positive discriminants
Skin disorders	
Acne	Scars, seborrhoea, cysts; back, chest involvement
Seborrhoeic dermatitis	Scaling, involvement of flexures
Perioral dermatitis	Micropapules; perioral involvement
Discoid lupus erythematosus	Irregular distribution; atrophy and scarring
Systemic disorders	
Systemic lupus erythematosus	Rash on other light-exposed areas, arthropathy, positive anti-nuclear factor, haematological findings
Dermatomyositis	Mauve—lilac rash around the eyes with swelling; rash on backs of fingers, muscle tenderness, pain and weakness; positive laboratory findings
Carcinoid syndrome	Marked telangiectasia, flushing attacks, hepatomegaly
Polycythaemia rubra vera	General facial redness and suffusion; possibly hepatosplenomegaly
Superior vena cava obstruction	Swelling and redness of face and neck; distended neck veins

rosacea, but there are symptoms of systemic disease. Dermatitis of the face (including seborrhoeic dermatitis) is marked by scaling which is not characteristic of rosacea.

Polycythaemia rubra vera and superior caval obstruction both give the face a plethoric appearance but should not be confused with rosacea as the redness is not confined to the facial convexities and is not accompanied by inflammatory lesions. The carcinoid syndrome is characterized by reddened areas on the face in the same distribution as in rosacea but the condition is accompanied by severe systemic symptoms.

Dermatomyositis is characterized by an odd mauvish erythema around the eyes as well as erythematous patches affecting the backs of the hands, elbows and knees. In addition the pain, tenderness and weakness of limb girdle muscles should quickly distinguish this disease.

COMPLICATIONS

Rhinophyma

This is mostly seen in middle aged and elderly men although it occasionally occurs in women too. The nose becomes irregularly enlarged and 'craggy' with accentuation of the pilosebaceous orifices (Figure 10.20). At the same time the nose develops a mauve or dull red discolouration with prominent telangiectatic vessels coursing over it (Figure 10.21). The bizarre appearance is popularly (though inaccurately) associated with alcoholism and because of this has been dubbed 'whisky drinker's nose', 'elephantiasis des buveurs' and 'grog blossom'. Rarely the paranasal areas, the chin and forehead are affected by the same process.

> Complications of rosacea include irregular craggy enlargement of the nose – known as rhinophyma, persistent lymphoedema and various types of ocular inflammation.

Lymphoedema

Persistent lymphoedema is another unpleasant though uncommon complication of rosacea seen predominantly in men. The swollen areas are usually a shade of red and may persist when the other manifestations of rosacea have remitted (Figure 10.22).

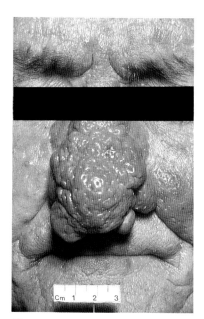

Figure 10.20 Severe irregular craggy enlargement of nose due to rhinophyma.

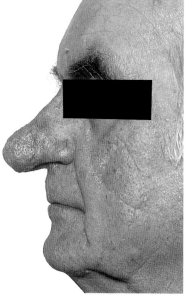

Figure 10.21 Rhinophyma with prominent telangiectasia.

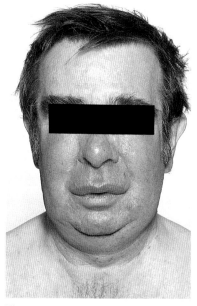

Figure 10.22 Persistent facial swelling due to lymphoedema.

164

PATHOLOGY AND PATHOGENESIS

When venous return is impeded, hypertension develops in the venous circulation behind the impediment. This results in the development of saccular dilatations of the small venules and because of the changed pressure relationships at the tissue level, exudation into the tissues and oedema.

This situation arises in the long veins of the legs when the venous valves are faulty so that blood leaks back through these faulty valves after being pushed towards the heart by the 'muscle pump' of the lower leg (Figure 11.2). The valves become faulty because venous thrombosis destroys their structure but sometimes they are congenitally faulty. The venous hypertension caused by the back pressure is transmitted back to the smaller superficial veins via the perforating veins. Visible varicosities and telangiectasia (Figure 11.3 and 11.4) are the direct result of this

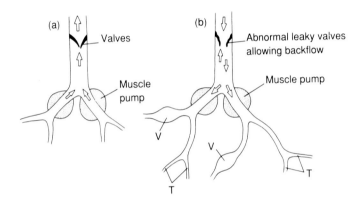

Figure 11.2 (a) Normal venous return from legs. (b) Venous hypertension due to leaky valves. V = varicosities. T = telangiectatic vessels.

Figure 11.3 The results of venous hypertension – 'the gravitational syndrome'. Note the pigmentation, telangiectasia and visible varicosities.

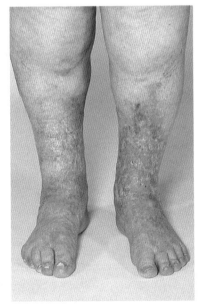

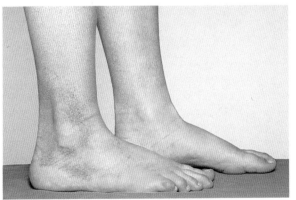

Figure 11.4 Telangiectasia seen in the early stage of venous hypertension.

173

transmitted increased venous pressure but are in themselves of little significance apart from their cosmetic effects and the message they convey of serious hypoxaemic problems at the tissue level. The visible varicosities may occasionally localize over perforating veins which, if the deep veins are incompetent, transmit the increased venous pressure to the superficial venous system.

The increased pressure at the venous end of the capillaries leads to transudation and the deposition of fibrin perivascularly (Figure 11.5). The tissue oedema and the fibrin cause hypoxaemia, inflammation and eventually fibrosis. Extravasation of red blood cells results in the deposition of haemosiderin pigment in dermal macrophages, imparting a brownish pigmentation to the skin.

The small blood vessels thicken and proliferate in response to the hypoxaemia (Figure 11.6), giving rise to a characteristic histological picture that can, because of the vascular proliferation, in extreme cases even resemble Kaposi's sarcoma (page 227).

> Venous thrombosis or trauma damages valves in the leg veins impeding venous return and causing venous hypertension. This results in visible varicosities and oedema as well as thickening of small blood vessels and perivascular deposition of fibrin.

CLINICAL FEATURES

The earliest signs are of pitting ankle oedema and prominently distended superficial long veins in the lower leg. A network of smaller veins also appears around the medial malleolus and elsewhere around the foot. At this stage there may be few complaints apart from discomfort and 'heaviness' of the lower leg. Somewhat later brownish discolouration of the skin develops and the swelling becomes firmer and eventually woody to the touch because of the fibrosis (Figure 11.7). Ulceration may occur at any stage, usually after a minor injury to the ankle which then does not heal but steadily enlarges.

Somewhat later brownish discolouration of the skin develops and the swelling becomes firmer and eventually woody to the touch because of the fibrosis.

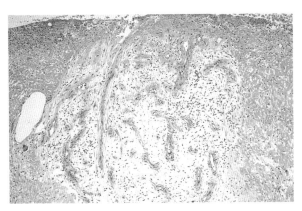

Figure 11.5 Pathology of venous hypertension showing thickening of and increase in number of small blood vessels in the dermis.

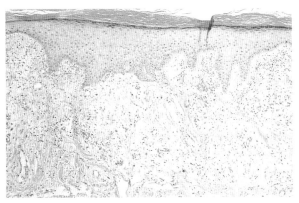

Figure 11.6 Pathology of venous hypertension showing marked inflammation with marked thickening of small blood vessels from fibrin deposition.

Venous ulcers are usually seen around the medial malleolus and are usually single (Figure 11.8) but multiple ulcers and locations elsewhere around the ankle (Figure 11.9) are by no means rare. Large ulcers may encircle the leg. The base of venous ulcers is often lined by a yellowish grey slough and the edges are for the most part flush with the skin surface and irregular in outline (Figure 11.10).

Venous ulcers are usually seen around the medial malleolus and are usually single.

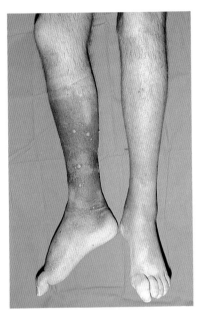

Figure 11.7 Venous hypertension. Note the pigmentation and appearance of the skin, suggesting that it is bound down to underlying tissues.

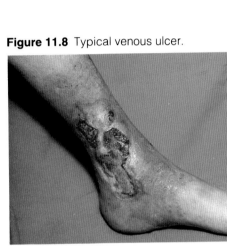

Figure 11.8 Typical venous ulcer.

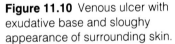

Figure 11.10 Venous ulcer with exudative base and sloughy appearance of surrounding skin.

Figure 11.9 Venous ulcer extending on to the foot.

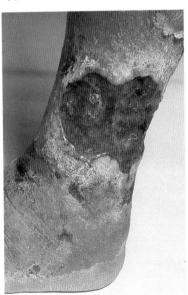

175

COURSE AND PROGNOSIS

Many ulcers heal either with treatment or for no apparent reason, but may take many months to do so. Unfortunately when healed they tend to recur. Some never completely heal but at times tend to improve and at other times seem to worsen.

COMPLICATIONS

1. ***Infection***. They may become severely infected with either Gram-positive cocci or Gram-negative micro-organisms.
2. ***Bleeding***. Uncommonly, large veins may rupture and cause severe bleeding.
3. ***Eczema***. An eczematous rash is common in patients with venous ulcers. In two-thirds to three-quarters of patients this is the result of allergic contact hypersensitivity to one of the medicaments used in treatment (e.g. neomycin, Vioform) or one of the constituents of the vehicle (e.g. lanolin or ethylene diamine) (page 120). In a few patients autosensitization is thought to occur in which sensitivity to the breakdown products from the ulcerated area develop. Venous eczema develops on the opposite leg, the lateral aspects of the thighs and the upper arms and at other scattered sites.
4. ***Malignant change***. Rarely squamous cell carcinoma or basal cell carcinoma may occur in long-standing lesions although it is difficult to know which comes first, the ulcer or the cancer (see Table 11.1).
5. ***Anaemia/malnutrition***. Patients with persistent ulcers often develop a normochromic anaemia and are generally debilitated. The loss of protein, salts and metabolites in the exudate from the open area and absorption of products of tissue degradation and bacterial activity are probably responsible.

TREATMENT

The aims of treatment must be matched to the patient. Younger, more affluent patients may demand that no effort is spared to heal their ulcer. Older, socially deprived patients may even regard their ulcer as a 'friend' which acts as a focus of sympathy and their only point of contact with the community. Between these extremes are most patients, who need simple, effective treatments.

The most useful approach is to try to improve venous drainage by:

1. Elevation of the legs above the head level for regular periods during the day (two 1-hour periods would be suitable).
2. Compression bandaging, using either specially made elasticated stockings or elasticated bandage. The pressure should be graduated so that it is greatest at the ankle and least at the top of the bandage or stocking. Care must be taken to ensure that there is no restriction of arterial blood supply.
3. Gentle regular exercise to ensure that the 'calf muscle pump' assists in the return of blood towards the heart.
4. Weight reduction.

An essential part of treatment for venous ulcers is improvement in venous drainage by periods of elevation of the leg and skillfully applied compression bandaging.

Dressings

Nonadherent, nontoxic, nonsensitizing dressings should be used. Antibacterial properties may be helpful. In addition ideally they should be partially absorptive and semiocclusive to provide high humidity at the wound interface. This promotes re-epithelialization. 'Hydrocolloid' dressing materials, gels and some paste bandages are suitable. Tulle dressings are also acceptable.

Non adherent, non toxic, non sensitizing dressings should be used.

Topical treatments

The ulcer base may be irrigated with normal saline, dilute potassium permanganate solution or very weak chlorhexidine or hypochlorite solutions. Many 'traditional' agents are damaging to the healing tissues and must not be left in contact with the wound surface.

Surgery

Split skin fragment grafts may speed ulcer healing in the short term but may not improve the long-term outlook. Grafts with skin cultivated *in vitro* have also been used. Surgical management of the incompetent veins may assist in some cases.

Ischaemic ulceration

Ulceration due to ischaemia is a frequent clinical problem though less often seen than that due to venous hypertension.

PATHOGENESIS

Atherosclerosis accounts for the majority of cases. This affects major vessels and mostly occurs gradually so that the ulceration occurs in an area of chronically ischaemic skin. Embolism may cause acute ulceration and gangrene.

Diabetes predisposes to atherosclerosis and impairs wound healing, making the problem particularly frequent in this group of patients.

Disease of the medium sized or small blood vessels may also cause ulceration as in allergic vasculitis or lupus erythematosus.

It should be noted that both 'ischaemic' and 'venous' ulcers are often due to both processes although one predominates, as both venous hypertension and atherosclerotic arterial disease often coexist.

It should be noted that both 'ischaemic' and 'venous' ulcers are often due to both processes although one predominates, as both venous hypertension and atherosclerotic arterial disease often co-exist.

CLINICAL FEATURES

Ischaemic ulcers occur anywhere around the feet or lower legs. The skin around the ulcerated area tends to be pale, cool, smooth and hairless. Light pressure with a finger on the skin easily makes it a deathly white and the pink colour takes longer to return than normal. The ulcers tend to be painful, irregular, and filled with a dark crust (Figure 11.11).

Ischaemic ulcers occur anywhere around the feet or lower legs. The skin around the ulcerated area tends to be pale, cool, smooth and hairless.

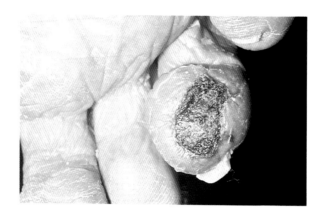

Figure 11.11 Ischaemic ulcer on toe.

PROGNOSIS
Such lesions tend to be progressive and gangrene often develops.

TREATMENT
Medical treatment is only helpful in the earliest and mildest cases. Keeping the affected part warm and protecting it from injury are important. Peripheral vasodilating drugs are only marginally useful (e.g. pentaerythritol tetranitrate, glyceryl trinitrate, isosorbide dinitrate, nifedipine) and other drugs promoting vascular flow and endothelial function such as hydroxyethyl rutosides and oxypentifylline may only be slightly more effective.

Sympathectomy (by surgical removal or by chemical destruction with injected alcohol) removes sympathetic vasoconstrictor tone and causes some vasodilatation which unfortunately rarely results in much clinical benefit. Of greater help is endarterectomy, either by open surgical technique or percutaneously, or arterial grafting.

Decubitus ulceration

These lesions are the result of localized ischaemia due to long-continued pressure on skin at contact points with bedclothes and occurs in the unconscious or paralysed patient.

Figure 11.12 Ischial ulceration in a paralysed patient.

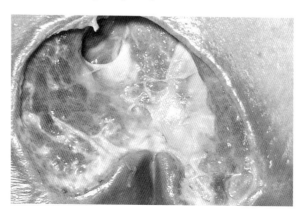

CLINICAL FEATURES

Classically ulcers occur over the sacrum or ischial regions (Figure 11.12), the heels, the back of the head, the scapulae and the elbows. The ulcers are often deeply penetrating and sloughy.

PROPHYLAXIS AND TREATMENT

Meticulously careful nursing with regular turning and the use of sheep's fleece, bedding or 'ripple' mattresses which constantly change pressure points help prevent decubitus ulcers. Maintenance of nutrition and general health as much as possible will also aid prevention of 'pressure sores'.

If established, the programme of 'turning' must be reviewed and improved. The individual ulcerated lesions need cleaning with nontoxic antibacterial solutions and dressing with nonadherent, nontoxic dressings (see under venous ulcers).

Neuropathic ulcers

Neuropathic ulcers result from repeated inadvertent injury to hypo- or anaesthetic areas of skin subsequent to nerve injury. They are most often seen in diabetes in the UK and Europe but leprosy is a common cause in some parts of the world.

CLINICAL FEATURES

These lesions may be very deeply penetrating. They occur mostly on the soles of the feet but may also be seen elsewhere on the foot (Figure 11.13).

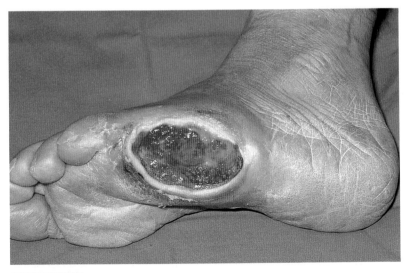

Figure 11.13 Neuropathic ulcer.

TREATMENT

Local treatment is unlikely to make any impact on these lesions. The only effective treatment is to protect the damaged area with padding and appliances and if possible restore sensation to the anaesthetic area.

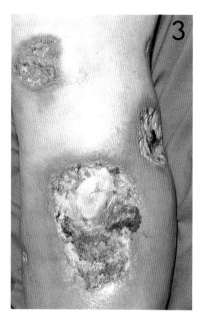

Figure 11.14 Multiple ulcers of leg in pyoderma gangrenosum. These developed over a three-day period.

Less common causes of ulceration

Pyoderma gangrenosum

A rare serious ulcerative disorder often due to serious underlying systemic disease.

AETIOPATHOGENESIS
The disorder may occur in the course of ulcerative colitis, Crohn's disease, rheumatoid arthritis, or myeloma, although in about half the cases no predisposing cause is found. It has been suggested that the tissue destruction is caused by a vasculitis although it is difficult to find evidence of this in the intense inflammation that characterizes this disorder.

CLINICAL FEATURES
The most frequent sequence is that of an acutely inflamed purplish nodule that rapidly becomes an ulcer which then spreads with frightening speed (Figure 11.14). The ulcer characteristically has bluish-mauve undermined margins. Such ulcers may be 'dinner plate' sized or even larger. Eventually they become static in size and may then spontaneously heal. Some patients have multiple lesions and may succumb to the disorder. Lesions may recur or new ones develop after a quiescent phase.

TREATMENT
Apart from the previously described regimen of cleansing and dressing and treatment directed to any underlying disease, some drugs, including minocycline and dapsone, have been reported as promoting the healing of pyoderma gangrenosum lesions.

Vasculitic ulcers

Ulcers may develop in the course of a disorder in which small blood vessels are inflamed and thrombosed (vasculitic). They often occur on the legs (Figure 11.15) but may develop anywhere. They may start from a patch of purpura. Treatment is directed towards the underlying illness.

Haematological causes

Leg ulcers are more common in patients with sickle cell disease and idiopathic thrombocytopaenic purpura.

Infective causes

Tuberculosis, tertiary syphilis and deep fungus infections can all result in persistent ulcers.

Arteriovenous malformation

Shunting of the blood at deeper levels may deprive the overlying skin and cause ulcers (Figure 11.16).

Malignant disease

This is an uncommon but important to recognize cause of persistent

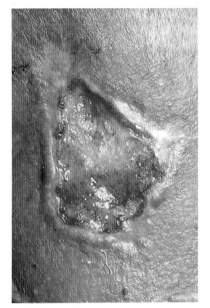

Figure 11.15 Vasculitic ulcer.

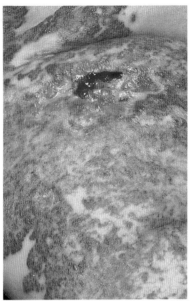

Figure 11.16 Ulcerated area in vascular birthmark.

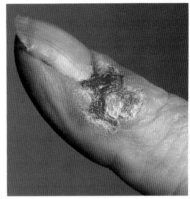

Figure 11.17 Ulcer due to squamous cell carcinoma on finger. The lesion had slowly extended over an 18-month period.

ulceration. The lesions are usually squamous cell carcinoma or basal cell carcinoma. They have raised edges and are slowly but relentlessly progressive (Figure 11.17).

Diagnosis and assessment of ulcers

Before treatment is planned it is important to reach a definitive diagnosis and assess the social background of the patient.

CLINICAL
The history, anatomical site and appearance of the lesion are the most important sources of diagnostic information. Also important is the condition of the surrounding skin.

LABORATORY
A biopsy from the margin may provide useful information and will do no harm. Bacterial swabs are not often helpful unless the ulcer is obviously clinically infected as an open wound will always harbour a large number of microbes. Haematological tests will identify underlying anaemia, a leukocytosis due to infection and rare haematological disorders.

SPECIAL VASCULAR TESTS
Venography, arteriography, measurement of blood pressure at the ankle and ultrasound Doppler blood flow studies are amongst the tests that may assist in assessment.

Benign tumours, moles, birthmarks and cysts

Introduction

The large number of cell and tissue types in skin is responsible for the enormous number of benign tumours that may arise from it. The biological position of many of these lesions is quite uncertain as it is difficult if not impossible to distinguish a benign acquired tumour from a lesion that results from a developmental anomaly. Despite the large number of such lesions they have a limited number of clinical appearances and because of this, accurate clinical diagnosis is difficult and requires experience and attention to detail. Many of these lesions are quite rare and don't belong in a book of this size. The treatment of all the lesions included is discussed together at the end of the chapter.

Tumours of epidermal origin

Seborrhoeic warts

Seborrhoeic warts are extremely common benign tumours of aging skin.

Also known as basal cell papillomas, seborrhoeic warts are extremely common benign tumours of aging skin. Most patients over the age of 40 years have one or two seborrhoeic warts – some have literally hundreds. They seem most common in Caucasians but similar lesions are seen in black-skinned and Asian peoples.

CLINICAL APPEARANCE

Their commonest clinical appearance is that of a brownish warty nodule or plaque on the upper trunk or head and neck regions.

Their commonest clinical appearance is that of a brownish warty nodule or plaque on the upper trunk (Figure 12.1) or head and neck regions. Their pigmentation varies from light fawn to black. They may occur as solitary lesions but mostly are multiple and quite often are present in vast numbers (Figure 12.2). They often have a greasy and 'stuck on' look. In black-skinned people they may appear as multiple blackish dome-shaped warty papules over the face, a condition known as dermatosis papulosa nigra. The differential diagnosis of warty lesions is given in Table 12.1. When deeply pigmented, they are sometimes mistaken for malignant melanoma.

Mostly they cause no symptoms, but patients complain that they

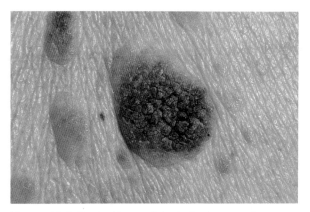

Figure 12.1 Typical brown/black stuck-on warty lesions known as seborrhoeic warts.

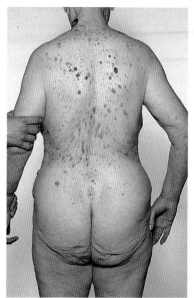

Figure 12.2 Large numbers of seborrhoeic warts.

catch in clothing and are unsightly. They may also irritate and, less frequently, become inflamed and cause soreness and pain.

Histologically there is epidermal thickening, the predominant cell being rather like the normal basal epidermal cell. Surmounting the thickened epidermis there is a warty hyperkeratosis whose arrangement has been likened to a series of church spires (Figure 12.3). Within the lesion are foci of keratinization and horn cysts.

Epidermal naevus

Epidermal naevus is the name given to a wide variety of uncommon localized malformations of the epidermis. Congenital in origin, they are classified as hamartomata and are mostly present at birth.

CLINICAL APPEARANCE
Many epidermal naevi are arranged linearly and are warty (Figure

> Many epidermal naevi are arranged linearly and are warty.

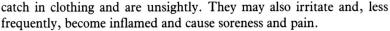

Table 12.1 Differential diagnosis of warty tumours

Lesion	Comment
Seborrhoeic wart	Mostly in elderly individuals and multiple; may have a greasy, stuck on appearance
Viral wart	Not usually pigmented; mostly in younger individuals on hands, feet, face and genitalia
Solar keratosis	Flat, pink and scaly mostly but can have a horny or warty surface; mostly on the backs of hands and face
Epidermal naevus	Mostly since birth; anywhere on body; often a linear arrangement

183

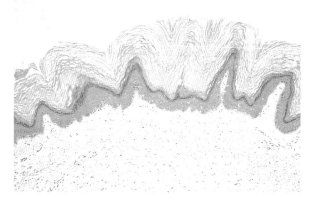

Figure 12.3 Pathology of flat seborrhoeic wart showing 'church spire' arrangement.

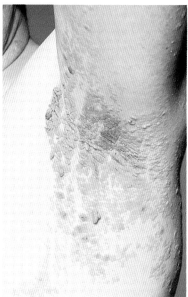

Figure 12.4 Epidermal naevus showing linear arrangement of warty lesions.

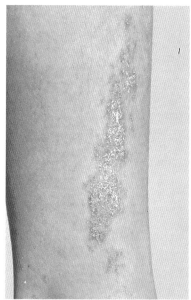

Figure 12.5 Naevus unius lateris – linear warty lesion.

12.4). Sometimes they track along a limb and adjoining trunk and are extensive and disfiguring. This type is known as naevus unius lateris (Figure 12.5). Histologically there is regular epidermal thickening and hyperkeratosis, often in a church spire pattern (Figure 12.6). In rare cases there is a degenerative epidermolytic change.

VARIANTS

Becker's naevus is an odd type of hamartomatous lesion that develops in adolescence or early adult life. It usually occurs around the shoulder or upper arms but is not unknown elsewhere. A comparatively large area of skin is affected by a brownish and sometimes hairy plaque (Figure 12.7). It consists of hypertrophy of all the epidermal structures including hair follicles and melanocytes.

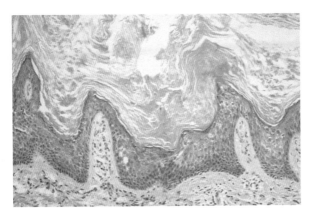

Figure 12.6 Pathology of epidermal naevus showing church spire arrangement.

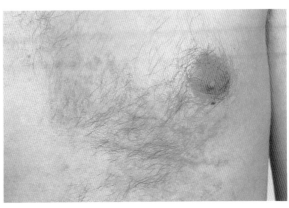

Figure 12.7 Becker's naevus on chest wall. The affected area is pigmented, thickened and hairy.

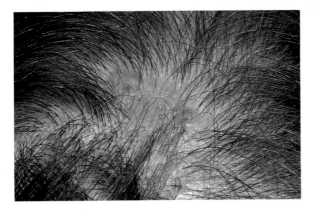

Figure 12.8 Typical orange plaque of naevus sebaceous on the scalp.

Naevus sebaceous also contains hypertrophied and deformed structures of epidermal origin in various amounts. This is either present at birth or shortly afterwards, and unlike Becker's naevus, may enlarge, thicken and develop other lesions in it, such as basal cell carcenoma in adult life. Most such lesions occur on the scalp as yellow or orange plaques (Figure 12.8).

Benign tumours of sweat gland origin

A summary of these lesions is given in Table 12.2. The following brief account describes a few of the most common lesions. The least uncommon of these is the *syringoma*. In most cases these are multiple small white or skin-coloured papules below the eyes (Figure 12.9) which may arise for no apparent reason quite suddenly in young adults. Uncommonly syringoma lesions are also evident on the arms and lower trunk. Histologically there are tiny comma-shaped epithelial structures, some of which appear cuticle lined, and microcysts (Figure 12.10) set in a more dense and less fibrillar connective tissue in the mid dermis.

Cylindroma is a benign tumour arising from apocrine sweat glands that, like syringoma, is often multiple. Smooth pink and skin-coloured

Table 12.2   Benign sweat gland tumours

Syringoma	Multiple white papules beneath eyes; composed of tiny cysts and comma-shaped epithelial clumps
Cylindroma	Solitary or multiple nodules on face or scalp; clumps of basaloid cells with eosinophilic colloid material
Syringocystadenoma papilliferum	Mostly develop in naevus sebaceous on scalp or on mons pubis
Nodular hidradenoma	Skin coloured or, rarely, pigmented solitary nodules of epithelial cells and ducts
Eccrine poroma	Solitary nodule on palms or soles or rarely elsewhere; basaloid clumps in upper dermis
Eccrine spiradenoma	Tender and painful solitary nodule

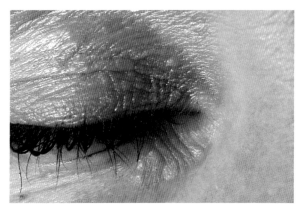

Figure 12.9 Syringoma lesions beneath the eye.

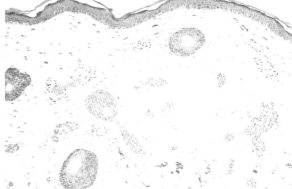

Figure 12.10 Pathology of syringoma showing many comma-shaped epithelial structures and tiny cysts.

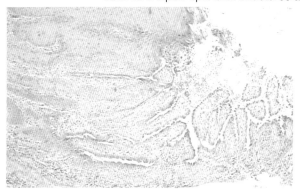

Figure 12.11 Pathology of syringocystadenoma papilliferum showing many ramifying channels lined by two layers of epithelial cells which form villi within the cavity.

nodules and papules occur over the scalp and face in young adults. Oval and rounded masses of basaloid epidermal cells surrounded by an eosinophilic band of a distinctive homogeneous connective tissue characterize the histological appearance.

Eccrine poroma describes an eccrine sweat duct-derived tumour that arises predominantly on the palms and soles in adults. Histologically the lesion appears contiguous with the surface epidermis and consists of basaloid cells in which there are cuticularly lined ductular structures.

Syringocystadenoma papilliferum is a fairly uncommon lesion derived from apocrine tissue. It develops either *de novo* on the scalp or mons pubis or arises from a pre-existing naevus sebaceous on the scalp. It consists of a central complex cavity that opens at the surface in a pore. The cavity forms numerous ramifying channels lined by two cell layers which form a series of villi within the cavity (Figure 12.11).

Benign tumours of hair follicle origin

A summary of these lesions is given in Table 12.3. The following brief account describes a few of the more common lesions.

Pilomatrixoma (calcifying epithelioma of Malherbe) is an extraordinary lesion developing around the head and neck and upper trunk in young adults mainly. Appearing as a solitary, smooth, skin-coloured or bluish nodule, it consists of large clumps of basal cells which progressively become calcified and eventually ossified, leaving behind their cell walls only (ghost cells) (Figure 12.12).

Trichoepithelioma is more often multiple than solitary and mostly occurs over the scalp and face. Histologically it consists for the most part of clumps of epithelial cells and horn-filled cysts.

Sebaceous gland hyperplasia is a common concomitant of aging, occurring in up to 20% of the population, although some have suspected that it is predominantly due to chronic solar damage rather than just the passing of the years. One, or more often several, yellowish skin-coloured papules develop over the cheeks, forehead, nose or chin, some of which have central puncta (Figure 12.13). They are often

> Sebaceous gland hyperplasia is a common concomitant of aging, occurring in up to 20% of the population. One, or more often several, yellowish skin coloured papules develop over the cheeks, forehead, nose or chin, some of which have central puncta.

Table 12.3 Benign hair follicle tumours

Trichoepithelioma	Solitary or multiple nodules on face or scalp containing cystic spaces
Trichofolliculoma	Solitary nodule on the face — may closely resemble follicular structures
Pilomatrixoma	Solitary skin-coloured or slightly bluish nodule on face or upper trunk with curious mummification of basaloid cells in clumps (ghost cells)

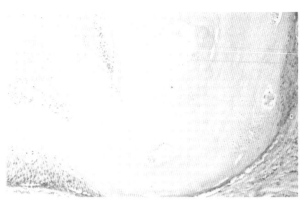

Figure 12.12 Pathology of pilomatrixoma showing cells undergoing transformation into 'ghost cells'.

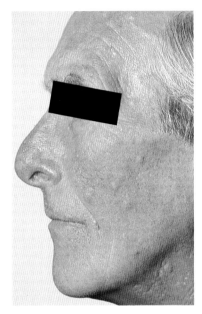

Figure 12.13 Sebaceous gland hyperplasia. Note multiple yellowish papules on the face.

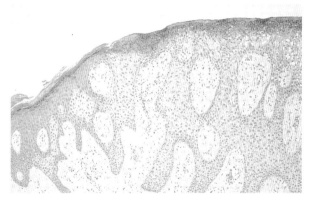

Figure 12.14 Pathology of clear cell acanthoma showing hypertrophied epidermis showing areas of large pale epithelial cells.

mistaken for basal cell carcinomata (page 217) or dermal cellular naevi (page 191). Histologically they consist of hypertrophied lobules of normal sebaceous gland tissue.

Clear cell acanthoma (*Syn.* Degos acanthoma) is described here only because of its odd and distinctive nature. Indeed it may well not be hair follicle derived. Clinically it is usually a moist, pink papule or nodule on the upper arms, thighs or trunk that has been present unchanging for several years. The name derives from the epidermal thickening composed of large clear cells that when stained with periodic acid–Schiff reagent are found to be stuffed with glycogen (Figure 12.14) and infiltrated with polymorphonuclear leukocytes.

Melanocytic naevi (moles)

> Melanocytic naevi are developmental anomalies consisting of immature melanocytes in abnormal numbers and sites within the skin. They are very common and on average, white skinned Caucasians have 16 over the skin surface.

These are developmental anomalies consisting of immature melanocytes in abnormal numbers and sites within the skin. They are very common and on average, white-skinned Caucasians have 16 over the

Table 12.4 Main varieties of melanocytic naevi

Type	Clinical features	Comment
Congenital		
Simple	Present since birth, tend to be larger than acquired naevi	Increased tendency for malignant transformation compared to acquired naevi
Girdle	Cover large areas around pelvic or pectoral zone (bathing trunk or cape naevus)	
Acquired	Develop predominantly in late childhood and early adolescence although a few continue to appear in early adult life	
Junctional	Macular, brown → black	Anywhere on skin or mucosae
Dermal cellular	Papular or nodular, may be hairy; colour is usually light brown but occasionally skin coloured	Very common on face and scalp
Naevus spilus	Large speckled light brown naevus	Uncommon
Dysplastic naevus syndrome	Many moles with irregular margins and pigmentation; may be sporadic but also familial	Increased tendency to malignant melanoma
Juvenile melanoma	Orange pink nodule or plaque in childhood	
Blue naevus	Blue appearance is due to depth of pigment in dermis	
Cellular blue naevus	Bluish nodule on scalp, hands or feet	
Mongolian spot	Large flat greyish blue macule	Present at birth over sacrum; may fade
Naevus of Ota or Ito	Facial and neck regions, flat blue-black areas	Predominantly in Asians

skin surface. Melanocytic naevi come in a wide variety of shapes and sizes and the main types are summarized in Table 12.4.

Congenital naevus

The congenital naevus is so named because it is present at birth. The more common variety is solitary and dark brown, and is more than 1 cm^2 in size. It is plaque-like or nodular (Figure 12.15). It shares with the limb girdle naevus the increased tendency to malignant transformation. It has been suggested that 10% of the larger congenital naevi develop malignant melanoma.

The most deforming congenital melanocytic naevi are those that cover large tracts of skin on the pelvic region and adjoining back (*bathing trunk naevus*) or over the shoulder region and upper limb (*cape naevus*) (Figure 12.16). Histologically these lesions consist of numerous 'packets' (theques) of naevus cells (Figure 12.17). Naevus cells may be small and basophilic (lymphocytoid), large and less intensely staining (epithelioid), or spindle shaped. They may also coalesce to form naevus giant cells or, after they have been present for many years, may show degenerate changes including fatty degeneration and calcification

189

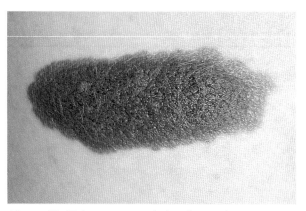

Figure 12.15 Large congenital melanocytic naevus.

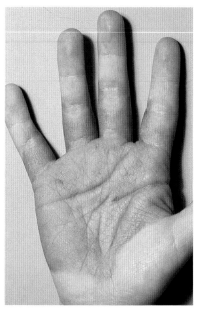

Figure 12.16 Congenital naevus affecting most of one hand.

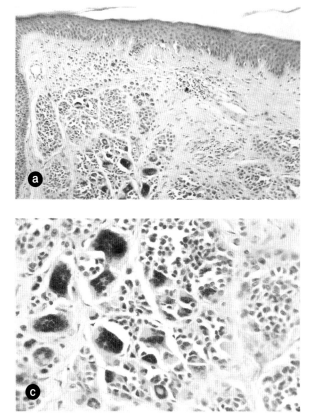

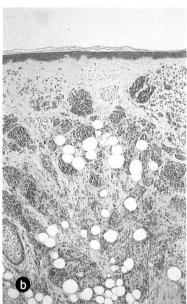

Figure 12.17 (a) Pathology of congenital melanocytic naevus showing packets or theques of naevus cells, some of which are 'naevus giant cells'. (b) Degeneration in naevus. (c) Many large naevus giant cells.

(Figure 12.17a and b). Naevus cells tend to be facetted together in a rather characteristic way.

> Congenital melanocytic naevi are present since birth and may be very large.

Acquired naevus
As the name suggests, acquired naevi make their appearance after birth, usually in late childhood, adolescence or young adult life. *Potential difficulty* arises when an adult notices a brown spot or papule for the first time. Was it there for many years before being noticed? Or is it a new benign mole, some other pigmented lesion, or a malignant melanoma? The differential diagnosis for this situation is given in Table 12.4.

Junctional naevus
Junctional naevus is the term used to describe a flat brown or black mole in which clumps of naevus cells can be observed at the dermoepidermal junction (Figure 12.18) nestling in dermal papillae. It is presumed that this is the first stage in the 'life cycle' of the ordinary mole.

Dermal cellular naevus
Clumps of naevus cells are found within the upper dermis, accounting for the papular or nodular nature of these lesions. Their pigmentation is variable – often they are fawn or light brown or just skin coloured. They are common on the face, and are often 'hairy' (Figure 12.19) accounting for the episodes of pain, redness and swelling occasionally observed in these lesions and due to folliculitis. In a few lesions there is a deep component with many spindle-shaped naevus cells that may superficially resemble the cellular component of a neurofibroma (page 200). *Potential difficulty arises* in the elderly when there is little pigment, as they are often misdiagnosed as basal cell carcinoma.

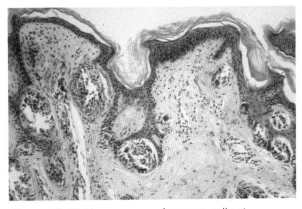

Figure 12.18 Many groups of naevus cells at dermoepidermal junction in 'junctional naevus'.

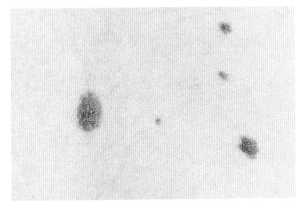

Figure 12.19 Common dermal cellular naevi.

Acquired melanocytic naevi develop in childhood and adolescence. They may consist of clusters of naevus cells at the dermoepidermal junction (junctional) or clusters within the dermis (dermal) or a combination of these two types (compound).

Compound naevus

This has the characteristics of a dermal cellular naevus but there are areas of 'junctional activity' with foci of naevus cells at the dermoepidermal junction. It is presumed that this lesion is intermediary in development between the junctional naevus and the dermal cellular naevus.

Degenerative changes in naevi

Naevus cell naevi gradually become fewer during the aging process and it is believed that moles develop involutional changes before disappearing. Some develop lipid vacuoles in their substance, others develop a type of foamy change, yet others appear to calcify before finally disappearing.

Blue naevus

Although it is believed that this type of mole is very similar to the ordinary naevus cell naevus, there are striking differences. In the first place, in the ordinary *cellular blue naevus* the melanin pigment and the bulk of the naevus cells are in the mid and deep dermis. This accounts for the striking blue colour given by the pigment in the lesion as the red wavelengths are filtered out by the superficial dermis and epidermis. This type of blue naevus is found over the scalp (Figure 12.20) and sometimes over the back of the hands or feet.

The *Mongolian spot* is another type of blue naevus which is extremely common in Asiatics. It occurs as an expanse of macular greyish discolouration over the sacral area in the newborn. Generally it becomes less prominent in later life and only persists in a small proportion.

Figure 12.20 Blue naevus.

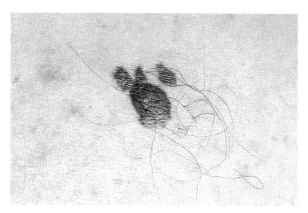

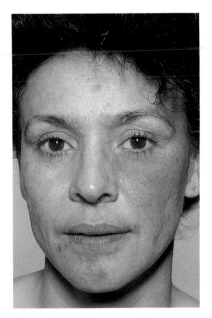

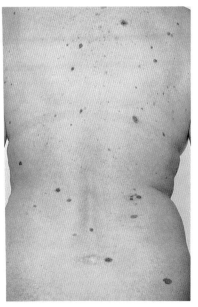

Figure 12.21 Naevus of Ota.

Figure 12.22 Multiple dysplastic moles with irregularity of shape and pigmentation.

Naevus of Ota is another form of blue naevus seen mostly in patients of Asian ancestry in which the spindle-shaped dermal naevus cells are over the side of the upper part of the face (Figure 12.21). *Naevus of Ito* is very similar, but over the side of the neck and lower part of the face. Both these lesions tend to persist and cause considerable distress because of the cosmetic disability produced.

Blue naevus and Mongolian spot appear 'blue or grey' because of the depth of the naevus cells within the skin.

Dysplastic naevus syndrome (B–K naevus syndrome; atypical mole syndrome).

Recognition of this disorder is particularly important because of greatly increased frequency of malignant melanoma in such patients. The condition may occur sporadically but is also familial in many patients accounting for the 'B–K naevus syndrome' as the surnames of the first two families described with the disorder began with a 'B' and a 'K'.

The individual lesions are quite large compared to ordinary moles, and have irregular margins and irregular brown pigmentation, some having an orange-red hue (Figure 12.22). They are often present in large numbers and may be scattered anywhere over the skin surface. It is said that the risk of a melanoma developing is approximately 1%, but it is certainly much more than that in the familial form if one of the affected members of the family has had a melanoma – perhaps 10%. It

In the dysplastic naevus syndrome individual lesions are large compared to ordinary moles, and have irregular margins and irregular brown pigmentation or an orange-red hue. They are often present in large numbers. The risk of a melanoma developing is approximately 1%.

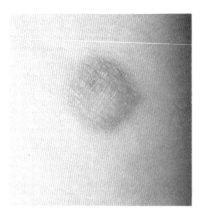

Figure 12.23 Juvenile melanoma. A red nodule on the arm of a nine-year-old boy.

is much greater again if the individual has already one melanoma, the chances of developing another approach 100%!

From the histological point of view these lesions often have what the dermatopathologists call a 'worrying appearance', meaning that many have one or another feature suggesting melanoma. There may be a degree of cytological atypia and excessive mitoses.

Juvenile melanoma

These are quite uncommon benign lesions of childhood and adolescence. Although usually solitary papules or small plaques, they are occasionally multiple (Figure 12.23). The individual lesions are pink or orange and may have a corrugated or *peau d'orange* surface. Their name derives from their histological appearance which may look frighteningly like a melanoma to the uninitiated. There are large spindle-shaped or strap-like naevus cells that seem to be 'raining down' into the dermis from marked collections of cells in the junctional zone. Juvenile melanoma lesions usually disappear spontaneously in adult life.

Vascular malformations (angioma)/capillary naevi

Stork mark

This is the popular name for the red discolouration at the back of the neck in a high proportion of the newly born. It fades in later childhood and seems to be due to vasodilatation rather than an excess of blood vessels.

Port wine stains

These common vascular malformations may occur anywhere but seem most frequent on the face and scalp. The deep crimson colour (of 'port wine') is distinctive and cosmetically very disturbing to those who carry the lesion (Figure 12.24). The lesions contain many dilated blood vessels but there is no obvious histological abnormality of the vasculature.

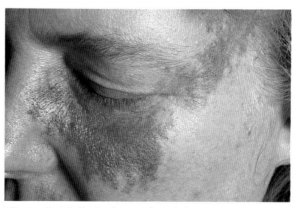

Figure 12.24 Typical port wine stain.

194

As the owner of the port wine stain ages the surface of the lesion becomes more thickened and rugose and even develops polypoid outgrowths, adding to the grotesque appearance. When the lesion occurs on a limb, deep vascular malformations may also be present which can cause limb hypertrophy. Over the ophthalmic region the obvious skin malformation of blood vessels may be associated with an underlying meningeal angiomatous malformation. When this combination of lesions is associated with epilepsy the disorder is known as the Sturge-Weber syndrome.

> Congenital vascular malformations include port wine stains in which there is capillary dilation and capillary angioma (strawberry marks) where there is marked endothelial proliferation.

Capillary angioma

This term is somewhat confusing as it is usually applied to what is popularly known as a strawberry mark, containing a mass of capillary endothelial channels, although senile angioma shares this histological appearance.

In most cases the lesion is present at birth but may develop in the first few months of life. They are raised purplish nodules and plaques whose surface is often lobulated (supposedly like a strawberry) and show an enormous range of sizes. The smaller lesions have little functional significance (Figure 12.25) and mostly flatten or even disappear without trace around the time of puberty. The larger lesions are very deforming and may cover quite a large area of skin (Figure 12.26). This type of lesion is associated with two sorts of complication. The first is ulceration, especially after minor trauma. This is particularly a problem of larger lesions and is presumably due to a 'poverty amongst plenty' situation in which the overlying superficial dermis and overlying epidermis are ischaemic because of the shunting of blood between the larger, deeper vessels of the angioma. The eroded areas sometimes bleed but the bleeding can be stopped with gentle pressure

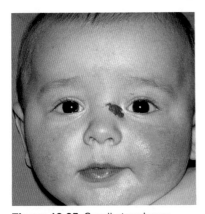

Figure 12.25 Small strawberry naevus on left side of nose.

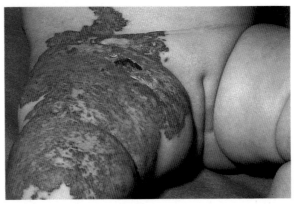

Figure 12.26 Large capillary naevus affecting thigh and lower abdomen.

and the eroded area gradually heals with routine care. The other complication is luckily quite rare and only occurs with the largest of capillary angiomas. For an as yet undiscovered reason, blood platelets become sequestered in the abnormal vascular channels of the angioma, creating a consumption coagulopathy and uncontrolled bleeding (Katzenbach-Merritt syndrome). The bleeding can be dealt with by administration of systemic steroids although the rationale for this is not clear.

Cavernous haemangioma

The cavernous haemangioma is composed of large vascular spaces but has elements with smaller blood vessels too. Generally it is a soft, compressible mauvish-blue swelling which may vary slightly in size from day to day. It is often connected to vascular malformations of large vessels deep in the soft tissues. This lesion shows little tendency to reduce in size in later life.

Lymphangioma circumscriptum

This lesion is a malformation of lymphatic channels although there may also be an associated blood vessel anomaly. Lymphangioma lesions tend to occur around the limb girdles and usually have a deep component which it is almost impossible to eradicate surgically. Clinically the malformation is recognized by the appearance of a diffuse skin swelling with what appears to be a cluster of tense vesicles at the skin surface. These often have a dark central patch within them and have a frogspawn-like appearance (Figure 12.27).

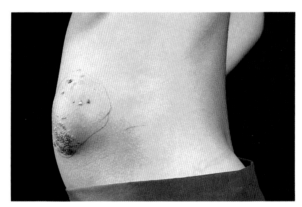

Figure 12.27 Lymphangioma circumscriptum affecting the abdomen. There is a deep component making eradication difficult.

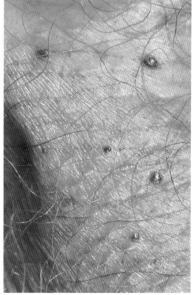

Figure 12.28 Angiokeratoma of the scrotum.

Angiokeratoma

There are several types of angiokeratoma. They all consist of a small subepidermal vascular malformation which is surmounted by a hyperkeratotic epidermis. They may occur as solitary red papules or occasionally as a crop of red spots over the scrotum (Figure 12.28). Rarely they are also seen over the labia majora. When literally hundreds of tiny red papules develop over the trunk in young men the possibility of a very rare inherited metabolic abnormality must be considered. The characteristic angiomatous lesion in this disease, known as angiokeratoma corporis diffusum is identical to that seen in the other types of angiokeratoma.

Senile angioma (Campbell de Morgan spot, cherry angioma)

As with seborrhoeic warts and skin tags, senile angioma is a frequent accompaniment of skin aging. Histologically it resembles the capillary angioma but clinically its smooth surfaced, dome-shaped purplish or cherry red appearance is quite characteristic (Figure 12.29). Many lesions may appear over a period of some months but apart from the distress that their appearance seems to cause they have no special significance for general health.

Venous lake

This term is used to describe a not uncommon bluish saccular dilatation of the lip seen in the elderly (Figure 12.30). It does not cause symptoms and has no special significance.

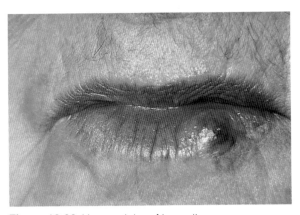

Figure 12.30 Venous lake of lower lip.

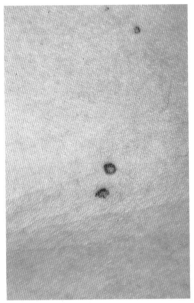

Figure 12.29 Senile angioma on the trunk in man aged 63 years.

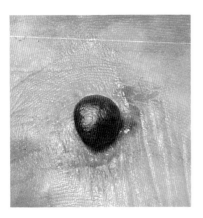

Figure 12.31 Dome-shaped, plum-red coloured shiny nodule of pyogenic granuloma.

Capillary aneurysm

Because the commonest presentation of this tiny vascular lesion is of a suddenly appearing black pinhead spot it is sometimes mistaken for an early malignant melanoma. If left it gradually fades.

Glomus cell tumour

This benign vascular tumour arises from the glomus cells controlling tiny vascular shunts between arterial and venous capillaries at the periphery. The constituent cells have a characteristic cuboidal appearance and the lesion, which often occurs around the fingertips, is often quite painful.

Pyogenic granuloma

The true status of this odd lesion is uncertain. It does not appear to be a hamartomatous malformation as it characteristically appears suddenly over a few days or a week or two and then disappears after several weeks or at the most a few months. Typically it is a red dome-shaped papule with a glazed or eroded surface (Figure 12.31). It may occur anywhere on the body surface but is particularly common around the fingers and toes. Its pathology is quite distinct, consisting of a matrix of what appears to be oedematous glassy connective tissue in which numerous thin-walled vascular channels can be seen. There is also a moderately dense mixed cellular infiltrate which presumably is responsible for the origin of the term 'pyogenic granuloma', although as far as is known, no infectious micro-organism appears responsible for its development.

> Pyogenic granuloma is a rapidly developing glazed red papule of unknown origin consisting of thin wall vascular channels in primitive connective tissue.

Dermatofibroma (histiocytoma; sclerosing haemangioma)

There are no true 'fibromas' of dermal connective tissue and it is not certain whether the dermatofibroma is a benign neoplasm or some form of localized chronic inflammatory disorder. It certainly does contain many spindle-shaped and banana-shaped mononuclear cells which may be fibroblast derived, and there is a variable amount of new collagenous dermal connective tissue. There are also many histiocytic cells present which often contain lipid or iron pigment, both of which may derive from the large number of small blood vessels also contained in the lesion.

Clinically they are firm or hard intracutaneous nodules. Mostly they are found on the limbs as solitary lesions but sometimes two or three or even more are found in the same patient. Generally they are brownish in colour (from the haemosiderin pigment) and have a rough or warty surface because this dermal nodule has the propensity of thickening up

> The dermatofibroma contains many spindle-shaped and banana-shaped mononuclear cells which may be fibroblast derived. New collagenous dermal connective tissue and many histiocytic cells present which often contain lipid or iron pigment are also seen.

the epidermis immediately above it (Figure 12.32). This epidermal thickening is of considerable interest as it suggests that the dermatofibroma releases some mediator or cytokine causing the change.

The lesion has no serious clinical significance but is sometimes mistaken for a melanoma.

Hypertrophic scar

Although this is a reactive lesion and not a neoplastic tumour it is appropriate to describe hypertrophic scar here as it is sometimes confused with true neoplastic lesions. The scar is a reparative response to injury of some kind, accidental or surgical, trauma, or tissue destruction from an inflammatory skin disorder such as acne, in which the tissue architecture cannot be entirely restored and the defect is made good with fibrous tissue. A hypertrophic scar describes the situation in which excess scar tissue is formed a short time after the initial injury. The lesion is usually pink, smooth and variably raised (Figure 12.33). It generally flattens after some months or can be encouraged to do so with topical corticosteroids and firm pressure bandaging.

Keloid scar

Like hypertrophic scar, this lesion arises in response to injury, but the response is totally inappropriate to the often minor degree of trauma. It tends to occur in young adults and adolescents, particularly women, and particularly around the shoulders, upper limbs and upper trunk. Some ethnic groups also appear more likely to develop these lesions – black-skinned individuals being particularly prone. Clinically the lesions are raised and appear to send extensions into neighbouring skin (Figure 12.34). They show little tendency to regress and surgical treatment alone is usually insufficient as they tend to recur in the scar. Corticosteroids, radiotherapy and topical retinoic acid have all been tried, with varying success. Nothing is known of their cause but their histological appearance, with oedematous pale connective tissue, suggests reversion to the embryonic type of collagen.

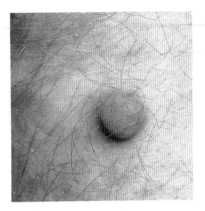

Figure 12.32 Dermatofibroma: brownish-red, firm, intracutaneous nodules.

In hypertrophic scar excess scar tissue is formed a short time after the initial injury, but this generally flattens after some months.

In Keloid scar the response is totally inappropriate to the often minor degree of trauma.

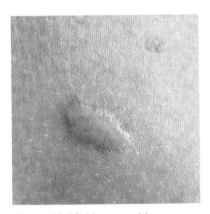

Figure 12.33 Hypertrophic scar.

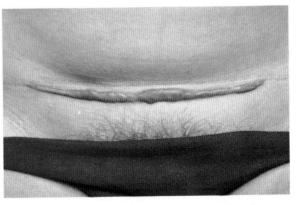

Figure 12.34 Keloid scar occurring at the site of a scar from a Caesarean section.

Leiomyoma

This is an uncommon benign tumour of plain muscle that arises either from arrector pilores muscle of hair follicles or from the smooth muscle of blood vessel walls. It is mostly smooth surfaced, oval and bluish red in colour, varying in size from 1 to 3 cm in length and 0.5 to 1.5 cm in breadth. This lesion has two claims to fame. The first is that it may be spontaneously painful, especially in the cold, and indeed can sometimes be seen to contract when cooled. The other notorious property is its ability to be confused histologically on account of its spindle- and strap-shaped plain muscle cells which may be taken for fibrous or neural tissue by the unwary.

Neural tumours

These are in fact tumours of the connective tissue accompanying the neural elements.

Neurofibroma and Von Recklinghausen's disease

The neurofibroma occasionally occurs as an isolated skin tumour but more often it is multiple and part of a not uncommon inherited syndrome known as neurofibromatosis or Von Recklinghausen's disease. The individual lesion is soft and compressible and skin coloured. It is often quite large, up to several centimetres across, and may be lobulated (Figure 12.35). Histologically the typical picture is of a

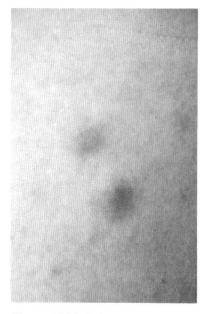

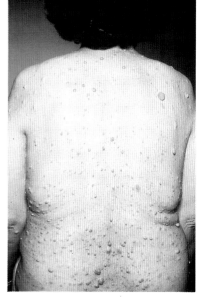

Figure 12.35 Soft mauve or pink compressible lesions of neurofibroma.

Figure 12.36 Multiple neurofibromata in Von Recklinghausen's disease.

nonencapsulated dermal mass composed of interlacing bundles of spindle-shaped cells often in a 'nerve-like' arrangement, set in a homogeneous matrix amidst which mast cells may be seen. Von Recklinghausen's syndrome is inherited as a dominant characteristic although some 30–50% of patients don't give a family history of the disorder and one must presume that there is a high rate of new gene mutation.

Neurofibromata start to appear in childhood and increase in numbers during adolescence and young adult life. They are cosmetically very disabling (Figure 12.36) and in the worst cases result in gross deformity. Ultimately large numbers may be present. Some become very large, soft diffuse swellings, others become pedunculated and pendulous. Alongside the neurofibromata, light brown uniformly pigmented macular patches appear (*café au lait* patches) over the trunk and limbs (Figure 12.37). These have quite distinct margins but are irregular in shape and variable in size. A useful diagnostic point is the presence of small pigmented macules at the apices of the axillae. During the life-time of the affected individual there is a greatly increased risk of tumours affecting both the central and peripheral nervous systems as well as of tumours of muscle and connective tissue. Phaeochromocytoma and tumours of sympathetic tissue are also found more often in patients with neurofibromatosis than in the general population.

The disorder causes a great deal of distress and disability and genetic counselling of affected individuals is of great importance.

> There is a greatly increased risk of tumours affecting both the central and peripheral nervous systems as well as of tumours of muscle and connective tissue.

> In neurofibromatosis multiple benign tumours of neural connective tissue develop alongside brown 'café au lait' macules during adolescence as adominantly feritable disorder.

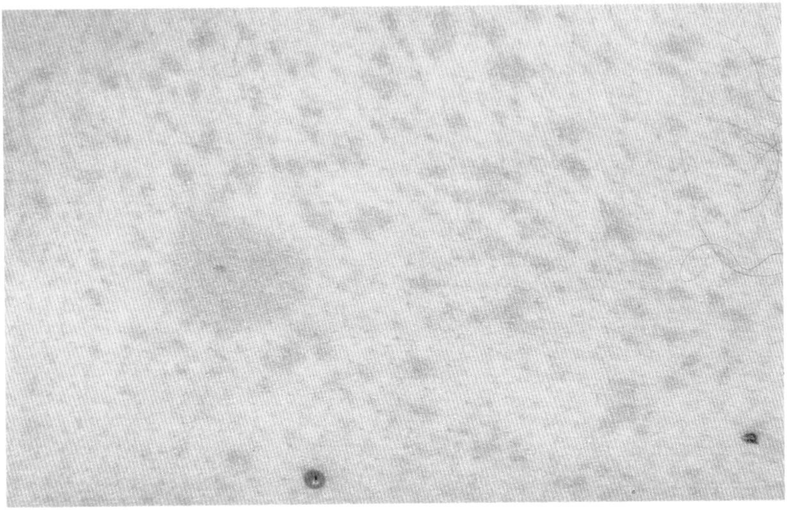

Figure 12.37 *Café au lait* patch in Von Recklinghausen's disease.

Neurilemmoma

The neurilemmoma is another benign tumour of neural connective tissue but is much less common than the neurofibroma. It is mostly a solitary lesion, varying in size from a pinhead to a golf ball, and may occur anywhere on the skin surface. Microscopically it can be seen to consist of thin spindle-shaped cells arranged in a stacked or 'storiform' manner.

Neuroma

This rare, benign neural tumour is the most differentiated of all the neural connective tissue tumours and consists of well-formed nerve elements. It occurs at the site of nerve injury and occasionally seems to arise spontaneously.

Lipoma

Lipomata are common, solitary or sometimes multiple, benign tumours of fat. They may be enormous in size or only 1–2 cm in diameter and can occur any where. They are soft, skin-coloured and have poorly defined edges. Histologically they are difficult to define as they consist of mature fat cells and have the most flimsy of connective tissue capsules separating them from the surrounding normal fat.

Collagen and elastic tissue naevi

These are rare intracutaneous plaques and nodules often with a knobbly or a corrugated skin surface and a difficult to discern edge. They are very difficult to identify histologically because they are composed of what appears to be normal connective tissue although in the case of elastic tissue naevus, special stains will identify the excess of elastic tissue. They may occur as 'shagreen patches' (due to a fancied likeness to shark skin) in the syndrome known as tuberose sclerosis.

Tuberose sclerosis (epiloia)

This recessively inherited syndrome is a neurocutaneous disorder. The cutaneous components include shagreen patches (see above), hypopigmented patches on the trunk often in the shape of an ash leaf, subungual fibroma, which is a fibrous nodule that develops beneath the toe and finger nails, and adenoma sebaceum. Adenoma sebaceum is a poorly named disorder that occurs on the cheeks and the central part of the face of patients with tuberose sclerosis. Pink or red, firm papular lesions characterize the condition (Figure 12.38) and when these are examined histologically only vascular fibrous tissue is found rather than an excess of sebaceous glands.

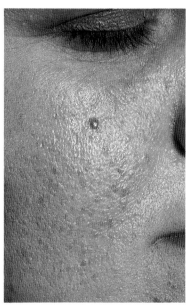

Figure 12.38 Pink nodules characterizing the disorder known as adenoma sebaceum.

Mast cell naevus and mastocytosis

All these lesions are characterized by an excess of mast cells that may or may not release histamine and occasionally heparin on stimulation.

Mast cell naevus (mastocytoma)

This lesion represents one, or occasionally several, localized collections of mast cells (Figure 12.39). It presents as a pink or red nodule 1–3 cm in diameter in infants and young children, but usually disappears spontaneously later in childhood. Rubbing it or heating it, as during bathing, may result in it swelling and developing a red halo in the surrounding skin – a sign known eponymously as Darier's sign.

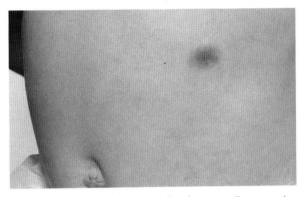

Figure 12.39 Solitary red nodule of mast cell naevus in a child of three years.

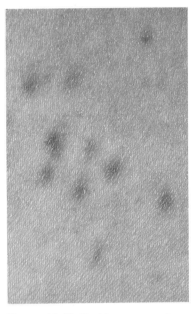

Figure 12.40 Red-brown papules of urticaria pigmentosa.

> Mastocytosis (urticaria pigmentosa) describes a group of disorder in which there may be excess mast cells in many tissues but is mainly manifest in the skin.

Mastocytosis (urticaria pigmentosa)

This term is used to describe a group of disorders in which there may be excess mast cells in many tissues but is mainly manifest in the skin. The term urticaria pigmentosa was formerly employed because it is not uncommon for the individual lesions to become pigmented although it is not certain why this should be. The juvenile form is the most common variety and in this form numerous pink or red-brown papules develop over the trunk and limbs (Figure 12.40). In some young patients the lesions are intensely itchy and they experience discomfort and erythema when bathing but for the most part the condition doesn't cause symptoms. Juvenile mastocytosis usually remits spontaneously during adolescence.

There are several adult types but only two need be described here. The first is the papular variety and is somewhat like the juvenile form save that it persists (Figure 12.41). The other form is very uncommon and rejoices in the old-fashioned descriptive name of telangiectasia macularis eruptiva perstans of Parkes Weber. Clinically it lives up to its name very well in that in early adult life pink or pink-brown telangiectatic macules start to appear, persist and increase in number as the years roll by.

In all the generalized varieties of mastocytosis, studies have shown

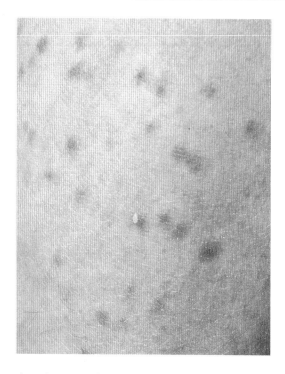

Figure 12.41 Adult mastocytosis.

that there are deposits of mast cells in visceral structures such as liver, spleen and bone in an appreciable number of cases – up to 20% in some series, but this seems to be of no particular consequence and does not appear to result in any functional deficit in the great majority of patients.

Potential difficulty in confirmation of the diagnosis stems from the small increase in the number of mast cells in the lesions in the adult variety. Special fixation (e.g. in alcohol) and special stains (e.g. toluidine blue) are necessary to show up the metachromatic granules of the mast cells.

Cysts

A cyst is an epithelium-lined cavity filled with fluid or semisolid material. The distinguishing features of the commonly encountered cysts of the skin are summarized in Table 12.5.

> A cyst is an epithelium-lined cavity filled with fluid or semisolid material.

Epidermoid cyst

> An epidermoid cyst is lined by epidermis and produces stratum corneum.

This lesion is lined by epidermis and produces stratum corneum. It is often surrounded by a tough fibrous capsule presumably stimulated by the leakage of the cyst contents. If these find their way into the dermis, considerable inflammation results. The horny content may eventually degenerate, forming a foul smelling semisolid material. The fancied resemblance of this to sebum has mistakenly led to the term 'sebaceous cysts' for these lesions. Epidermoid cysts may occur anywhere but are most common over the head and neck and upper trunk.

Table 12.5   Differential diagnosis of common skin cysts

Cyst type	Body site	Clinical features
Epidermoid	Virtually anywhere	Smooth walled, firm lesions may become inflamed if leaks; common
Milium	At sites of blistering Spontaneously on upper cheeks	Pinhead sized, white hard lesions
Pilar	Scalp and scrotum	May be inherited, often multiple; less common than epidermoid cysts; smooth walled but not as firm as epidermoid cysts
Sebocystoma multiplex	Anywhere but especially the upper trunk	May be inherited; always multiple; usually small, smooth walled; contents less firm than other types; may become inflamed and develop acne-like lesions; uncommon
Dermoid	Face, particularly around the eyes	Deep set in skin; may be oval and less mobile than other cyst types

Milia

Milia are tiny epidermoid cysts that occur at the sites of subepidermal blistering as in porphyria cutanea tarda (page 262) or spontaneously over the upper cheeks and beneath the eyes. They are usually no larger than a pinhead and are white, so that they are often mistaken for xanthelasmata by the inexperienced. They contain tiny accretions of horn which can be expressed by slitting the thin epidermis over them with a needle tip.

Pilar cysts (tricholemmal cysts)

The lining epithelium of these less common cysts is derived from a portion of the hair follicle neck and shows a quite characteristic type of keratinization in which there is abrupt formation of a glassy-appearing type of horn without a granular cell layer. Pilar cysts are usually multiple and are often genetically determined as an autosomal dominant trait. They occur on the scalp and on the scrotum in particular. Rarely the lining epithelium seems to 'lose control' and proliferates wildly, even becoming malignant on rare occasions, particularly in elderly women for some odd reason. As with epidermoid cysts, inflammation occurs if the cyst contents leak out.

> The lining epithelium of pilar cysts is derived from a portion of the hair follicle neck and shows a quite characteristic type of keratinization in which there is abrupt formation of a glassy-appearing type of horn without a granular cell layer.

Sebocystoma multiplex (steatocystoma multiplex)

These cystic malformations are formed from sebaceous gland tissue and other hair follicle derived epithelium. They are always multiple, often being present in very large numbers. They are inherited as an autosomal dominant trait. Their content is sometimes pure sebum. In fact these cysts are the only real source of real sebum, as sebum on the skin surface is contaminated by epidermal lipid. Large numbers of small cysts are distributed over the body but particularly over the upper trunk.

Dermoid cysts

Dermoid cysts are uncommon lesions that seem to contain embryonic epithelium capable of forming a wide spectrum of tissue types. They may occur anywhere but are especially often found around the eyes as oval, firm, smooth-walled swellings.

Follicular retention cysts

When large hair follicles develop a hard immovable comedonal plug in the follicular neck or at the skin surface the follicle distends because of the continuing secretion of sebum and production of horny material. Often these cysts rupture, causing inflammation, but sometimes this doesn't happen and quite large swellings are produced. This seems to happen particularly frequently over the back in the elderly, when they are sometimes known as giant comedones.

Treatment of benign tumours, moles and birthmarks

Surgical excision or some other form of surgical ablation is appropriate for the large majority of patients with small benign lesions. However, this may not be the case in young children or the very old or where are large numbers of such abnormalities. It should be remembered that on many occasions it is the appearance of the lesion that is the predominant concern of the patient and it is not helpful, for example, to substitute a simple facial mole with an ugly surgical scar. One overriding principle is important to remember. If any form of surgical removal or destruction is planned, histological evidence of the nature of the lesion is required. Even the most experienced dermatologist is not more than 65–70% accurate in the clinical diagnosis of not typical pigmented lesions and is only a little better with nonpigmented tumours. Knowing the true nature of the lesion destroyed prevents embarrassment and inappropriate and even tragic mistakes in management.

Minimally scarring procedures such as curettage and cautery and shaving off small benign dome-shaped lesions flush with the skin may be quite adequate to remove the lesion and prevent unpleasant scar formation. Cryotherapy may also be useful for some superficial lesions. Treatment by lasers is indicated for some vascular malformations but requires specialized instrumentation and personnel with experience and skill which are only available in a few centres.

Malignant disease of the skin

Introduction

All forms of malignant disease of the skin are becoming more frequent. The reasons for this are:

1.   increased exposure to solar ultraviolet irradiation;
2.   an increasingly 'elderly' population;
3.   increasing exposure to an increasing number of carcinogenic substances;
4.   an increasing number of people who are immunosuppressed. The likelihood is that these trends will continue, making this subject increasingly important.

Nonmelanoma skin cancer

Under this heading we will deal with premalignant epidermal lesions, malignant lesions of interfollicular epidermis and the much less common malignant lesions of adnexal structures.

Solar keratoses (senile keratoses)

DEFINITION
Solar keratoses (SK) are common localized areas of epidermis due to chronic solar exposure in which epidermal growth and differentiation are irregular and abnormal.

CLINICAL FEATURES
The typical solar keratosis (SK) is a raised pink or grey, scaling or warty hyperkeratotic plaque or papule (Figure 13.1). They are mostly 2–5 mm in diameter but sometimes reach much larger proportions (Figure 13.2). They are mostly found on the exposed areas of skin of elderly, fair-skinned subjects who show other signs of solar damage. Multiple lesions are the rule, and when a solitary SK is found it may be assumed that there is widespread solar damage to the epidermis and that other very small SK are present and that further SK will appear.
   Differential diagnosis of small scaling or warty lesions of exposed

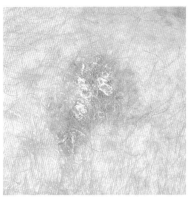

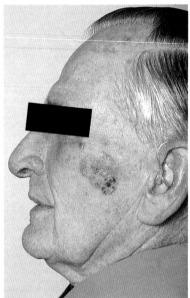

Figure 13.1 Typical solar keratosis.

Figure 13.2 Large solar keratosis affecting left cheek.

Table 13.1 **Differential diagnosis of scaling/warty lesions on exposed skin**

Lesion	Comment
Solar keratosis (page 207)	Mostly multiple, accompanied by other signs of solar damage; virtually confined to fair complexioned elderly subjects
Seborrhoeic keratoses (page 182)	Generally pigmented; not confined to exposed sites; very variable in size
Bowen's disease (page 211)	Generally larger than SK and more plaque-like, but otherwise quite similar
Superficial BCC (page 217)	Flat scaling slightly raised plaque, with slightly raised well-defined edge
Discoid lupus erythematosus (page 74)	Evidence of scarring often present; mostly younger subjects, and more females than for SK
Psoriasis/ seborrhoeic dermatitis	Usually also other sites involved; scaling not warty; lesions more extensive than SK

BCC = basal cell carcinoma; SK = solar keratoses

skin sites is given in Table 13.1. Clinical diagnosis of solar keratosis may be quite difficult and with 'not quite typical' lesions an accuracy of more than 65% is exceptionally good, even for experienced clinicians. However, biopsy is simple and for this group of disorders it is helpful in distinguishing lesions that look similar clinically.

> Solar keratoses are common small scaly or warty areas of epidermal irregularity on exposed skin due to chronic solar exposure.

PATHOLOGY: AETIOPATHOGENESIS OF SOLAR KERATOSES AND NON MELANOMA SKIN CANCER

The affected epidermis is generally slightly irregularly thickened, although 'atrophic SK' may have a thinner epidermis. Parakeratosis and/or hyperkeratosis surmounts the lesion which demonstrates heterogeneity of epidermal cell and nuclear size, shape and staining (epidermal dysplasia) (Figure 13.3). These changes may be quite subtle, requiring some practice to identify them with certainty, although in other lesions the abnormalities are striking, resembling those of Bowen's disease (Bowenoid SK). The edges of the epidermal abnormality are usually quite distinct and sloped. Sweat ducts are conspicuously uninvolved. There is always a subepidermal inflammatory cell infiltrate of lymphocytes which occasionally is a dense 'lichenoid band' (Figure 13.4). Occasionally other features of lichen planus (page 142) are imitated.

Chronic exposure to solar ultraviolet irradiation (UVR) is thought to be the most important causative agency although chronic heat damage (page 30), X-irradiation and chemical carcinogens (such as arsenic) may also be responsible in some subjects. The fact that SK occur alongside other forms of solar damage on light-exposed skin in fair-skinned subjects who have had much sun exposure, and that similar lesions can

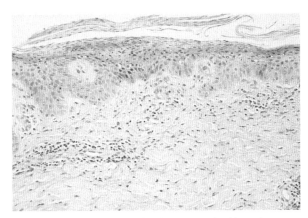

Figure 13.3 Pathology of solar keratosis. Note the heterogeneity of cell size, shape and depth of staining as well as the parakeratosis.

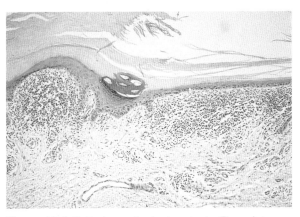

Figure 13.4 Pathology of solar keratosis. There is marked inflammation with many lymphocytes in the subepidermal region.

be produced experimentally by UVR in mice, is persuasive evidence that solar UVR is of major importance.

It is thought that SK represent one premalignant phase on the path to frank neoplasia in the form of squamous cell carcinoma, even though they hardly ever transform to malignant lesions.

The role of papilloma viruses in the causation of skin cancer has long been debated. Modern techniques (e.g. *in situ* hybridization) now indicate that some antigenic types of human papilloma (HP) virus (e.g. HPV16 and 18) are particularly likely to provoke neoplasia. In addition, the high prevalence of non metanoma skin cancer (NMSC) in renal transplant patients and in certain genodermatoses is believed to be at least in part due to papilloma viruses.

Immunological factors are of importance in the development of SK and other forms of NMSC. As mentioned above, patients who have had renal transplants and who are immunosuppressed by administration of steroids, azathioprine and/or cyclosporin have a greatly increased incidence of SK and NMSC, depending on the length of time that they have been immunosuppressed. Patients with acquired immune deficiency syndrome (AIDS) are also at increased risk of skin cancer (page 94).

EPIDEMIOLOGY AND NATURAL HISTORY

Recent surveys have highlighted just how common are these lesions. In the subtropical parts of Australia, SK have been found in more than 50% of the population over the age of 40 years. In the equable (if somewhat damp) climate of South Wales, approximately 20% of the population of more than 60 years have been found to have SK. They gradually become more common after the age of 50 years. As mentioned previously, they are much more common in fair-skinned subjects, particularly those with reddish hair and blue eyes, and such individuals who live in sunny climates are acknowledged as being greatly at risk. Men seem at greater risk than women, but it is not known whether this is due to an increased dose of UVR in men. Subjects with Celtic ancestry seem peculiarly sensitive to NMSC from solar exposure and although part of their susceptibility is due to their light complexions this is not believed to be the whole story, and it may well be that they also have some metabolic abnormality akin to xeroderma pigmentosum (see below, page 221). Notwithstanding the degree of pigmentation, no racial types are immune to SK or other forms of NMSC. For example, albino black-skinned Africans are very prone to develop such lesions, and dark-skinned subjects from Egypt and elsewhere in the Middle East develop profuse SK and all forms of skin cancer.

A very small proportion of SK progress to squamous cell carcinoma (SCC), perhaps as low as 0.2%, and the main significance of SK, apart from their intrinsic inconvenience, is that they indicate that the patient has received a significant amount of solar-induced UVR damage and that frankly neoplastic lesions are more likely to arise.

A small proportion of SK actually disappear spontaneously.

44444444444444

Exposure to heat, certain papilloma viruses, chemical carcinogens and immunosuppression from drugs or disease may also be factors in epidermal neoplasia.

TREATMENT

Clearly, solitary lesions or small numbers of SK may be surgically excised or curetted off, depending on their size and site. When greater numbers are present and the diagnosis has been confirmed, they may be removed by cryotherapy with liquid nitrogen.

Chemotherapy is sometimes appropriate when there are very large numbers of lesions present, as is often the case in individuals who are seriously 'photodamaged' (Figure 13.5) and three types are available for patients with multiple, large SK or SK and other forms of NMSC. The first is topical 5-fluorouracil as a 5% ointment (Efudix, Roche). This agent is applied daily or twice daily to the lesions over a 10 or 14 day schedule. The lesions often become sore and inflamed, and the patient should be alerted as to this possibility and given a topical corticosteroid to improve the symptoms. This treatment is effective in perhaps 50 or 60% and often saves considerable inconvenience and discomfort for elderly patients.

Systemic retinoids (either etretinate or isotretinoin) may be used for patients with multiple SK or other types of NMSC of several sites in whom other types of therapy are unsuitable for one or another reason and who can tolerate the uncomfortable side effects (page 316). They are given in the same doses as for disorders of keratinization for periods of between three and six months. They reduce the size and number of lesions and reduce the rate of appearance of new lesions.

Intralesional injections of alpha-2β or gamma interferon, two or three times weekly (1000 000 units of alpha-2β on each occasion) for three or four weeks causes resolution in 70–100% of lesions of SK or other types of NMSC. This treatment is only suitable for very large lesions for which surgical or other destructive types of therapy are unsuitable.

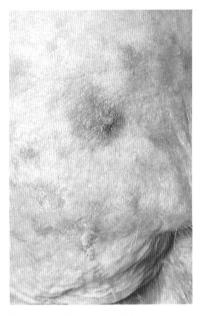

Figure 13.5 Multiple solar keratoses and marked photodamage on the forehead of a man of 68 years.

RECOGNITION OF SOLAR KERATOSES

- Commonest on exposed skin of elderly white males
- Scaling or warty plaques or papules
- Usually accompanied by other signs of photodamage
- Mostly multiple, persistent lesions, but a tiny proportion progress to SCC and others disappear

Bowen's disease (intraepidermal epithelioma)

DEFINITION

Bowen's disease is a localized area of epidermal neoplasia remaining within the confines of the epidermis for long periods.

Bowen's disease is a localized area of epidermal neoplasia remaining within the confines of the epidermis for long periods.

CLINICAL FEATURES

The most typical type of lesion of Bowen's disease is a raised red scaling plaque, and lesions are often very psoriasiform in appearance. They are mostly present on light-exposed areas of skin and are a not uncommon problem on the lower legs of women (Figure 13.6) which receive both incident UVR and UVR reflected from the pavement. Single lesions are most common but multiple lesions may occur. Lesions on the trunk were seen more commonly when arsenic was used as a treatment for psoriasis, epilepsy and sundry other 'chronic ailments'. Individual lesions gradually enlarge and thicken and may eventually transform to squamous cell carcinoma.

The main differential diagnoses are the same as for solar keratoses, and are set out in Table 13.1, but they tend to be larger and more psoriasiform.

> Lesions tend to be larger and more psoriasiform than solar keratoses.

HISTOLOGY AND AETIOPATHOGENESIS

The histological appearance could be described as an exaggerated version of an SK in which there is marked thickening and marked heterogeneity of the epidermal cells. The epidermal thickening and marked parakeratosis may give a superficial appearance of psoriasis (Figure 13.7). Bizarre large keratinocytes (cellules monstreuses) complete the distinctive appearance. Bowen's disease is caused by the same set of factors as SK (see above).

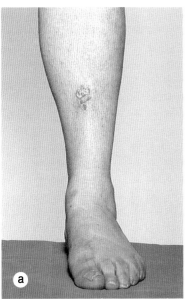

Figure 13.6 (a) Psoriasiform patch of Bowen's disease on the lower leg of an elderly woman. (b) Bowen's disease.

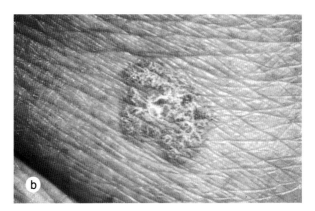

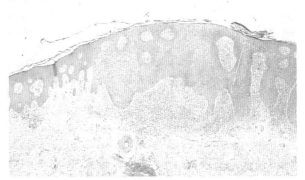

Figure 13.7 Pathology of Bowen's disease with area of irregularly thickened epidermis. Note accompanying inflammation.

Erythroplasia of Queyrat

This is the term used for Bowen's disease affecting the glans penis. It presents as a red velvety patch that slowly progresses, eventually transforming into a squamous cell carcinoma if left untreated. Surgical excision of the affected area is the best form of treatment.

EPIDEMIOLOGY

They occur in the same segments of the population as do SK, but are somewhat less common.

TREATMENT

Excision, curettage and cautery, liquid nitrogen cryotherapy and topical 5% fluorouracil ointment are used, as for SK. Intralesional interferon for very large lesions and systemic retinoids for multiple lesions may be needed for some patients (as for SK, see above).

Squamous cell carcinoma/squamous cell epithelioma

DEFINITION

Squamous cell carcinoma (SCC) is a malignant neoplasm of interfollicular epidermis.

CLINICAL FEATURES

The majority of lesions of SCC are warty nodules or plaques that gradually, or in some cases, rapidly, enlarge to form exophytic eroded nodules or ulcerated plaques (Figure 13.8 and 13.9). The lesion of SCC is in most cases solitary, although it often occurs against a background of solar damage with multiple SK.

> The majority of lesions of squamous cell carcinoma are warty nodules or plaques that gradually, or in some cases, rapidly, enlarge to form exophytic eroded nodules or ulcerated plaques.

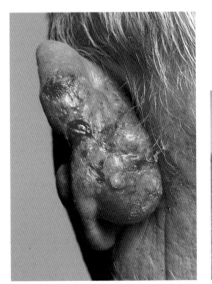

Figure 13.8 Irregular nodular plaque on ear due to squamous cell carcinoma.

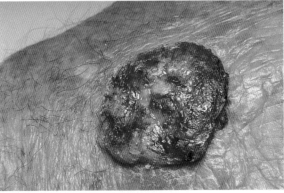

Figure 13.9 Eroded nodule of squamous cell carcinoma.

213

Metastases are late to occur but certainly do so if the primary lesions are left untreated, spreading to local lymph nodes, local skin sites and ultimately lungs, bone and brain.

Suspicion as to the development of SCC should be particularly high in areas of:
1.   severe photodamage;
2.   X-ray dermatitis;
3.   chronic heat injury such as erythema ab igne;
4.   chronic inflammatory skin disease such as chronic discoid lupus erythematosus and chronic hypertrophic lichen planus.

PATHOLOGY AND AETIOPATHOGENESIS
The histological features of SCC may be difficult to identify but always include marked epidermal thickening with clumps of epidermal tissue within the dermis. There is usually cellular and nuclear heterogeneity and atypia with evidence of abnormal mitotic activity. There is also evidence of focal and inappropriate keratinization so that so-called 'horn pearls' are formed (Figure 13.10). There is usually evidence of invasion of surrounding tissue by epithelial clumps and columns.

> There is usually cellular and nuclear heterogeneity and atypia with evidence of abnormal mitotic activity. There is also evidence of focal and inappropriate keratinization so that so-called 'horn pearls' are formed.

There is a variable amount of inflammation beneath and within the abnormal epidermal tissue. Care has to be taken in distinguishing SCC from the massive but benign epidermal thickening known as pseudoepitheliomatous hyperplasia occasionally seen in hypertrophic lichen planus, prurigo nodularis and lichen simplex chronicus.

The factors in the aetiology of SCC are as discussed for SK with some additions. These are as follows:

• Chronic UVR radiation damage from solar exposure
• *X-irradiation damage* to the skin
• *Persistent heat injury* to the skin (as in erythema ab igne)
• Chronic *inflammatory and scarring disorders* of the skin such as discoid lupus erythematosus, hypertrophic lichen planus and dystrophic epidermolysis bullosa
• *Certain genodermatoses* and localized congenital malformations such

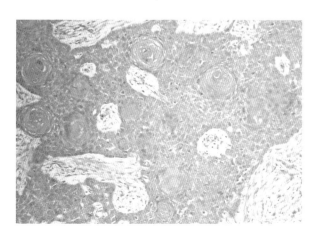

Figure 13.10 Pathology of squamous cell carcinoma showing mass of abnormal epithelium with scattered areas of differentiation (horn pearls).

as xeroderma pigmentosum (page 221), epidermodysplasia verruciformis (page 221) and epidermal naevus (page 183)
- *Papilloma virus infection* – certain antigenic types (e.g. HPV5,
  HPV16 and HPV18) seem particularly likely to cause malignant
  transformation in particular clinical settings such as in immunosuppressed renal transplantation patients, epidermodysplasia verruciformis and in giant warty tumour of the genitalia
- Exposure to *chemical carcinogens* such as industrial contact with tars
  and pitch or systemic administration of arsenic

Of the above factors, solar UVR exposure is by far the most important
numerically although it is true that some of the other factors may play
subsidiary roles.

EPIDEMIOLOGY AND NATURAL HISTORY

Squamous cell carcinoma predominantly occurs in the same population
groups as already described for SK. It also occurs in others due to the
other causative factors noted above. Regrettably it is difficult to obtain
accurate figures for the incidence of the disease as reporting is not as
complete as it should be. In one survey in subtropical Australia,
approximately 2% of the population over the age of 40 years had one
SCC when examined. Whatever the exact figures at present, studies
indicate that SCC as well as other forms of NMSC are increasing in
incidence.

The large majority of lesions of SCC are removed before they
metastasize but some patients are not so lucky and die from the spread
of their SCC lesion (Figure 13.11). Unfortunately accurate figures are
not available.

TREATMENT

Excision with an adequate margin to ensure inclusion of all neoplastic
tissue and some healthy tissue all around the lesion is sufficient for cure
in more than 95% of patients. Grafting may be required in some cases.
For the very elderly with solitary, large, difficult to remove lesions,

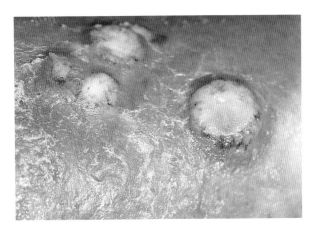

Figure 13.11 Metastatic nodules of
squamous cell carcinoma.

treatment by radiotherapy may be the kindest and most efficient method. Cryotherapy may also be used in these circumstances although it is often uncertain how deep the freezing reaches. Systemic retinoids may be appropriate when there are multiple SK and other signs of photodamage as well as the index lesion and intralesional interferon may be suitable for large lesions.

When the SCC has metastasized, chemotherapy and radiotherapy may be required.

Keratoacanthoma (molluscum sebaceum)

> Keratoacanthoma is a suddenly-appearing epidermal tumour with some of the characteristics of an SCC but which resolves after a short period.

DEFINITION

This term describes a suddenly appearing epidermal tumour with some of the characteristics of an SCC but which resolves after a short period.

CLINICAL FEATURES

Keratoacanthoma (KA) usually appears within a week or two on light-exposed skin as a solitary crateriform nodule (Figure 13.12). It then gradually enlarges for a few weeks and then stays at that size for a variable period before finally remitting after a total of three to four months. Lesions that are more persistent should be suspected of being an SCC. The most important differential diagnosis is SCC. If left to resolve spontaneously, scarring often remains.

A rare clinical variant of KA is known as self-healing epithelioma of Ferguson Smith. It occurs as an inherited (autosomal dominant) trait in which odd irregular sinus containing epitheliomatous nodules appear on the trunk and limbs which eventually resolve.

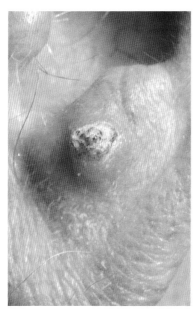

Figure 13.12 Solitary crateriform nodule of keratoacanthoma.

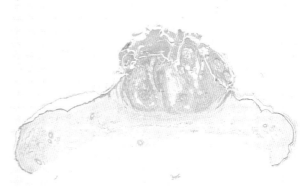

Figure 13.13 Pathology of keratocanthoma. Note the cup-shaped epidermal invagination.

PATHOLOGY AND AETIOPATHOGENESIS

Keratoacanthoma has a characteristic symmetrical cup or flask-shaped structure (Figure 13.13). There is a minor degree of epidermal dysplasia and little evidence of tissue invasion by the epithelium. Keratoacanthoma seem to be provoked by the same stimuli that cause solar keratoses but they are much less common and much less predictable. Some very photodamaged individuals will never develop a KA but other less injured individuals may develop several such lesions. It has been suggested that they develop from hair follicle epithelium.

TREATMENT

Excision is recommended. If the lesion is quite small curettage and cautery may be more suitable.

Basal cell carcinoma (basalioma; basal cell epithelioma)

DEFINITION

Basal cell carcinoma (BCC) is a locally invasive but rarely metastasizing malignant epithelial tumour of basaloid cells without the tendency to differentiate into horny structures.

> Basal cell carcinoma is a locally invasive but rarely metastasizing malignant epithelial tumour of basaloid cells without the tendency to differentiate into horny structures.

CLINICAL FEATURES

There are several clinical types (see Table 13.2):

1. **Nodulocystic.** This is by far the commonest variety. Translucent or skin-coloured dome-shaped nodules (2–15 mm in diameter) slowly appear on the skin and remain static for long periods, often for several years, before ulcerating (Figure 13.14). They often have a telangiectatic overlying skin and may be flecked with pigment. They mostly occur as solitary lesions but it is not uncommon to find that there are one or two other similar lesions present as well. They are most common on the exposed areas of the skin of the head and neck (they are uncommon on the limbs)

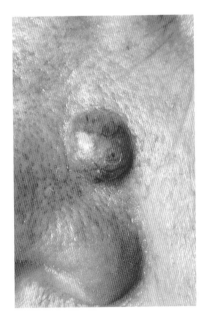

Figure 13.14 Typical nodulo-cystic basal sarcoma.

Table 13.2 Clinical types of basal cell carcinoma

Clinical type	Comment
Nodulocystic	Solid or cystic nodule; commonest.
Ulcerative	Usually a later stage of nodulocystic lesion; has a rolled margin; this type is known as rodent ulcer
Pigmented	Darkly pigmented nodule; may be confused with melanoma
Morphoeic	Flat, white scar-like – often difficult to diagnose
Superficial	Flat scaling pink patch – often with a fine 'hair-like' margin

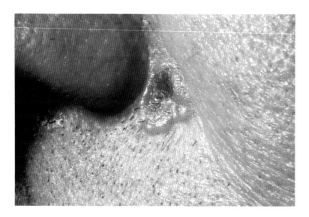

Figure 13.15 Ulcerated plaque of nodulocystic basal cell carcinoma (rodent ulcer).

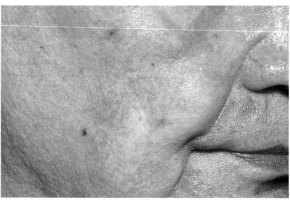

Figure 13.16 Several small black nodules of pigmented basal cell carcinoma on the face of a patient with basal cell naevus syndrome.

but an appreciable proportion (perhaps 20%) occur on the trunk. Differential diagnosis of nodulocystic BCC includes dermal cellular naevus (page 191), sebaceous gland hypertrophy (page 187) and benign hair follicle tumours (page 187).

2. *Ulcerative*. The nodulocystic type eventually breaks down to form an ulcer with raised everted edges (Figure 13.15). This type is known colloquially as 'rodent ulcer'.

3. *Pigmented*. Nodulocystic lesions may become quite darkly pigmented and are then quite often mistaken for melanomatous lesions (Figure 13.16).

4. *Morphoeic*. These are often whitish, scar-like, depressed firm plaques, and are so named because of their supposed resemblance to localized scleroderma (Figure 13.17).

5. *Superficial*. This type of BCC is clinically quite unlike the other varieties. It takes the form of a variably sized, thin, pink scaling plaque with a well-defined edge (Figure 13.18). If the edge is examined with a hand lens a fine 'hair-like' raised margin can be discerned. This form may be mistaken for Bowen's disease or even a patch of psoriasis. They occur on the trunk and limbs more often than the other types.

> The commonest type of BCC is the nodulocystic but ulcerative and pigmented types are not unusual. 'Superficial' red scaling types and sclerotic 'morphoeic' are less frequent.

All types of BCC gradually expand and invade and destroy local tissue structures. They cause most problems because of this tendency to compromise and eventually destroy local structures such as the ear, nose and eye. They metastasize rarely. It is difficult to know how frequently this occurs. But when it is realized that BCC is one of the commonest of human tumours and that metastasis has been recorded in

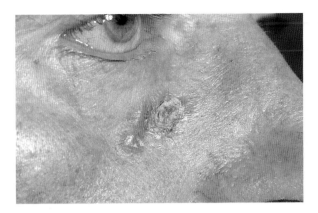

Figure 13.17 Eroded sclerotic plaque of morphoeic basal cell carcinoma.

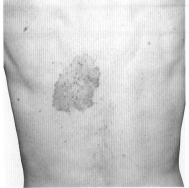

Figure 13.18 Large superficial basal cell carcinoma affecting the back. Note the psoriasiform appearance with the well-defined edge.

Clumps of small basophilic epidermal cells occupy the upper dermis, the outermost cells often being more columnar than the rest and arranged in a neat palisade around the nodule.

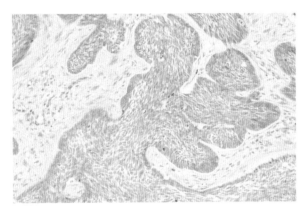

Figure 13.19 Pathology of basal cell carcinoma showing well-defined clumps of basaloid cells.

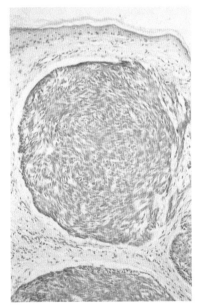

Figure 13.20 Pathology of basal cell carcinoma. Note the prominent palisading at the edge of clumps of cells and space between the cells and the surrounding dermal connective tissue.

the literature only 500 times approximately, the proportion of lesions that do metastasize must be extremely small.

PATHOLOGY AND AETIOPATHOGENESIS

Histologically BCC does not usually produce a challenge to the pathologist's diagnostic skill. Clumps of small basophilic epidermal cells occupy the upper dermis, the outermost cells often being more columnar than the rest and arranged in a neat palisade around the nodule (Figure 13.19). Many mitotic figures may be seen amongst the mass of basal cells as may many degenerate cells – it is thought that the slow rate of growth is explained by cell death keeping pace with cell proliferation in the tumour (Figure 13.20). In routine histological sections it is common to find a gap between the clumps of tumour cells and the surrounding dermis due to the dissolving out of soluble glycoprotein-like material. There may also be empty areas within the clumps that in life contained similar material. The dermis usually contains some inflammatory cells and a variable degree of fibrosis, this latter being greater in the morphoeic type.

There is usually no evidence of differentiation but occasionally there are foci of what appear to be more mature cells and even horn formation (squamous metaplasia).

It is quite clear that most lesions of BCC are due to chronic solar exposure and UVR damage as they occur on light-exposed sites in photodamaged subjects. However, a larger proportion of BCC occurs in younger, nonlight-exposed, nonphotodamaged subjects than SK or other forms of NMSC. The explanation for this is uncertain but it may be that some lesions arise from congenital malformations and are unrelated to UVR exposure.

It is suspected that BCC lesions arise from hair matrix type epithelium, whatever the exciting cause, but little is known concerning the evoking stimulus to the development of BCC.

> Most BCC are caused by chronic UVR exposure but some may arise from congenital malformations.

EPIDEMIOLOGY
The occurrence of BCC mirrors that of SK (page 209), but as mentioned above differs in that in an appreciable proportion, lesions occur in younger individuals in nonlight-exposed sites. As with SCC and other forms of photodamage, BCC appears to be increasing in incidence.

TREATMENT
The majority of lesions can easily be excised. Smaller lesions can be curetted off and the base cauterized. Both these surgical ablative techniques result in a 95% cure. Larger lesions may be treated by radiotherapy or cryotherapy after confirming the diagnosis by biopsy. Basal cell carcinoma lesions also respond to systemic retinoids (page 316) and to intralesional interferons (page 211).

Basal cell naevus syndrome (Gorlin's syndrome)

DEFINITION
This is a rare autosomally inherited condition in which multiple pigmented BCC lesions develop as part of a multisystem disorder.

CLINICAL FEATURES
Multiple BCC may start to develop in the second decade of life and erupt in large numbers in succeeding years. Less severely affected individuals start to develop BCC later in life and develop fewer lesions. The BCC lesions are mostly pigmented and may occur anywhere on the skin surface. Small pits may be found on the palms but otherwise there are no skin abnormalities.

A series of skeletal anomalies are also present in the majority of patients, including mandibular cysts and bifid ribs. In addition patients have a high incidence of ovarian, central nervous system and spinal tumours.

PATHOLOGY AND AETIOPATHOGENESIS
The BCC lesions are no different histologically from other types of BCC. In recent years considerable progress has been made in identifying the gene responsible for this disorder.

TREATMENT
When there is no doubt as to the diagnosis, genetic counselling is advisable. Individual lesions should be removed as necessary. When there are large numbers present and new lesions are continuing to appear, administration of systemic retinoids will reduce the numbers of lesions and the rate of appearance of new BCC (page 316).

Xeroderma pigmentosum

DEFINITION
Xeroderma pigmentosum (XP) is the name given to a group of rare inherited disorders in which there is faulty repair of damaged DNA and the development of numerous skin cancers.

> Xeroderma pigmentosum (XP) is the name given to a group of rare inherited disorders in which there is faulty repair of damaged DNA and the development of numerous skin cancers.

CLINICAL FEATURES
The phenotypic expression depends on the particular genetic abnormality responsible, but in all types, preneoplastic and neoplastic lesions including SK, SCC, BCC and melanoma develop from childhood, and in the worst cases cause death in later adolescence or early adult life. The development of skin cancers is accompanied by severe photodamage resulting in a characteristic and pitiful appearance (Figure 13.21). In one severe recessive variety known as the de Sanctis-Cacchione syndrome there are also crippling neurological defects, including cerebellar ataxia and intellectual impairment.

PATHOLOGY AND PATHOGENESIS
When skin is exposed to UVR, damage occurs to the nuclear DNA of epidermal cells, causing linkage between adjoining DNA helices and the formation of abnormal 'pyrimidine dimers'. In normal individuals these are 'excised' and the continuity of the helices is restored by a repair sequence dependent on a series of enzymes. Simple biochemical tests are available to determine whether there is a problem in DNA repair after UVR damage dependent on the incorporation of the DNA precursor, thymidine. More complicated 'complementation' tests are also available to determine which particular genetic type is responsible but as these tests are extremely specialized, and the conditions are very rare, only a very few centres are currently able to perform such tests.

EPIDEMIOLOGY AND NATURAL HISTORY
It has been estimated that overall the incidence of XP is 1 in 250,000. It

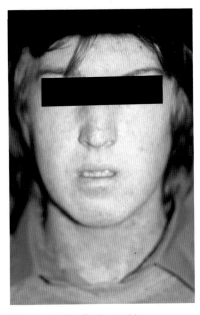

Figure 13.21 Patient with xeroderma pigmentosum. Reproduced with thanks to Dr Dafydd Roberts.

appears that in some areas, such as parts of the Middle East, the condition is unusually frequent.

TREATMENT
Management is directed to genetic counselling, removal of neoplastic lesions as they occur and prevention of further photodamage by advice and sunscreens. Recently the use of systemic retinoids have been shown to reduce the rate of development of new cancers and is now an important aspect of the management of these patients.

Melanoma skin cancer

Under this heading the various neoplastic disorders affecting melanocytes (pigment-producing cells) will be described.

Lentigo maligna (Hutchinson's freckle)

DEFINITION
Lentigo maligna (LM) is a slowly progressive preneoplastic disorder of melanocytes in which malignant melanoma often develops.

> Lentigo maligna is a slowly progressive preneoplastic disorder of melanocytes in which malignant melanoma often develops as a pigmented macule on exposed skin.

CLINICAL FEATURES
Lentigo maligna develops insidiously on exposed areas of skin particularly the skin of the face. The lesion itself is a pigmented macule with a well-defined, rounded or polycylic edge which may be up to 5 cm in diameter or even larger (Figure 13.22). Older lesions may become slightly raised and warty. a characteristic feature is the varying shades of brown and black contained within the lesion – a feature known as variegation. Differential diagnosis includes seborrhoeic wart, simple senile lentigo and pigmented solar keratosis (see Table 13.3).

The disorder is usually slowly progressive over a period which may be in excess of 20 years. If left untreated a true malignant melanoma (MM) develops within the LM which then has the characteristics of a typical MM (see below).

PATHOLOGY
The most striking features are the presence of large numbers of abnormal, often spindle-shaped, melanocytic clear cells at the base of the epidermis and clumps of melanin pigment in the upper part of the dermis. As the disease progresses, clumps of abnormal melanocytes appear projecting into the dermis and a dense infiltrate of mononuclear cells develops superepidermally (Figure 13.23).

TREATMENT
This is dictated by the size and exact site of the lesions. Often they are of size and site precluding surgical removal. In these instances, other locally destructive measures have been used, including curettage and cautery and cryotherapy. Radiotherapy has also been used with good

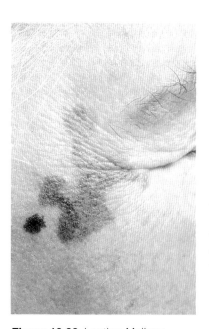

Figure 13.22 Lentigo Maligna. Note variegated pigmentation and irregular margin.

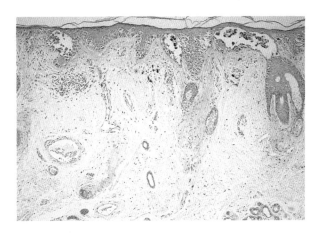

Figure 13.23 Pathology of lentigo maligna. There are many abnormal melanocytic cells along the base of the epidermis and large clumps of cells in places.

effect in some patients. Careful follow-up is required to detect the earliest signs of development of a frank melanoma.

Malignant melanoma

DEFINITION
Malignant melanoma (MM) is an invasive neoplastic disorder of melanocytes in which the tendency is either for invasion horizontally and upwards into the epidermis (superficial spreading MM or SSMM) or vertically downwards (nodular MM or NMM).

> Malignant melanoma (MM) is an invasive neoplastic disorder of melanocytes.

Table 13.3 Differential diagnosis of melanoma

Type of lesion	Main differentials	Comment
LM	Seborrhoeic wart, senile lentigo, pigmented solar keratosis	Seborrhoeic wart tends to be warty; Senile lentigo is not variegated; SK tends to be scaly and pink/brown
SSMM	Seborrhoeic wart, pigmented BCC, vascular malformation, melanocytic naevus	Seborrhoeic wart tends to be warty; BCC has a pearly look; Malformation may blanch if not thrombosed; Melanocytic naevus is less variegated
Acral lentiginous melanoma	Melanocytic naevus, vascular malformation	Melanocytic naevus is less variegated; Malformation may blanch if not thrombosed
NMM	Seborrhoeic wart, pigmented BCC, vascular malformation, melanocytic naevus, pyogenic granuloma	Seborrhoeic wart tends to be warty; BCC has a pearly look; Malformation may blanch if not thrombosed; Melanocytic naevus is less variegated; Pyogenic granuloma tends to be redder and smaller than MM

LM = lentigo maligna. SSMM — superficial spreading malignant melanoma. NMM = malignant melanoma growing vertically downwards. BCC = basal cell carcinoma. SK = solar keratoses. MM = malignant melanoma.

Table 13.4   Clinical features of malignant melanoma

Recent:	Growth in size, or appearance of new pigmented lesion
	Change in colour (mostly increased pigmentation)
	Change in shape (development of irregular margin)
Development of itchiness in lesion	
Irregularity of margin/pigmentation	
Erosion and/or crusting	
Appearance of satellite nodules	
Enlargement of regional lymph nodes	

Some 50% of lesions of MM develop from a pre-existing melanocytic naevus.

Any pigmented lesion that suddenly develops or any change in the size, shape or colour of a pre-existing lesion should be suspected of being an MM.

Irregularity in the margin, and in the degree of pigmentation, and erosion or crusting of the skin surface are important features.

CLINICAL FEATURES

Some 50% of lesions of MM develop from a pre-existing melanocytic naevus and the other 50% develop *de novo* on any part of the skin surface. Any pigmented lesion that suddenly develops or any change in the size, shape or colour of a pre-existing lesion should be suspected of being an MM. Particular signs that are valuable in recognition of MM are irregularity in the margin, irregularity in the degree of pigmentation, and erosion or crusting of the skin surface (Figure 13.24) (Table 13.4). Itchiness of the lesion is a not uncommon symptom in MM.

One way in which MM may present is as a rapidly growing non-pigmented nodule with an eroded surface looking somewhat like a pyogenic granuloma (Figure 13.25).

Another unusual variety of MM is the so-called acral lentiginous melanoma which develops around the fingers or toes and sometimes subungually. This form seems to have a particularly poor prognosis.

Late local signs are the development of satellite pigmented nodules and enlargement of the regional lymph nodes. Redness and other signs

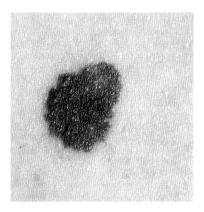

Figure 13.24 Nodular malignant melanoma. This lesion enlarged and darkened over a period of three months.

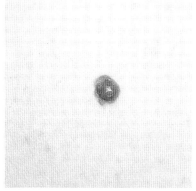

Figure 13.25 Red shiny nodule due to malignant melanoma that was initially diagnosed as a pyogenic granuloma.

of inflammation may be present in MM but benign compound moles may also become inflamed and inflammatory change **by itself** is not common in MM.

Although MM is a potentially fatal disorder the early stages are easily curable and it is vitally important that every physician learns the signs of MM. Pigmented lesions can be very difficult to diagnose and there is no shame in requesting another opinion. The differential diagnosis includes melanocytic naevus (page 188), pigmented basal cell carcinoma (page 217), histiocytoma (page 198) and vascular malformation (page 194).

The rate of progress of the disease seems largely determined by the inherent biology of the MM. When the lesion tends to spread horizontally (SSMM) it tends to be noted and treated earlier than when the predominant direction of growth is vertically downwards (NMM). It is therefore not surprising that the overall prognosis is much better for SSMM than for NMM. The single most important determinant of prognosis appears to be depth of invasion into the dermis (see below). Thus patients with small lesions of less than 1 mm invasion into the dermis have an expectancy of a five-year survival rate in excess of 95%. Because of the significance of prognosis of depth of invasion into the dermis, various classifications based on microscope measurements have been developed. The two most common are the Breslow's thickness technique and the Clark staging method. In the Breslow technique, three categories are recognized – less than 1.5 mm, 1.5–3.5 mm and more than 3.5 mm. Clark's staging method recognizes five stages dependent on where the tumour reaches: one being confined to the epidermis, and five where there is infiltration of the subcutaneous fat. Stages 2, 3 and 4 describe progressively deeper levels within the dermis.

> Lesions that spread horizontally (superficial spreading MM) have a better prognosis than lesions that spread vertically (nodular MM).

Spread of MM is local, regional and distant. Distant metastases occur by haematogenous spread. Haematogenous metastases may occur anywhere but quite commonly they develop in the lungs, liver and brain. Regional spread is via lymphatics to regional lymph nodes. When regional lymph node metastases have been found the five-year survival rate is less than 25%, and when distant metastases have occurred the comparable figure is around 5%.

Secondary satellite lesions develop around the primary MM in many instances. When metastases are widespread the production of melanin pigment and its subsequent release into the circulation may be sufficiently great to result in a generalized darkening of the skin and even excretion of melanin in the urine (melaninuria), although this is quite rare. Occasionally regression of part of the lesion occurs and rarely the entire lesion, and metastases, may undergo spontaneous resolution.

Overall, men have a worse prognosis than women. Back lesions in men and leg lesions in women have the least favourable prognoses.

225

> The cardinal histological feature is the presence of clumps of abnormal melanocytes at the dermoepidermal junction.

> Solar UVR is believed to be the single most important causative factor but as up to 50% of lesions of MM occur on non sun-exposed sites, other factors may play a role. The propensity for patients with the dysplastic mole syndrome and large congenital melanocytic naevi to develop MM suggest that developmental factors may also be involved in some instances.

PATHOLOGY AND AETIOPATHOGENESIS

The cardinal histological feature is the presence of clumps of abnormal melanocytes at the dermoepidermal junction. In SSMM abnormal melanocytes tend to invade upward into the epidermis and horizontally along the epidermis. In NMM there are groups of abnormal cells invading vertically downwards (Figure 13.26). There is usually some accompanying inflammatory cell infiltrate. It has to be said that the histological diagnosis of melanoma may be difficult and should be left to the expert.

Solar UVR is believed to be the single most important causative factor but as up to 50% of lesions of MM occur on nonsun-exposed sites, other factors may play a role. The propensity for patients with the dysplastic mole syndrome (page 193) and large congenital melanocytic naevi to develop MM suggest that developmental factors may also be involved in some instances. There is some evidence that episodes of intense sun exposure over short periods, with sunburn, may be very harmful. This could explain why MM is comparatively frequent on areas of skin that are only occasionally exposed to the sun.

EPIDEMIOLOGY

Malignant melanoma is extremely rare before puberty but can occur at any age after that. It is seen in all racial types but is more common in fair-skinned Caucasian types. Acral lentiginous melanoma seems most frequent in black-skinned individuals and subjects of Japanese or other Asian descent. The incidence has increased in all countries which keep accurate figures and increases have been noted since records first began. The rate of increase seems to be of the order of 7% per annum. The incidence is greatest in Queensland, Australia and tends to be high in the hot sunny areas which have a large fair-skinned population of European descent.

TREATMENT

The treatment of choice is excision with a generous margin of normal skin. There is debate concerning the width of the margin but it should be at least 2 cm around the lesion for MM of 1 cm diameter. There is also debate as to whether regional lymph nodes should be removed

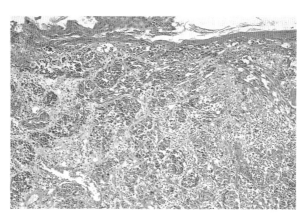

Figure 13.26 Pathology of malignant melanoma. Note irregular clumps of abnormal naevus cells throughout the upper dermis.

prophylactically or not. The balance of opinion suggests not, provided that there is no clinical evidence of spread.

Metastatic disease responds poorly if at all to chemotherapy, but some decrease in size of metastatic deposits and occasional temporary remission has been noted with combinations of antimetabolites and other anticancer drugs as well as retinoids, interferons and interleukin-2.

Neoplastic disorders of mesenchymal elements

Kaposi's sarcoma (idiopathic haemorrhagic sarcoma)

DEFINITION
Kaposi's sarcoma is a rare multifocal malignant vascular tumour of skin and other organs which occurs either as an endemic, slowly progressive disease or as a rapidly progressive disorder in the immunosuppressed.

CLINICAL FEATURES
The endemic type occurs predominantly in elderly males of either Jewish origin from central Europe or of Italian origin from around the Po valley. Mauve or purplish-red nodules and plaques and brownish macules (Figure 13.27) develop over the dorsa of the feet and the lower legs. These lesions are usually accompanied by swelling of the lower legs. They are slowly progressive and may not appear in other sites for very many years. It has been estimated that the mean survival time after the appearance of the first lesions is approximately 12 years. Eventually lesions disseminate to other parts of the skin and to the viscera.

The rapidly progressive type occurs in patients with AIDS, particularly male homosexuals, renal transplant patients and in areas of Africa – notably Uganda.

The clinical manifestations are similar to those of endemic Kaposi's sarcoma but are very much more extensive and much more rapidly progressive. A very rare, similar disorder occurs in lymphoedematous limbs postradical mastectomy, known as Stewart Treves disease.

PATHOLOGY AND PATHOGENESIS
The lesions consist of abnormal slit-like vascular channels lined with spindle-shaped cells, a mixed inflammatory cell infiltrate, haemorrhage and fibrosis. The true nature of this disorder is uncertain but it has been suggested that it is virally induced.

TREATMENT
As the disorder appears multifocal, cure does not appear possible at the moment. However, radiotherapy keeps localized areas in check and systemic interferon produces partial regression and remission in many patients.

> Kaposi's sarcoma is a rare multifocal malignant vascular tumour of skin and other organs which occurs either as an endemic, slowly progressive disease or as a rapidly progressive disorder in the immunosuppressed – particularly those with AIDS.

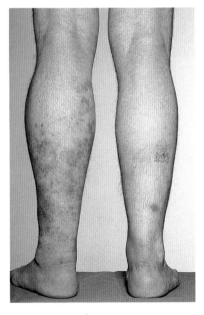

Figure 13.27 Classical Kaposi's sarcoma with brown macules and mauve plaques on the lower legs.

227

Dermatofibrosarcoma protuberans (DFSP)

DEFINITION
This disorder is a rare, slowly progressive, locally invasive neoplasm of dermal fibroblasts.

CLINICAL FEATURES
The most frequent site is the trunk. A firm irregular intracutaneous plaque is the characteristic picture. The lesion gradually expands both laterally and into the fat and rarely metastasizes, and only then late in the disease.

TREATMENT
The treatment of choice is excision.

Other sarcomas

Other sarcomas of the skin and subcutis that rarely develop include liposarcoma (from fat cells), neurofibrosarcoma (from nerve sheath cells – often in Von Recklinghausen's disease) and leiomyosarcoma (from plain muscle cells).

Lymphomas of skin (cutaneous T-cell lymphoma)

Mycosis fungoides

DEFINITION

Mycosis fungoides (MF) is a multifocal neoplastic disorder of T lymphocytes that primarily affects the skin.

Mycosis fungoides (MF) is a multifocal neoplastic disorder of T-lymphocytes that primarily affects the skin.

CLINICAL FEATURES
This uncommon disorder starts off as a series of red macules and scaly patches over the trunk and upper limbs. These gradually extend and become more prolific but cause little in the way of inconvenience apart from their appearance and mild pruritus (Figure 13.28). The red patches persist although they may fluctuate in intensity and eventually start to thicken to become plaques and later still, eroded tumours (Figure 13.29). The ringworm-like appearance of some of the early patches and the fungating plaques in the late stages presumably were responsible for the term mycosis fungoides. In the later stages of the disorder, lymph node enlargement, hepatosplenomegaly and infiltration of other viscera occur. At the time of writing the disorder is inevitably fatal although the rate of progress is quite variable, with survival ranging from two or three years in some patients to 20 years in others.

The above sequence is the 'classical' type of MF, and other less common variants are occasionally seen.

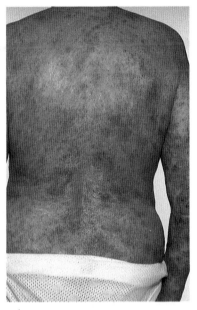

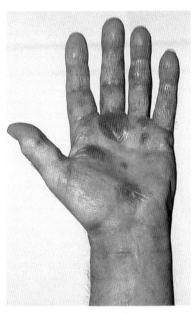

Figure 13.28 Multiple infiltrated red plaques on the trunk of a patient with mycosis fungoides.

Figure 13.29 Eroded nodules on the palm of a patient with terminal mycosis fungoides.

Sézary syndrome

This is marked by an erythroderma which has a particular intense erythematous colour, a picture sometimes referred to as *l'homme rouge*. It is accompanied by thickening of the tissues of the face, neck and palms. It is also characterized by the appearance of abnormal mononuclear cells circulating in the peripheral blood. These cells, which are identified in the 'buffy coat', are large and have a large dense reniform nucleus.

Worringer-Kollop disease

This is a very rare localized form of the disease – at least it stays localized to one plaque for long periods before disseminating as does classical MF.

Other forms of T-cell lymphoma

In addition to the above declared forms of cutaneous T-cell lymphoma, there are a number of uncommon precursor disorders which were known collectively (and inappropriately) as **parapsoriasis**. These by no means always progress to T-cell lymphoma, and their true nature is uncertain. In addition they are not well characterized clinically and are known individually by different names by different groups of dermatologists. For this reason little space will be devoted to them and for detailed descriptions the larger textbooks should be consulted.

14

Skin problems in infancy and old age

Every age of life has particular medical problems but those of infancy and old age are sufficiently distinctive in presentation and management that they warrant separate commentary.

Infancy

Functional differences

In the neonatal period and early infancy the skin's defences are not yet fully developed, and it is much more vulnerable to chemical, physical and microbial attack. Apart from the depressed skin defences, the surface area to weight ratio is higher than at other times and there is a greater hazard from increased absorption of topically applied medicaments. For example, serious systemic toxicity can result from application of corticosteroids or a salicylic acid preparation. There is also a greater rate of 'normal' water loss through intact, nonsweating skin (transepidermal water loss) in the newborn compared to the adult, indicating immaturity of the skin's barrier function. This is easily confirmed by the use of a special water sensor device known as the evaporimeter.

The vascular network in the skin seems more labile than in the adult. A rash may change from a vivid scarlet to a pale pink within a few hours. During the early weeks of life the newborn child possesses the blood levels of hormones found in the mother at the time of birth. This may be of special significance for the sebaceous glands, which react to circulating androgenic compounds by enlargement and increased sebum secretion.

Management problems in infancy

As already pointed out, there are important differences in the structure and function of infant skin, and these need to be remembered when designing treatment. Medicaments appear to be absorbed more easily and are more likely to cause systemic toxicity. Topical agents which are well tolerated by adults may cause quite severe reactions in infancy because of the lack of maturity of the barrier.

The ability to scratch doesn't seem to develop till around the age of six months, and when scratching is possible, the appearance of the rash may alter substantially because of the presence of excoriations and the physical effects of persistent scratching on the skin (lichenification, page 102) as well as the presence of infective lesions (Figure 14.1a and b). The inability of the infant to complain of discomfort, pain and irritation in specific terms leads to general irritability and persistent crying. When this continues for long periods, parents can't sleep and the intrafamilial emotional tension spirals upwards within the family home, necessitating attention to all those involved.

Widespread rashes may lead rapidly to dehydration in infancy because of the greatly increased rate of water loss through the abnormal skin, and a watchful eye must be kept open for this unnecessary and potentially dangerous complication. The same is true of heat loss from the inflamed skin. Hypothermia can develop very rapidly in young infants who have a widespread inflammatory skin disorder and, like dehydration, is a dangerous complication. These two complications, dehydration and hypothermia, may be prevented by:

1. anticipating their development, and monitoring water loss from the skin with an instrument known as an evaporimeter and body temperature by taking the rectal temperature;
2. nursing infants with severe widespread skin disease in an incubator or supplying the necessary extra heat and fluid.

> Infant skin provides a less efficient barrier than in more mature years. Drugs penetrate more easily and water loss occurs more readily.

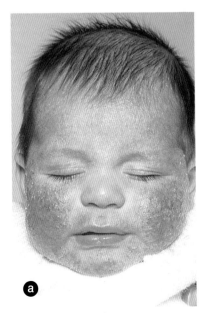

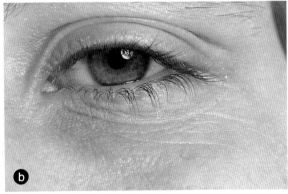

Figure 14.1 (a) Atopic dermatitis of face at age four months. There is marked inflammation but excoriations. (b) Lichenification around the eyes in an older child due to rubbing.

Napkin rash

Several different skin disorders localize to the napkin area which is perhaps not surprising when the physical assault that the wearing of napkins provides is considered.

Erosive napkin dermatitis

This is the commonest type of napkin dermatitis. Red, glazed, fissured and even eroded areas develop on the skin at sites in contact with the napkin (Figure 14.2). The flexures are mostly spared with the worst areas appearing on the convexities. There is often a strong ammoniacal smell when the napkin is removed. This is due to the release of ammonia from the action of the urease released from the faecal bacteria on the urea in the urine.

The condition responds as if by magic when the child is nursed without napkins for two or three days, but this is rarely possible, and other measures have to be adopted. This should include encouraging more frequent napkin changes and the use of soft muslin napkins rather than abrasive towelling napkins, or the use of disposables that leave the skin surface dry. As far as topical applications are concerned, all that is required is an emollient washing agent and an emollient used two or three times per day (page 310). Topical 1% hydrocortisone ointment twice daily could be used if the condition proves resistant.

Seborrhoeic dermatitis

Scaling red areas develop mainly in the folds of the skin although the eruption 'overflows' on to other areas in the napkin area. When the condition is severe and 'angry', skin outside the napkin area may be

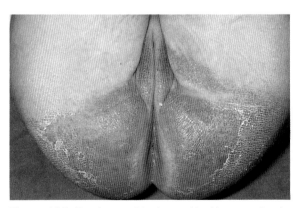

Figure 14.2 Erosive napkin dermatitis. Note sparing in the flexures.

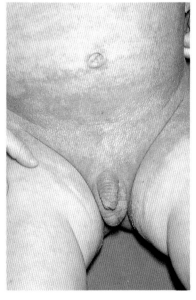

Figure 14.3 Napkin dermatitis of seborrhoeic dermatitis type.

affected – particularly the scalp, face, neck and sometimes elsewhere (Figure 14.3). The involved sites may also crack, and become exudative. The same kind of care of the napkin area as outlined above for erosive napkin dermatitis should be advised. In addition, the use of hydrocortisone (or other weak topical corticosteroids) in combination with broad-spectrum antimicrobial compounds such as the imidazoles (e.g. miconazole or clotrimazole) should be used twice daily. The involvement of the yeast *Candida albicans* in this form of napkin dermatitis has been claimed but not confirmed.

Napkin psoriasis

This is an uncommon, odd psoriasis-like eruption that develops in the napkin area and may spread to the skin outside (Figure 14.4). It is not clear whether infants who develop this are more likely to have psoriasis in later life. It probably starts off with irritation of the skin in the area and treatment should once again be directed to better hygiene and care of the skin under the napkin. Weak topical corticosteroids and emollients used as indicated above usually improve the condition quite quickly.

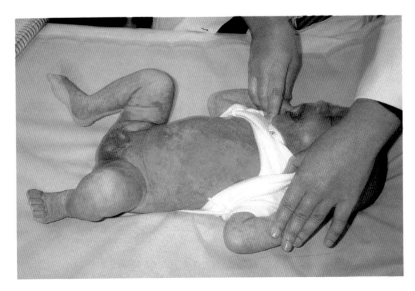

Figure 14.4 Napkin psoriasis. Psoriasiform lesions spread from napkin area to involve other areas of skin as well.

Napkin rashes may be erosive due to primary irritation at the points of contact on the convexities or flexural as in infantile seborrhoeic dermatitis.

Atopic dermatitis

This is mainly covered in Chapter 8, but several points need to be made here. The condition rarely starts before four to six weeks of age and mostly begins between two and three months. The disorder may first show itself on the face but it spreads quite quickly to other parts of the body, although the napkin area is conspicuously spared. This is presumably the result of the area being kept moist. The ability to scratch develops after about six months of age and the appearance of the disorder alters accordingly, with excoriations and areas of lichenification. At this time the predominantly flexural distribution of the disorder makes itself apparent with thickened, red scaly and excoriated (and sometimes crusted and infected) areas behind the knees and in front of the elbows.

The treatment of the disorder in early infancy doesn't differ substantially from its treatment in older groups (page 108) although particular care must be taken not to cause undesirable toxic side effects in infants. Emollients are important and mothers should be carefully instructed on their benefit and how to use them. Similarly, bathing should be frequent quick 'dunks' in lukewarm water, with patting dry, rather than long-lasting hot scrubs with vigorous towelling afterwards. Weak topical corticosteroids only should be used – 1% hydrocortisone and 0.1% clobetasone butyrate are appropriate. Preparations of 1% hydrocortisone containing urea seem to confer some extra benefit.

Cradlecap

The newborn often develop yellowish scale over the scalp with very little else abnormal to see. It has no special significance and usually disappears after a few weeks. Application of olive oil or arachis oil with 2% salicylic acid, and shampooing with 'baby shampoos' hastens the removal.

Infantile acne (page 151)

It is not uncommon for infants a few weeks or a few months old to develop seborrhoea, comedones superficial papules and pustules over the cheek, forehead, nose and chin (Figure 14.5). This infantile acne is extremely alarming to the parents but has no special significance other than that maternal androgens have crossed the placental barrier and caused the sebaceous glands to enlarge and become more active. When the disorder develops in later infancy and is severe, the possibility of virilization due to an endocrine tumour or adrenocortical hyperplasia has to be considered. Other signs of androgen overactivity, such as precocious muscle development and male distribution of facial and body hair, should be sought.

Although the disorder subsides without sequelae within a few weeks, in most instances it can be unpleasantly persistent. Rarely, deep nodules and even cysts develop, as in ordinary adolescent acne.

Treatment with mild topical agents is usually sufficient (e.g. 0.05% tretinoin gel, 5% benzoyl peroxide gel or 3% sulphur in calamine lotion). It would be unusual for systemic antibiotics to be needed.

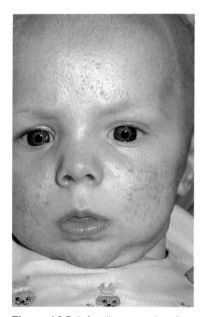

Figure 14.5 Infantile acne showing numerous acne spots affecting the cheeks and forehead.

Toxic epidermal necrolysis (Staphylococcal scalded skin syndrome)

There are two different severe disorders that share some features and the name *toxic epidermal necrolysis*. The first is covered in Chapter 6 and is a reaction to certain drugs. The other is seen in early infancy and is better termed the *Staphylococcal scalded skin syndrome*, and will be described here. The disorder affects very young infants in the first few weeks of life, although uncommonly it can occur in older children. There is a widespread erythematous eruption characterized by striking desquamation of large areas of skin, just as in a scald or burn. There may be a slight fever and some systemic disturbance but usually the children are not severely ill. However, it has been said that there is a 2–3% mortality. The disorder appears to be due to a particular phage type of *Staphylococcus aureus* (phage type II) which releases an erythematogenic exotoxin. This toxin can be shown experimentally to cause shedding of the most superficial part of the epidermis and stratum corneum (just below the granular layer) in the skin of the newborn.

Treatment should be with an appropriate systemic antibiotic such as flucloxacillin. The skin should be managed as for a burn, and concern over heat loss, dehydration and severe infection is necessary. Topically, emollients and mild antibacterial agents should be employed.

> The *staphylococcal scalded skin syndrome* affects very young infants in the first few weeks of life, with a widespread erythematous eruption characterized by striking desquamation of large areas of skin, just as in a scald or burn. It is due to a particular phage type of staphylococcus aureus (phage type II) which releases an erythemogenic exotoxin.

Lip licking cheilitis

Children aged four to eight years are most commonly affected by this minor but sometimes puzzling problem. An area around the mouth becomes sore, red, scaly and cracked (Figure 14.6). It is due to a common habit of licking the lips and skin around the lips, which become irritated and dry and are then licked to moisten them, making the situation worse. The treatment is patiently to explain the nature of the problem to mother and child and to use an emollient on the affected area.

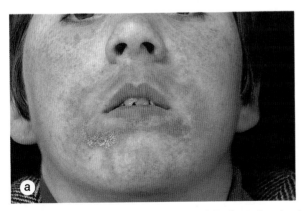 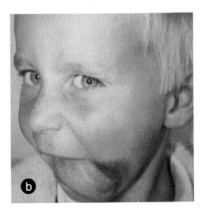

Figure 14.6 (a) Lip-licking cheilitis. (b) Patient showing how far his tongue can reach to produce the rash!

Juvenile plantar dermatosis

This disorder has apparently become more common in recent years, affecting children aged 6–12 years predominantly. It seems to be a form of eczema that affects the soles of the forefeet and, rarely, elsewhere. The affected skin becomes 'glazed', scaly and cracked, and the condition tends to be very persistent. Treatment with emollients, topical corticosteroids and weak tar preparations is recommended but the disorder tends to resist treatment and eventually remits spontaneously.

Letterer-Siwe disease (page 269)

This rare disorder is included here so as to remind readers of the possibility of this grave disorder occurring in infants and young children, when a persistent and progressive red and scaling rash occurs in the flexures. It is a form of malignant histiocytosis, and affected children require specialized management.

Old age

There is a growing acreage of elderly skin. Because of global increased affluence and health measures there has been a staggering increase in the proportion of the population over the age of 60 years. It has been said that the increase in longevity since the beginning of the twentieth century is approximately that seen in the human race in the previous 5000 years. We can no longer afford to be ignorant of either the aging process and its effects on the skin or the disorders that are particularly frequent in the elderly.

The aging process

Very little is known as to why organs and tissue age. Generally we distinguish between intrinsic aging and extrinsic aging. The latter is not true aging, i.e. the effects of the passage of time alone on the tissues, but the results of cumulated environmental trauma. As far as the skin is concerned the most significant environmental trauma stems from solar radiation in the form of ultraviolet radiation (UVR) (pages 20–29).

There are many hypotheses to account for intrinsic aging that range from a kind of built-in obsolescence within the DNA molecule itself to the cumulated results of metabolic damage from active oxygen species and free radicals. Whatever the explanation, at present there is very little that can be done to stem the tide of the passing years other than by carefully choosing long-lived parents. Thin mice on restricted diets live longer than fat mice on unrestricted diets – whether there is a message in this for human beings is at present uncertain. Another inexplicable aspect of aging is its variability. There are enormous variations in the rates at which different individuals age, as well as major differences in the rates at which individual organs and systems age within one individual.

> The physical appearances of aging are due to both intrinsic (inevitable aging) and cumulated environmental trauma – mostly the affects of solar UVR.

Skin changes in the elderly

Structural changes

All skin components and regions alter in the process of intrinsic aging. Both the epidermis and the dermis become thinner on nonlight-exposed sites with the passing of the years. The degree of thinning is variable but between the ages of 20 and 80 years the thickness of the dermis on the flexor aspect of the forearm changes from a mean of approximately 1.1 mm thickness in men to a thickness of 0.8 mm. The epidermis thins from a structure some four to five cells thick at the age of 20 to one of approximately three cells thick at age 80. The individual keratinocytes also shrink with age, although the horn cells at the surface inexplicably increase in area. Interestingly, the stratum corneum does not appear to change substantially in thickness in the skin of the aged.

These changes are much less evident on sun-exposed parts of the skin and are dependent on the cumulated dose of UVR and the skin's response to the UVR (and other environmental influences).

Blood vessels share in the attrition of age and become less in number and thicker. Adnexal structures also decrease in size and numbers with increasing age. This applies particularly to the hair (page 276) but not always to the sebaceous glands as on the face they may, paradoxically, enlarge, which is sometimes clinically evident in the condition of sebaceous gland hyperplasia (page 187).

The dermal connective tissue loses much of its proteoglycan ground substance and the collagen fibres become mainly tough, insoluble and heavily cross-linked biochemically.

Pigment cells become fewer in number and smaller, and Langerhans cells are also less in evidence in the skin of the elderly.

> Both epidermis and dermis become thinner with increasing age.

Functional changes

The most important alterations are perhaps in the ways in which the skin responds to injuries and other damaging stimuli. Wound healing is slower and may be less complete in the elderly. The aged also respond less vigorously to chemical and physical trauma – the erythema and swelling is less marked and slower to develop. Delayed hypersensitivity also is depressed and this applies to other aspects of the immune response, although this aspect of the aging process is complex and less well characterized than many others.

The activity of the smaller and less in number pigment cells is depressed, and nonexposed areas of skin are in general paler in the elderly than in young and mature subjects. On exposed areas of skin, melanocytes show irregular increases in pigmentation.

Sweat gland responses to heating decrease, and the rate of sebum secretion also decreases, although this is less marked than many other functions in the elderly.

Sensory discrimination decreases in the elderly but unfortunately not the sensations of itch or pain!

> Sebum and sweat secretion rates, pigment production and immunological defences are all decreased in the aged.

Skin disease in the elderly

There are very few skin disorders that are specific to the elderly. But there are many disorders that are more frequent in the aged, and others that have a somewhat different natural history and appearance. Management of skin disease also differs somewhat in the elderly. Only a few areas have been selected as examples of the differences.

Dry and itchy skin in the elderly

> As the skin ages, it becomes drier and tends to become itchier.

As the skin ages, it becomes drier and tends to become itchier. This tendency is heightened by:

1. low relative humidity;
2. frequent hot bathing and vigorous towelling;
3. low ambient temperature;
4. systemic illness.

The itchiness can in particular be disabling and it is important to try to reduce the desiccating stimuli to which the skin is exposed. The generous use of emollients (Chapter 21) as topical applications and as cleansing agents, and bath additives, is mandatory.

Although itchiness due to dry skin in the elderly is quite common, it has to be remembered that scabies and the other causes of generalized pruritus also occur in the elderly and should be diligently sought.

Eczema in the elderly

Eczema is a common problem in one form or another in the elderly. It is dealt with in Chapter 8, but some points are worth emphasizing here.

1. **Atopic dermatitis** is uncommon but by no means unknown in the elderly and is as trying and uncomfortable for patients as at other times of life.
2. **Discoid (nummular) eczema** is a form of constitutional eczema that seems more common in the elderly than in any other age group.
3. **Eczema craquelée** is an eczematous disorder that is virtually specific to the skin of the elderly, occurring against a background of generalized xerosis (or drying of the skin surface).
4. **Photosensitive eczema** is more common in elderly men and

when, as it often is, it is very persistent, it can cause enormous difficulties in diagnosis and management.

5. Minor degrees of *seborrhoeic dermatitis* are very common in the elderly and occasionally the disorder can spread to become generalized.

6. Eczema can spread extremely rapidly in the elderly and become extremely disabling. While in some patients seborrhoeic dermatitis may be the underlying cause, a reason for the development of eczema is not found in many.

> Eczematous rashes are common in the elderly. Eczema cracquelée is specific to the elderly.

TREATMENT

Treatment of eczema in the elderly is no different from that in any other age group, save for two issues. Firstly, emollients are even more important in this age group than in younger patients. Secondly, because the healing processes are slower in the elderly there should be greater readiness to use systemic remedies, including cyclosporin, azathioprine and corticosteroids.

Skin tumours

Skin tumours of one sort or another are the most frequent reason for the elderly consulting the physician. Seborrhoeic warts are found in virtually everyone over the age of 60 years, and, although benign, often result in minor symptoms and embarrassment because of the cosmetic disfigurement they cause. When few in number they can easily be removed by curettage and cautery. When present in large numbers (page 182) they can present an insoluble problem for management. Solar keratoses (page 207) are another frequent cause of presentation – some 4% of all new patient consultations in the dermatology department of the University Hospital of Wales are for solar keratoses. Although very few of these lesions progress to squamous cell cancer they are important as an indication that serious solar damage has occurred and that more significant lesions may develop. They are uncommon below the age of 45 years and very common over the age of 60 years. As with seborrhoeic warts, solar keratoses may also cause minor symptoms and some cosmetic problems.

More serious are the lesions of basal cell carcinoma (page 217) which are almost as common as solar keratoses. Because of their capacity for local invasion and tissue destruction they cause considerable morbidity. Squamous cell carcinoma (page 213) is much less common but can metastasize as well as cause local tissue destruction. Malignant melanoma (page 223) is slightly more common in the elderly compared to young age groups but lentigo maligna is virtually restricted to the elderly.

> Seborrhoeic warts are found in virtually everyone over the age of 60, and although benign, often cause minor symptoms and embarrassment.

> Solar keratoses are uncommon below the age of 45 and very common over the age of 60.

> Basal cell carcinoma are almost as common as solar keratoses.

The elderly are often physically, socially and economically deprived and cannot find the necessary resources for adequate treatment of their skin disorder.

Management of skin disorders in the elderly

Through no fault of their own, the elderly are often physically, socially and economically deprived. Their housing, hygiene, nutrition, clothing and means of heating may all be deficient and this should be taken into account when designing treatments. If they live alone, as is often the case, they may well be unable to find anyone to help with applications of ointments to body parts they cannot reach themselves or to assist with bandages.

For the most part the elderly will not be able to afford or cope with stringent diets or be able to buy adjuvant materials such as cleansing agents or sunscreens.

It must be remembered that the elderly may also find difficulty in hearing, understanding and/or remembering instructions, especially if these are complex and involve more than one medicament. If possible, instructions on the medications should also be given to an accompanying relative or legibly written out.

Difficulty may also be experienced in applying topical applications because of lack of mobility or simply because they can't adequately see the affected area.

All of the above potential difficulties will become obvious by simple enquiry and observation and need to be taken into account when trying to help an elderly patient with a skin problem.

Pregnancy and the skin

Pigmentation

Changes in the degree of pigmentation are very common during pregnancy. Most women develop a generalized increased pigmentation of the skin. Darkening of the skin occurs quite regularly in the midline of the abdomen, converting the linea alba into the linea nigra. The areolae of the breasts change in colour from pink to brown and the skin of the external genitalia also darkens. The face also darkens in a rather characteristic manner. Dark areas appear symmetrically across the cheeks, around the eyes and over the forehead, giving a mask-like appearance (Figure 15.1). This is known as melasma (or chloasma) and seems much more common and troublesome in darker, Mediterranean and Asian skin types. The same problem is sometimes seen in nonpregnant women and it is claimed that it is more common in those

> Most women develop a generalized increased pigmentation of the skin during pregnancy.

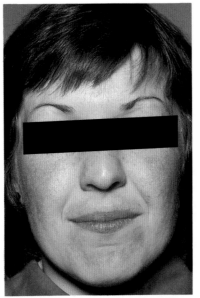

Figure 15.1 'Mask of pregnancy' also known as melasma or chloasma.

who take the contraceptive pill. Some 60% of pregnant women develop some melasma, while 30% of women on the pill do so.

The pattern of melasma varies. The commonest type is centrofacial (about 65%). The 'malar' type with pigmentation on the cheeks and the mandibular pattern with pigmentation along the lower jaw is less common.

> The increase in blood levels of melanocyte stimulating hormone and the consequent stimulation of melanocyte activity and the increase in oestrogen and progesterone may be responsible for melasma.

The underlying reason for the increase in pigmentation during pregnancy is not certain but it has been suggested that it is the increase in blood levels of melanocyte-stimulating hormone and the consequent stimulation of melanocyte activity. The increase in oestrogen and progesterone may also play a role.

Pigmented moles also darken during pregnancy and sometimes cause concern because of this. In addition, new moles may appear during pregnancy.

Striae gravidarum

Striae distensae (or stretch marks) are linear areas of apparent atrophy of the skin due to disruption of dermal connective tissue fibres (Figure 15.2) as a result of ruptured dermal elastic fibres. They occur at the sites of skin stretching when there is excess ambient glucocorticoid activity. They occur as a normal phenomenon in early adolescence, in Cushing's syndrome after both systemic and topical corticoid therapy, and in pregnancy. In the latter case they are called striae gravidarum.

> In pregnancy striae occur predominantly over the lower abdomen and over the breasts during the third trimester.

In pregnancy they occur predominantly over the lower abdomen and over the breasts during the third trimester and are of major cosmetic concern to some women. It has been claimed that topical tretinoin preparations and formulations of organic hydroxyacids remove or reduce these lesions.

Cutaneous vascularity

One of the oddest of phenomena that occur in pregnant women is the appearance of small vascular malformations known as spider naevi (Figure 15.3). These only occur on the face, upper trunk and arms, i.e.

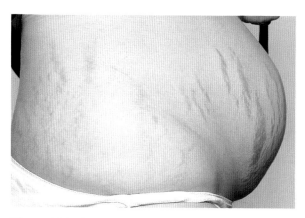

Figure 15.2 'Stretch marks' or striae distensae on the abdomen six months postpartum.

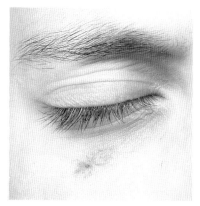

Figure 15.3 Spider naevus.

the area of drainage of the superior vena cava. As with liver disease, in which these lesions also occur, it may be that in pregnancy there is a relative excess of oestrogenic activity that provokes these vascular anomalies.

Interestingly, the palms in pregnancy may become redder and feel warmer, resembling the changes that occur in liver disease (Figure 15.4). Both the spider naevi and the palmar changes usually but not invariably gradually fade following delivery. Rarely, pyogenic granuloma-like tumours develop during pregnancy.

Pruritus in pregnancy

Generalized itching is sometimes a problem for pregnant women. In some instances there appears to be intrahepatic cholestasic leading to biliary retention in the last trimester. There is little that can be done concerning this problem save the use of emollients and mentholated calamine preparations.

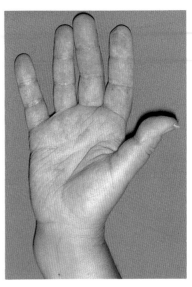

Figure 15.4 Reddened palms seen in liver disease and in pregnancy.

Effects of pregnancy on intercurrent skin disease

Common inflammatory skin disorders such as psoriasis and atopic dermatitis often improve during pregnancy but this is by no means invariable, as some patients seem to deteriorate and others do not change much. Amongst the conditions reputed to worsen during pregnancy, the condition of systemic lupus erythematosus ought to be mentioned. Apparently patients may be precipitated into an acute and severe attack by the stress.

Regardless as to whether the pre-existing disorder improves during pregnancy, worsens, or stays the same, a different approach to treatment is required. This is especially true for conditions such as acne and rosacea, where many patients would be receiving systemic antibiotics and even antiandrogens or retinoids. Such systemic medications should be stopped because of the risk of harming the foetus (teratogenicity). This particularly applies to isotretinoin (page 159) where some 30–50% of foetuses exposed to the drug are born with a serious malformation. It applies to a lesser, but still significant, extent to the tetracycline group of antibiotics and cyproterone acetate.

Topical treatments must also be assessed for their teratogenic potential. Most topically applied materials are absorbed to a greater or lesser extent and, at least theoretically, could constitute a risk to the foetus. The possibility that topical tretinoin could be responsible for foetal malformations after usage for acne has been extensively investigated but discounted as insufficient is absorbed through the skin.

This is the case for most skin medications unless very large areas of skin are being treated. Even if this is the case, there does not appear to be a significant foetal risk for pregnant women with psoriasis being treated with tars or dithranol preparations. It has to be remembered that women in the last trimester of pregnancy may find topical treatments more difficult to apply or tolerate.

> Effects of pregnancy on intercurrent inflammatory dermatoses is unpredictable but treatments must be modified as drugs may harm the foetus.

Effects of intercurrent maternal disease on the foetus

The foetus is only occasionally affected by skin disorders in the mother. The three major types of skin disease that cause congenital foetal disease are:

1. *The inherited genodermatoses*. It is obvious that genetic faults may be passed on and phenotypically expressed in the child. This may be obvious with some dominant disorders such as in some of the ichthyoses (page 249) but with many conditions the disorder doesn't become evident until later in childhood.

2. *Immunologically mediated diseases*. In some disorders, pathogenetic antibodies cross the placenta and cause disease in the foetus. This may be the case in lupus erythematosus and, in one rare variety of this, congenital heart block can be induced in the child. It may also occur in the rare blistering condition of pemphigus. In most of these cases the foetal skin disorder only lasts as long as the transplacentally transmitted antibodies last in the newborn child's circulation.

3. *Infections*. This is of most concern now with regard to human immunodeficiency virus (HIV) infection, and frighteningly high rates of HIV positivity have recently been found in pregnant women in some communities (1% in New York, for example). Syphilis may still be a problem if undiagnosed and untreated, and may then be transmitted congenitally. Other infective skin disorders that may be passed from mother to foetus include chicken pox, herpes simplex, candidiasis and warts, although these last two are better classified as 'intranatal' infections as the infection is caught from the birth passages.

Skin disorders occurring in pregnancy

Itchy rashes in the last trimester

> Several patterns of itchy, erythematous rash occur in the last trimester of pregnancy.

Several patterns of itchy, erythematous rash occurring in the last trimester of pregnancy have been described. They share several characteristics. For the most part their causes are unknown, they are transient, remitting spontaneously before delivery or at worst shortly afterwards, and they produce very considerable discomfort. In some cases they are associated with pre-eclamptic toxaemia but by no means is this so in the majority.

The rash mostly occurs over the abdomen and flanks but also appears on the upper limbs. The lesions are for the most part maculopapules

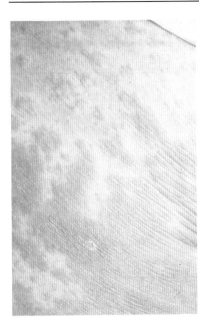

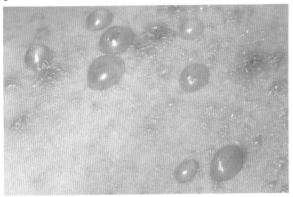

Figure 15.5 Common itchy erythematous eruption of pregnancy.

Figure 15.6 Blistering rash due to pemphigoid gestationis.

but in some patients red urticaria-like plaques develop (Figure 15.5). Annular and odd figurate lesions also develop in some patients. Treatment is symptomatic with emollient or weak topical corticosteroids.

Herpes gestationis (syn. pemphigoid gestationis)

This is an uncommon, extremely irritant blistering rash occurring in the last trimester of pregnancy. The eruption starts on the flanks or over the abdomen with itchy urticarial papules and vesicles and blisters (Figure 15.6). The blistering is subepidermal and is quite similar to that seen in senile pemphigoid (page 83). There is often a circulating antibody directed to the dermoepidermal junctional area although this is present in 'low titre'.

The rash usually remits shortly after birth but may recur in subsequent pregnancies or even after taking oral contraceptives. Treatment should be confined to topical applications in the first place. If this does not help, dapsone may be tried for short periods.

> A rare itchy blistering rash with similarities to pemphigoid is seen in the last trimester and is known as herpes gestationis.

Impetigo herpetiformis

This is a very rare and serious form of generalized pustular psoriasis seen in late pregnancy. It seems to be precipitated by low levels of serum calcium but really very little is known of the pathogenesis of this serious disorder.

CHAPTER
16

Disorders of keratinization

Epidermal differentiation

During epidermal differentiation (keratinization), plump cuboidal or spheroidal, hydrated, highly metabolically active cells gradually become tough, hardened, biochemically inactive, thin shield-like structures which are programmed to desquamate off the skin surface. During keratinization a tough, chemically resistant cross-linked protein band is laid down just inside the plasma membrane and the whole cell flattens to a thin disc (corneocyte). A characteristic feature of the normal stratum corneum is the presence of an intercellular cement material that contains polar lipid and glycoprotein.

The differentiation process in which basal epidermal cells gradually mature and transform into stratum corneum cells is known as keratinization. In this process, which takes about 14 days, plump cuboidal or spheroidal, hydrated, highly metabolically active cells gradually become tough, hardened, biochemically inactive, thin shield-like structures which are programmed to desquamate off the skin surface (Figure 16.1). This process is biochemically complex and it is not surprising that it is subject to genetically determined errors. During keratinization a tough, chemically resistant, cross-linked protein band is laid down just inside the plasma membrane and the whole cell flattens to a thin disc (corneocyte) (Figure 16.2). The corneocyte's water content is reduced from the usual 70 to 30% and most of the cellular organelles, including its nucleus, are eliminated. The keratinous tonofilaments become organized in bundles and are spatially orientated. A further characteristic feature of the normal stratum corneum is the presence of an intercellular cement material that contains polar lipid and glycoprotein.

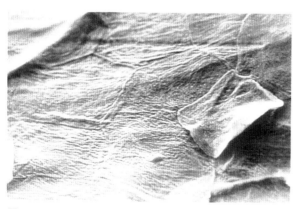

Figure 16.1 Corneocyte desquamating from skin surface as seen by scanning electron microscope.

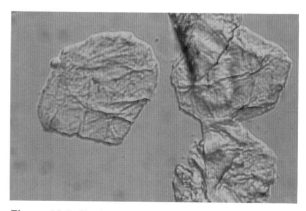

Figure 16.2 Single corneocytes as seen by phase contrast microscopy.

Stratum corneum function

It is believed that:

1. mechanical protection is provided by the keratinous tonofilaments and the retention of desmosomal contacts;
2. chemical protection is provided by the protein band around the corneocyte;
3. percutaneous penetration of materials applied to the skin surface is inhibited by the intercellular cement;
4. water movement in and out of the skin is inhibited by the intercellular cement at the base of the stratum corneum;
5. desquamation is probably controlled both by desmosomal contacts and by the intercellular cement.

Scaling

All the disorders of keratinization and many inflammatory skin diseases such as psoriasis are characterized by the formation of scale or hyperkeratosis at the skin surface. A scale is merely an aggregate of horn cells that have failed to separate one from the other in the horizontal plane and the condition of hyperkeratosis is an exaggeration of this problem in which there is a vertical as well as a horizontal dimension to this process. Thus regardless of the particular metabolic fault ultimately responsible, the final common pathogenetic pathway is a failure in the normal loss of intercorneocyte binding forces (cohesion) in the superficial portion of the stratum corneum (Figure 16.3).

> A scale is merely an aggregate of horn cells that have failed to separate one from the other in the horizontal plane and the condition of hyperkeratosis is an exaggeration of this problem.

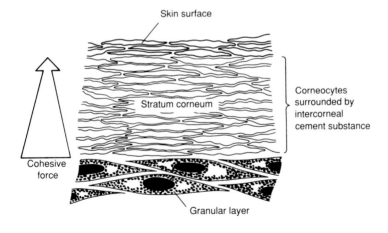

Figure 16.3 There is a drop in intracorneal cohesion as the skin surface is approached by the ascending corneocytes, allowing them to desquamate off.

DEFINITION

Ichthyosis is derived from the Greek *ichthyos*, meaning a fish. The term is unfortunate for a number of reasons – not the least is that the scale of 'modern' fish is in fact mesodermal rather than ectodermal in origin. The term ichthyosis is used to describe generalized noninflammatory disorders of keratinization and implies a congenital origin. There are some conditions that are localized, inflammatory, or are acquired, and clearly do not satisfy the above definition but retain a position within this category of skin disorders for convenience.

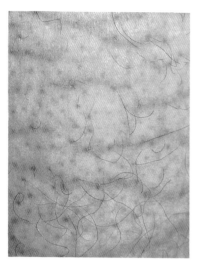

Figure 16.4 Fissuring of skin in ichthyosis. This is painful and limits movement.

> Xeroderma does not represent a single disease process. The term just means dry skin.

> Xeroderma tends to be worse in the winter time and when accompanied by itching is known, logically enough, as 'winter itch'. This is particularly a problem in low relative humidity.

> Xeroderma is seen in approximately 30% of patients with atopic dermatitis.

Disability in disorders of keratinization

Contrary to popular (both lay and medical) belief, skin diseases can be very disabling. There is a primitive revulsion at a disordered skin surface which results in significant isolation and social and emotional deprivation. Patients with chronic skin disorders often become severely depressed and find relationships difficult to sustain. They are also occupationally at a severe disadvantage. These factors are of particular significance for patients with congenital disorders who have life-long scaling skin disease. Apart from these issues it is not often appreciated just how severely physically disabled are some patients with skin disease. The abnormal scaling and hyperkeratotic skin does not have the normally excellent resilience and compliance of normal skin so that when it is stretched during normal limb or digit movements it may crack, causing a fissure (Figure 16.4). These fissures are painful and may limit further movement.

Xeroderma

Xeroderma does not represent a single disease process. The term derives from the Greek *xeros*, meaning dry, and xeroderma just means dry skin. In fact xeroderma is used to describe scaliness rather than water content. Because the appearance of scaling transiently disappears if the abnormal skin is hydrated, it has mistakenly been believed that scaling is the manifestation of water deficiency. This is just as logical as believing that because water puts out fire that fire is a manifestation of water deficiency! Unfortunately it is very difficult to measure water content of the stratum corneum directly so that it is impossible to know the true relationship between water content and scaling.

CAUSES

There are some normal individuals who tend to have a 'dry' skin and these are more susceptible to stimuli that provoke scaling of the skin surface. Aging tends to make the surface of the skin feel 'drier' and this seems to be associated with pruritus in susceptible individuals. A low relative humidity aggravates the problem as does repeated vigorous washing, especially in hot water with some soaps and cleansing agents. Presumably the toilet procedures leach out important substances that are vital to the integrity of the stratum corneum. Xeroderma tends to be worse in the winter time and when accompanied by itching is known, logically enough, as 'winter itch'. This is particularly a problem in the north eastern USA because of the low relative humidity.

Xeroderma is seen in approximately 30% of patients with atopic dermatitis. It has been suggested that this is a manifestation of autosomal dominant ichthyosis but there is more evidence in favour of the disorder being the result of the eczematous process itself. Xeroderma is also seen during the course of severe wasting diseases such as carcinomatosis, intestinal malabsorption and chronic renal failure, but should not be confused with acquired ichthyosis which is much more severe and seen in quite specific circumstances (page 286).

Keratosis pilaris

The status of this condition is not clear. The term signifies horny plugs in the hair follicles of the outer aspect of the upper arms, forming sheets of pink horny papules (Figure 16.5) and occasionally on the thighs. It is seen in 'ordinary xeroderma', in the course of autosomal dominant ichthyosis, and sometimes in normal young women for no apparent reason.

TREATMENT

Patients should be instructed to shower rather than bath, to use luke warm water rather than hot water, to use emollient cleansing agents rather than ordinary soaps and to pat dry rather than using vigorously towelling after bathing. If the patient lives in centrally heated rooms, humidifiers should be employed to raise the relative humidity. Emollients are a mainstay of treatment (page 310). These act by supplying an oily film on the skin surface to prevent evaporation of water and encourage a build-up of this in the skin. They contain a variety of oils and other lipids either as single phase substances or more frequently as emulsions. Some also contain materials known as humectants which are meant to encourage the retention of water in the skin. These include urea, glycerine, lactic acid and pyrrolidone carboxylic acid. Emollients act for a short time only – up to two to three hours at most – and need to be frequently applied. Their action can be supplemented by bath oils which deposit a film of lipid on the skin surface, or emollient cleansers that do a similar job.

Figure 16.5 Keratosis pilaris. Horny red papules on upper arms.

> Emollients act by supplying an oily film on the skin surface to prevent evaporation of water and encourage a build-up of this in the skin.

Autosomal dominant ichthyosis

DEFINITION

A common disorder of keratinization characterized by mild generalized scaliness clinically and reduction of the granular cell layer histologically which is inherited in an autosomal dominant manner.

> In autosomal dominant ichthyosis there is generalized scaling worse over the extensor surfaces.

CLINICAL FEATURES

There is widespread fine scaling over the skin surface which tends to be worse in the winter time when the humidity is low. It spares the flexures and is most noticeable over the extensor aspects of the limbs and trunk, being most noticeable over the back, the lateral aspects of the upper arms, the anterolateral thighs and particularly the shins (Figure 16.6 and 16.7). Keratosis pilaris may be seen over the outer aspects of the upper arms in a few subjects. The condition is hardly

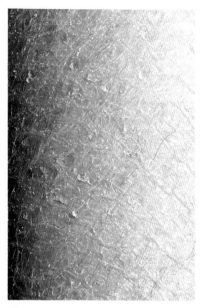

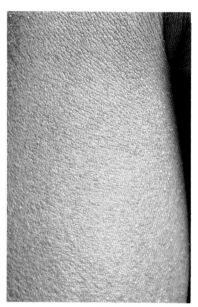

Figure 16.6 Moderately severe scaling in autosomal dominant ichthyosis.

Figure 16.7 Moderately severe scaling in autosomal dominant ichthyosis.

noticeable in most but quite marked and disabling in a few. In the worst affected, large polygonal dark scales form on the shins.

The condition is often mildly itchy and in the badly affected can cause some disablement because of the limitations imposed by the abnormal horny layer (page 308). The disorder is life long but may worsen in old age.

PATHOLOGY AND AETIOPATHOGENESIS
The condition is inherited as an autosomal dominant disorder but the biochemical basis is unclear. It has been estimated that the gene occurs with a frequency of 1 in 500. Histologically the only abnormality detectable is a much diminished granular cell layer (Figure 16.8).

Figure 16.8 Pathology of autosomal dominant ichthyosis. Note virtual absence of granular cell layer.

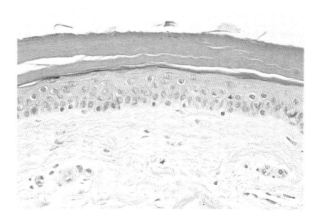

Ultrastructurally and biochemically there is decreased content of a basic histidine-rich protein known as filaggrin which is important in the orientation of the keratin tonofilaments. It is not known, however, how this abnormality leads to the increased binding between corneocytes, leading to scaling.

TREATMENT

Generally, little is required in the way of treatment other than emollients. Patients who have very severe scaling may be helped by the use of topical keratolytic agents to some body sites. These include preparations containing urea in concentrations of 10–15% and salicylic acid in concentrations of 1–6%. The latter is particularly effective in encouraging desquamation but may not be used on large body areas for any length of time as concentrations of more than 2% when applied to abnormal skin may cause salicylate intoxication (salicylism). It is most unusual that a patient is so affected severely as to require the use of retinoids (page 316).

> Emollients are usually sufficient to control the disorder but keratolytic preparations may be needed in some.

Sex-linked ichthyosis

DEFINITION

This is an uncommon, moderately severe disorder of keratinization which is inherited as a sex-linked characteristic in which the underlying metabolic fault is either a deficiency of steroid sulphatase or is closely linked to this.

> Sex linked ichthyosis is similar to but more severe than A.D.I.

CLINICAL FEATURES

The male children that are born with this disorder are often the products of postmature pregnancies and difficult labours. The reason for this appears to be a placental deficiency of the steroid sulphatase and a consequent failure of the usual splitting of circulating maternal oestrone sulphate in the last trimester of pregnancy. The free oestrone is thought to have a role in priming the uterus to oxytoxic stimuli.

The generalized scaling is usually more severe than in autosomal dominant ichthyosis (Figure 16.9). It is also more marked over the extensor aspects of the body surface but does not always spare the flexures and often affects the sides of the neck and even the face. The individual scales are often quite large, particularly over the shins (Figure 16.10) and appear pigmented with a dark brownish discolouration. Patients with sex- (or X-) linked ichthyosis may be significantly disabled by their disorder, especially in winter time when their condition tends to worsen.

251

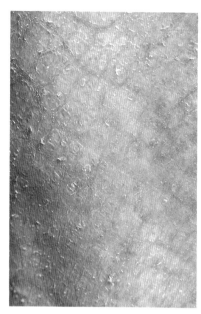

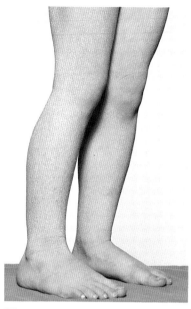

Figure 16.9 Skin scaling in sex-linked ichthyosis.

Figure 16.10 Typical scaling on shins in sex-linked ichthyosis.

> The trait is carried on an X-chromosome and is marked by steroid sulphatase deficiency.

ASSOCIATED DISORDERS

There is an association with cryptorchidism and even of testicular cancer on the basis of this, although this is quite rare. There is also an association with a form of cataract, although this does not usually result in functional impairment.

PATHOLOGY AND AETIOPATHOGENESIS

The trait is carried on an X-chromosone and is recessive so that it is not manifest in women (XX) who become carriers, but it is in male offspring (XY). In fact the carrier female may demonstrate patchy scaling which is consistent with the 'random deletion' (or Lyon) hypothesis. The disorder is quite uncommon, having a gene frequency of approximately 1 in 6000.

Histologically there is a minor degree of epidermal thickening and mild hypergranulosis (Figure 16.11). Biochemically all cells tested of affected male subjects show a steroid sulphatase deficiency but for diagnostic purposes either fibroblast, lymphocyte or epidermal cell cultures are tested. The steroid sulphatase abnormality results in excess quantities of cholesterol sulphate in the stratum corneum with diminished free cholesterol. This altered ratio of cholesterol sulphate to cholesterol has also been used as the basis of a diagnostic test and has been suggested as the underlying basis for the abnormal scaling.

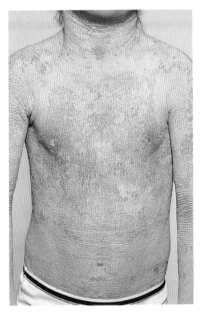

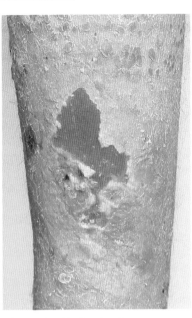

Figure 16.13 Epidermolytic hyperkeratosis showing typical severe hyperkeratosis and scaling.

Figure 16.14 Erosion in epidermolytic hyperkeratosis following minor injury to this area.

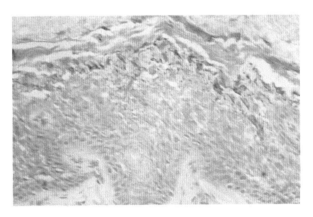

Figure 16.15 Pathology of epidermolytic hyperkeratosis with reticulate degenerative change.

high rate of epidermal cell production. Recent evidence suggests that there is a defect in the action of a keratin gene responsible for the production of keratin 10.

> Epidermolytic hyperkeratosis is a rare dominantly inherited disorder of keratinization characterized clinically by erythema, scaling and thick hyperkeratosis and blistering and histologically by reticular epidermal degeneration.

TREATMENT

Patients require particularly sympathetic management because of their disabilities. Topical emollients and keratolytics are not often very

255

helpful. The oral retinoids may improve their appearance considerably although the dose has to be carefully regulated as these drugs may temporarily increase the blistering as well as decreasing the hyperkeratosis! Dosages and toxicity are as for NBIE.

Lamellar ichthyosis

This is a rare autosomal recessive disorder of keratinization.

> Lamellar ichthyosis is a rare autosomal recessive disorder of keratinization characterized by a striking degree of hyperkeratosis but not much erythema.

CLINICAL FEATURES
The disorder is characterized by a striking degree of hyperkeratosis but not much erythema. As with NBIE and EH, some patients develop the condition after being born in a collodion membrane. The hyperkeratosis may be discoloured brown for reasons that are unclear, and the horny lamellae may overlap in a characteristic manner (Figure 16.16). As with the other severe disorders of keratinization there may be marked ectropion and ear deformities (Figure 16.17).

PATHOLOGY AND PATHOGENESIS
There is marked hyperkeratosis and hypergranulosis. Nothing is known about the underlying biochemical defect.

TREATMENT
This is similar to that for NBIE and EH, with oral retinoid drugs being the only available agent that can produce any substantial improvement.

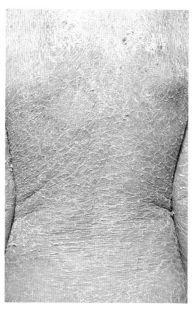

Figure 16.16 Lamellar ichthyosis. Marked hyperkeratosis and scaling.

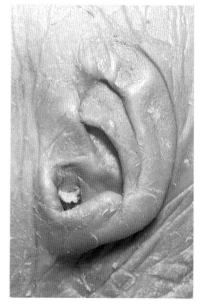

Figure 16.17 'Crumpled ear' seen in many severe disorders of keratinization.

Collodion baby

This is an odd condition in which babies are born covered by a shiny transparent membrane (Figure 16.18). This gradually peels off after a week or so, the peel looking like 'collodion' – hence the name. Ultimately the child may develop normally or may develop one of the severe disorders of keratinization discussed above.

Nothing is known of the cause. Collodion babies need to be carefully nursed as their skin barrier function may be abnormal so that they lose much water and become dehydrated.

Harlequin foetus

This is a rare and mostly fatal disorder in which the child is born encased in thick, abnormal, fissured hyperkeratotic skin. This disorder is also due to abnormalities of keratin synthesis. Survival of a few of these unfortunate children has been reported with the use of oral retinoids.

Refsum's syndrome (heredopathia atactica neuritiformis)

This is a very rare autosomal recessive metabolic disorder in which there is defective oxidation of certain branch chained fatty acids. This results in the accumulation in all tissues of phytanic acid found in green vegetables. This fatty acid substitutes for other fatty acids in membrane lipids which is probably responsible for many of the clinical manifestations of the disorder. These include cerebellar ataxia, polyneuritis, retinitis pigmentosa, nerve deafness and generalized ichthyosiform scaling.

Sjögren–Larsson syndrome

This rare recessive disorder is more common in some areas of Sweden. Affected individuals have an ichthyosiform skin disorder resembling NBIE and a spastic diplegia.

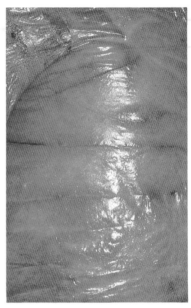

Figure 16.18 Shiny membrane covering skin in collodion baby.

Table 16.1   Precipitating causes of acquired ichthyosis

Hodgkin's disease and other reticuloses	Rarely, other neoplastic diseases
Essential fatty acid deficiency	Due to dietary deficiency, blind loop syndrome, or intestinal bypass operation
Serum lipid lowering drugs	For example, nicotinamide, butyrophenones
Leprosy	Usually subsequent to treatment
AIDS	Accompanied by severe pruritus

Acquired ichthyosis

Generalized skin scaling without accompanying inflammation develops in adult life in this disorder. Table 16.1 categorizes the precipitating factors. The most important cause of acquired ichthyosis is underlying malignant disease – particularly Hodgkin's disease. Essential fatty acid deficiency and some lipid lowering drugs are other causes.

Other disorders of keratinization

Darier's disease (keratosis folliculitis)

Darier's disease is an uncommon disorder that appears to be inherited as an autosomal dominant disorder but also occurs sporadically.

> Darier's disease is an uncommon disorder that appears to be inherited as an autosomal dominant disorder but also occurs sporadically.

CLINICAL FEATURES

A characteristic feature is the appearance of groups of brownish horny papules over the central trunk, shoulders, face and also elsewhere (Figure 16.19a and b). These easily become irritated and/or infected and become exudative and crusted. There is considerable variation in severity. Other features include the presence of tiny pits on the palms and a nail dystrophy in which there is a vertical ridge starting at an indentation at the nail free border (Figure 16.20).

PATHOLOGY AND PATHOGENESIS

There is a curious loss of cohesion between keratinocytes above the basal layer – a little like the acantholysis seen in pemphigus (page 87).

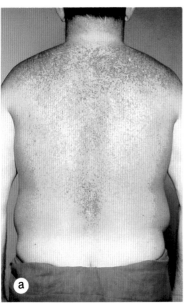

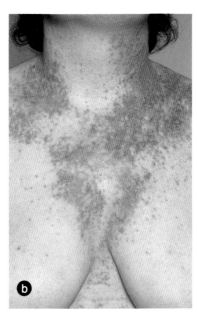

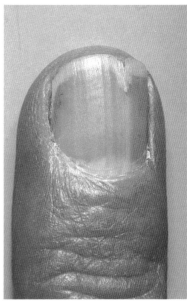

Figure 16.19 (a) Brown keratotic papules on trunk in Darier's disease. (b) Red exudative papules on chest in Darier's disease.

Figure 16.20 Typical nail change in Darier's disease with longitudinal ridge starting at V-shaped 'nick'.

258

The suprabasilar clefting that results is accompanied by an odd form of premature keratinization in which eosinophilic bodies (corps ronds) and small dense basophilic bodies (grains) are formed to be carried upwards by the epidermis (Figure 16.21). There is an abnormality in the synthesis of desmosomal components but the details are not clear.

TREATMENT
Topical treatment with mild keratolytics such as 2% salicylic acid or 0.025–0.05% tretinoin may be helpful. Oral retinoids are often of considerable assistance (page 316).

Hailey-Hailey disease (chronic benign familial pemphigus)

This is a rare familial disorder with some similarities to Darier's disease. Fissured, exudative, infected lesions develop in the groins, the axillae and around the neck in particular. It doesn't usually start before early adult life and is much worse in summertime. Histologically there is marked loss of cohesion between keratinocytes, giving the appearance of a 'crumbling brick wall'. Treatment is for the most part symptomatic but treatment with anti-infective agents may produce some clinical benefit.

Tylosis

This term describes a group of disorders in which there is marked thickening of palmar and plantar skin due to some localized abnormality of keratinization (Figure 16.22). The disorder is clearly heterogenous with autosomal dominant, autosomal recessive and sex-linked recessive types being described. There is also a wide range of clinical features with involvement of the dorsa of the hands and feet in some patients and an odd 'punctate' palmar pattern in others. The skin of the elbows and knees is affected in some patients and the disorder may also be an integral part of generalized ichthyosis. In one dominantly

> Tylosis describes a group of disorders in which there is marked thickening of palmar and plantar skin due to some localized abnormality of keratinization.

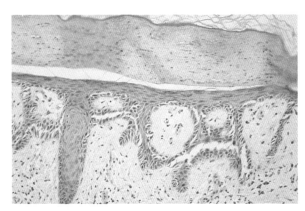

Figure 16.21 Pathology of Darier's disease with suprabasular clefting and parakeratosis.

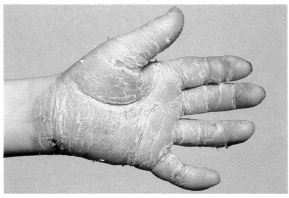

Figure 16.22 Massive palmar hyperkeratosis in one variety of tylosis.

259

inherited variety there is a close association with the development of carcinoma of the oesophagus. There is usually marked hyperkeratosis and epidermal thickening only but in a few patients are the changes of epidermolytic hyperkeratosis noted histologically.

TREATMENT
Luckily most patients are not as disabled as much as may be thought from the clinical appearance. As long as they keep their skin surface flexible and smooth with emollients and keratolytics they can manage everyday activities quite well. Oral retinoids (pages 315–316) may be helpful in some but in others the thinning of the affected skin produced is uncomfortable.

Erythrokeratoderma variablis
Erythrokeratoderma variablis (EKV) is a rare disorder whose inheritance is poorly characterized. Erythematous brownish hyperkeratotic plaques occur which gradually move across the skin surface. Treatment with oral retinoids is usually helpful.

Pachyonychia congenita
This is a rare autosomal recessively inherited disorder in which there is striking thickening of the nails. There are also hyperkeratotic areas over the palms and sometimes elsewhere.

Other genodermatoses

Tuberous sclerosis is a rare autosomal dominantly inherited disorder in which defects occur in many organ systems.

Tuberous sclerosis
Tuberous sclerosis is a rare autosomal dominantly inherited disorder in which defects occur in many organ systems.

CLINICAL FEATURES
Major skin abnormalities include the appearance of pink-red papules around the nose and cheeks which increase in number during adolescence, known inappropriately as adenoma sebaceum (Figure 16.23). Firm whitish plaques (shagreen patches) with a cobblestone surface, depigmented leaf-shaped macules and subungual fibromata are other skin signs. Cerebral malformations often result in epilepsy. Renal hamartomas occur in 50% of patients and bone cysts are common. Retinal malformations (phakomas) and muscle tumours (rhabdomyomas) are other problems found in this syndrome. Mental deficiency is seen in many patients with this disease.

Abnormalities include pink-red papules on cheeks (adenoma sebaceum), depigmented macules and firm whitish plaques (shagreen patches).

Von Recklinghausen's disease (neurofibromatosis)

This is a not uncommon autosomal dominant disorder but a high frequency of new gene mutations (50% cases) and variable expression of the disorder make its occurrence difficult to predict.

CLINICAL FEATURES
Main features:

1. Brown macules appear varying in size from a few millimetres in diameter to several centimetres. These are aptly described as *café au lait* patches and are characterized by the presence of giant melanosomes. The appearance of such freckle-like lesions in the axillae is diagnostic of the disorder.
2. Skin-coloured to pink-mauve compressible soft skin tumours, some of which are pedunculated, are also a typical feature (Figure 16.24). These are neurofibroma and may be present in large numbers, causing a considerable cosmetic disability.
3. Larger tumours on the limbs occur. These are plexiform neuromas.

The numbers of lesions increase with age. Patients are also subject to the development of a wide range of neoplastic lesions including acoustic neuroma, phaeochromocytoma and fibrosarcoma.

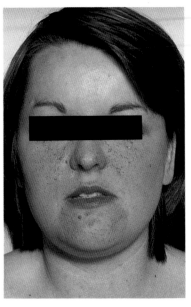

Figure 16.23 Adenoma sebaceum with many pink papules in the paranasal areas.

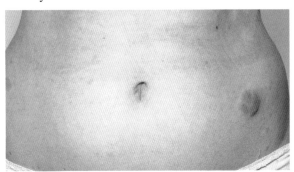

Figure 16.24 Mildly affected patient with neurofibromatosis. There is both a neurofibroma and a *café au lait* patch on the abdomen.

Anhidrotic ectodermal dysplasia

In this rare disorder there are characteristic frontal bosses on the skull as well as a saddle deformity of the nose. There are no eccrine sweat glands present so that individuals are subject to hyperpyrexia in hot weather. The hair may be sparse and fine and there are multiple abnormalities of the teeth. The most frequent type of anhidrotic ectodermal defect is inherited as a sex-linked recessive characteristic.

There is also a condition of *hypohidrotic ectodermal defect* in which there is some sweat gland development, palmoplantar hyperkeratosis and nail abnormalities.

In dominantly inherited neurofibromatosis numerous brownish macules (café au lait patches) co-exist with soft pedunculated neurofibromata.

17

Metabolic disorders and reticulohistiocytic proliferative disorders

Porphyrias

> The porphyrias are a group of disorders of metabolism of the haem. molecule.

The porphyrias are a group of disorders of metabolism of the haem molecule. Acute intermittent porphyria has no skin manifestations. Porphyrias that demonstrate skin disorder as a component are summarized in Table 17.1.

Porphyria cutanea tarda

Porphyria cutanea tarda (PCT) is a so-called 'hepatic porphyria'. There is a genetic component to the disorder although it has not been completely characterized. It is much more common in those with alcoholic liver disease but has also been seen in patients with liver tumours and those with hexachlorbenzene poisoning.

> In Porphyria cutanea tarda there is a defect in the action of the enzyme uroporphyrinogen decarboxylase resulting in accumulation of uroporphyrins and coproporphyrins in the blood, stools and urine.

METABOLIC BASIS

There appears to be a defect in the action of the enzyme uroporphyrinogen decarboxylase resulting in accumulation of uroporphyrins and coproporphyrins in the blood, stools and urine.

Table 17.1 Enzyme defects in porphyrias with cutaneous manifestations

Disorder	Enzyme affected	Inheritance
Porphyria cutanea tarda (cutaneous heptic porphyria)	Uroporphyrinogen decarboxylase	Autosomal dominant/ acquired
Variegate porphyria	Protoporphyrinogen oxidase	Autosomal dominant
Erythropoietic porphyria (Gunther's disease)	Uroporphyrinogen cosynthetase	Autosomal recessive
Erythropoietic photoporphyria	Ferrocheletase	Autosomal dominant

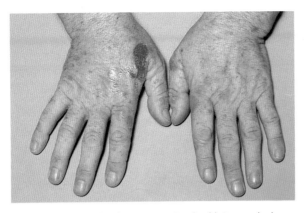

Figure 17.1 Porphyria cutanea tarda. Note eroded areas in light-exposed areas of the backs of the hands.

CLINICAL FEATURES

When associated with alcoholic liver disease the disorder is more often seen in middle-aged men. The characteristic features are seen in the light-exposed areas. In the early stages of the disease, blistering and fragility of the skin on the face and backs of the hands are noted (Figure 17.1). The affected areas also develop an odd pigmented and mauve suffused appearance (Figure 17.2). Later, increased hair growth occurs on the involved skin and a sclerodermiform thickening of the skin occurs. The diagnosis is made by finding increased uroporphyrins and coproporphyrins in the stools and urine. If available, monochromator testing (to irradiate the skin with very narrow bands of light or ultraviolet radiation) will reveal photosensitivity at 404 nm.

PATHOLOGY AND PATHOGENESIS

The enzyme defect results in abnormal amounts of the metabolites uroporphyrin III and coproporphyrin III accumulating in the tissues. These substances are responsible for the photosensitization. Histologically the blistering is subepidermal and in the long-standing case fibrosis develops and deposits of immunoglobulin are found perivascularly.

TREATMENT

The objective is to reduce the circulating levels of porphyrins. This is achieved by regular venesection – removing a pint at a time (every two or three weeks), or by the use of chloroquine orally resulting in accretion of large amounts of porphyrins in the urine.

Porphyria variegata

This is a very rare combination of PCT and acute intermittent porphyria. The latter is caused by a deficiency of delta-aminolaevulinic acid synthetase and is precipitated by certain drugs and anaesthesia, amongst other things. It will not be discussed further here other than to say that it often presents as attacks of abdominal pain and is potentially fatal. The condition is inherited as a dominant characteristic.

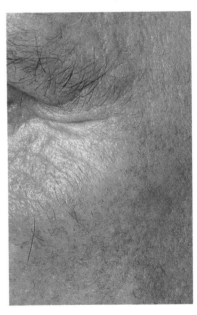

Figure 17.2 Suffused, slightly pigmented and hairy area on upper cheek and area lateral to orbit in a patient with porphyria cutanea tarda.

263

Erythropoietic protoporphyria

EPP is a very rare autosomal dominant disorder in which excess protoporphyrins are produced.

Erythropoietic protoporphyria (EPP) is a very rare autosomal recessive disorder in which excess protoporphyrins are produced. These are detectable in the blood and this forms the basis of diagnostic tests. Clinically the disorder often presents in childhood as episodes of skin soreness and extreme discomfort when exposed to the sun. Swelling, redness and urticarial lesions may develop in exposed skin. Later, fine pitted scarring is found on exposed sites. Pigment gall stones may develop.

Erythropoietic porphyria (Gunther's disease)

This is another very rare abnormality of porphyrin metabolism inherited as an autosomal recessive disorder. Affected individuals are extremely photosensitive and shun the light. They develop dreadful facial scarring, with hirsutes. This combination of clinical features has suggested to some that these patients provoked the fable of 'were wolves'.

Haemochromatosis (bronzed diabetes)

In primary haemochromatosis there is excessive gastrointestinal absorption of iron, resulting in iron deposition in the liver, testes, skin and pancreas. The brown-grey pigmentation is due to both the iron and increased melanin.

There are primary and symptomatic forms of this disorder. In the primary form there appears to be excessive gastrointestinal absorption of iron, resulting in iron deposition in the liver, testes, skin and pancreas. Involvement of the skin causes a brown-grey pigmentation due to both the iron and increased melanin in the skin. There is diabetes due to deposition of iron in the pancreas and cirrhosis from liver involvement. The condition seems to be inherited as a recessive characteristic but is much more common in men.

Secondary forms are found in conditions necessitating repeated blood transfusion and in conditions in which there is chronic haemolysis (e.g. sickle cell disease). It is also found in some African groups whose ingestion of iron is excessive alongside excess alcohol intake.

Anderson-Fabry disease (angiokeratoma corporis diffusum)

DEFINITION

This is a metabolic disorder inherited as a sex-linked recessive characteristic in which abnormal glycophingolipid is deposited in endothelial cells in particular.

CLINICAL FEATURES

There are myriads of tiny (1–2 mm) angiomata on the skin surface that develop gradually during adolescent years and early manhood. Neural involvement causes shooting pains in the lower half of the body. Renal involvement causes progressive renal failure and then death.

PATHOGENESIS

There is a deficiency in the lysosomal enzyme alpha-galactosidase resulting in the accumulation of neutral glycosphingolipids, such as trihexosylceramide, within small blood vessel walls.

Amyloidosis

Amyloidosis is the term used for a group of disorders in which an abnormal protein is deposited in tissues. Generalized amyloidosis is divided into the primary and secondary forms. The latter develops after long-standing inflammatory disease including infections such as chronic tuberculosis and chronic osteomyelitis. It may also occur in patients with long-standing severe rheumatoid arthritis. There are no skin manifestations in secondary amyloidosis. In primary amyloidosis the abnormal protein components are synthesized by clones of abnormal plasma cells and the condition is sometimes associated with multiple myeloma. In primary amyloid disease amyloid is deposited in the heart, nerves and skin as well as in the organs in which it is found in secondary amyloidosis. In the skin it is deposited in and around the dermal capillary blood vessels which become fragile and leaky. Swollen mauve-purple areas develop around the eyes and around the flexures.

> In primary amyloidosis abnormal protein components are synthesized by clones of abnormal plasma cells.

> Amyloid is deposited in the heart, spleen, kidneys, nerves and skin. In the skin it is deposited in and around the dermal capillary blood vessels which become fragile and leaky.

There are also 'amyloid' disorders which are restricted to the skin. In the rare macular amyloid, itchy, 'rippled' brown macular areas appear over the trunk (Figure 17.3). It seems more common in women and in patients of Asian origin. Histologically the deposits of amyloid are detectable subepidermally. Lichen amyloidosis is another rare cutaneous form of amyloid in which lichen planus-like lesions occur.

Amyloid can be detected in tissue using various histochemical tests including birifringence with Congo red and fluorescence with thioflavine T, as well as immunocytochemical tests.

TREATMENT
There is no effective curative treatment for amyloidosis.

Xanthomata

Xanthomata are deposits of lipid in histiocytes in skin and may be associated with normal levels of lipids in the blood (normolipaemic) or with elevated levels of serum lipids (hyperlipidaemia). The lipidized histiocytes have a characteristic 'foamy' appearance. The main hyperlipidaemic conditions are set out in Table 17.2.

> Xanthomata are deposits of lipid in histiocytes in skin.

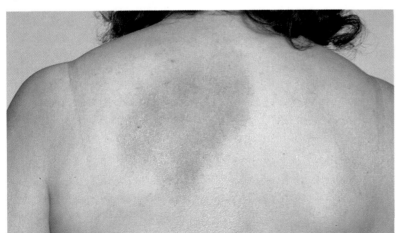

Figure 17.3 Pigmented area on the back in macular amyloid.

Table 17.2   The hyperlipidaemias (World Health Organization classification)

Type	Plasma cholesterol	Plasma triglycerides	Lipoproteins elevated	Inheritance	Skin lesions	Systemic manifestations	Some precipitating causes
I	N ↑	↑↑↑	Chylomicrons	Autosomal recessive (Burger-Grutz disease)	Eruptive xanthomas	Pancreatitis; Hepatosplenomegaly; Lipaemia retinalis	Dysglobulinaemia; Systemic lupus erythematosus and dermatomyositis
II	↑↑ / ↑↑	N / ↑	LDL / LDL, VLDL	Autosomal dominant (familial hyper-choleste-reraemia)	Xanthelasma; Tendon/tuberous xanthoma	Corneal arcus; Accelerated atherosclerosis	Excess dietary cholesterol; Hypothyroidism; Acute intermittent porphyria; Nephrotic syndrome; Multiple myeloma; Obstructive liver disease; Cyclosporin
III	↑↑	↑↑	Chylomicron remnants IDL	Uncertain	Planar xanthoma, Eruptive and tendon xanthoma	Accelerated atherosclerosis	Dysglobulinaemia Hypothyroidism
IV	N ↑	↑↑	VLDL	Uncertain	Eruptive xanthoma	Accelerated atherosclerosis Glucose intolerance Hyperuricaemia	Dermatomyositis Excess alcohol Pregnancy Nephrotic syndrome Isotretinoin
V	N ↑	↑↑↑	VLDL Chylomicrons	Uncertain	Eruptive xanthoma	Pancreatitis Hepatosplenomegaly Sensory neuropathy Lipaemia retinalis Hyperuricaemia Glucose intolerance	Alcoholism Diabetes mellitus Dysglobulinaemia

LDL = low density lipoproteins, VLDL = very low density lipoproteins.

Xanthalasma

Xanthelasma is a common form of xanthoma in which lesions appear as papules and arcuate or linear plaques around the eyes (Figure 17.4). The condition is not associated with hyperlipidaemia in 60–70% of patients. If their presence is cosmetically displeasing they can be removed by excision or topical treatment with trichloracetic acid. The latter should only be used with great care as the acid can produce serious burns if it is used incorrectly. The area around the lesion should be protected with Vaseline and the surface of the lesion lightly wiped with a cotton wool swab moistened with the acid. In a few seconds the area treated turns white and later a scale/crust forms.

> Xanthelasma is a common form of xanthoma in which lesions appear as papules and arcuate or linear plaques around the eyes.

Xanthoma tuberosum

The lesions of xanthoma tuberosum are large nodules of lipidized histiocytes and giant cells that develop around the tendons and extensor aspects of the joints in familial hyperlipidaemia (Table 17.2). Frequently affected sites include over the achilles tendon and the knees and elbows (Figure 17.5).

> Xanthoma tuberosum are nodules of lipidized histiocytes that develop around the tendons and extensor aspects of the joints in familial hyperlipidaemia.

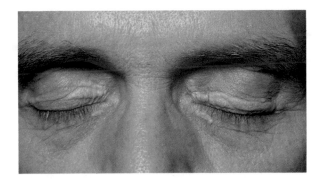

Figure 17.4 Yellowish plaques on eyelids in xanthalasma.

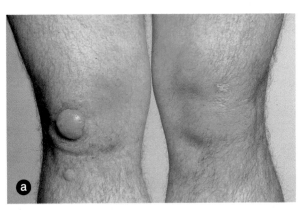
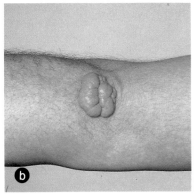

Figure 17.5 (a) Xanthoma tuberosum affecting the knee. (b) Xanthoma tuberosum affecting the elbow.

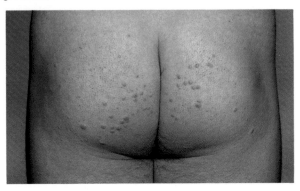

Figure 17.6 Yellowish-pink papules on buttocks in eruptive xanthoma.

Eruptive xanthomas

These mostly develop in diabetes but are also seen in congenital deficiencies of lipoprotein lipase (Burger Grütz disease) (Table 17.2). Large numbers of yellowish-pink papules develop all over the skin surface in a relatively short period of time (Figure 17.6).

TREATMENT

Treatment of these xanthomatous disorders is based on treatment of any underlying disease, diet and the use of lipid lowering agents (such as clofibrate, bezafibrate or gemfibrozil) in some cases.

Necrobiotic disorders

The term 'necrobiosis' is unfortunate in that it means literally 'death–life' but has come to be applied to a particular histological change in the dermal connective tissue. The necrobiotic areas are foci of damage where the dermal structure is 'blurred' and more eosinophilic than usual. It is surrounded by inflammatory cells – lymphocytes, histiocytes and occasional giant cells (Figure 17.7).

Granuloma annulare

This not uncommon inflammatory disorder is characterized by papules and plaques that adopt a ring-like pattern (Figure 17.8). It is quite common in children and young adults in whom it is most often seen as one or several lesions on the extensor aspects of the fingers, dorsa of the feet, hands and wrists.

Granuloma annulare tends to last for a few months and then disappear as mysteriously as it came. Treatment is generally not indicated but individual lesions respond to intralesional corticosteroids.

A much less frequent type is known as generalized superficial granuloma annulare in which the raised ring-like structure is not evident but is characterized by macular dull red or mauve areas (Figure 17.9) that have a necrobiotic structure histologically.

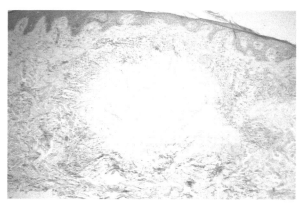

Figure 17.7 Pathology of granuloma annulare demonstrating central necrobiotic area surrounded by inflammatory cells.

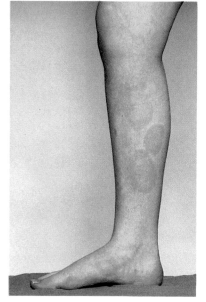

Figure 17.9 Flat pink patches due to diffuse granuloma annulare. This patient also had diabetes.

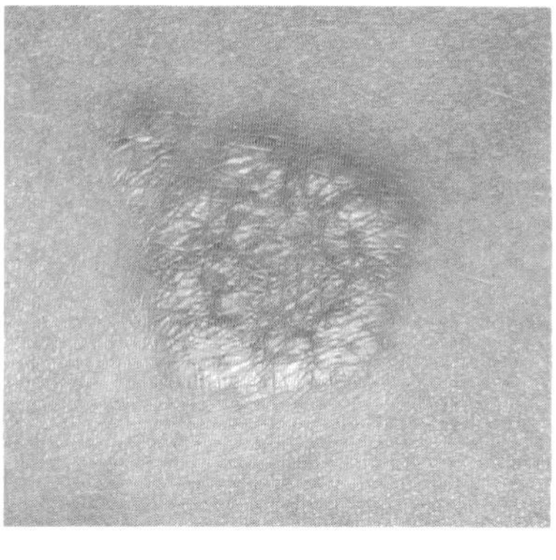

Figure 17.8 Typical ring of pale pink papules in granuloma annulare.

Granuloma annulare is a quite common inflammatory disorder in which granulomatous inflammation occurs around degenerate dermal collogen causing rings of papules on extensor surfaces.

Necrobiosis lipoidica diabeticorum

This condition is seen in 0.3% diabetics and is strongly associated with the diabetic state. It occurs mainly on the lower legs as yellowish-pink papules which persist and become atrophic (page 289). It is also characterized by necrobiotic foci histologically.

Reticulohistiocytic proliferative disorders

There is a group of poorly understood disorders which include Letterer-Siwe disease (LSD), Hand Schüller Christian disease (HSCD), eosinophilic granuloma (EG), xanthoma disseminatum (XD) and juvenile xanthogranuloma (JX). Letterer-Siwe disease, HSCD and EG seem to belong to the same 'family of diseases' in which there appears to be a reactive proliferation of Langerhans cells. It has been suggested that the proliferation of Langerhans cells is neoplastic, but the evidence for this is thin.

Letterer-Siwe disease is a very uncommon disorder of infants and young children, characterized by a papular and scaling eruption of flexures, trunk and scalp, with some resemblance to seborrhoeic dermatitis. In the skin there is a dense infiltrate of cells having the ultrastructural and immunocytochemical characteristics of Langerhans cells. There may be severe malaise and hepatosplenomegaly and some patients succumb. Treatment with corticosteroids and cytotoxic agents may be required.

Hand Schüller Christian disease is a rare disorder of young adults in which abnormal Langerhans cell deposits occur in the lung, pituitary, bone and orbit mostly. In EG the deposits are for the most part limited to the bony skeleton.

Xanthoma disseminatum and JX do not belong to the same 'Langerhans cell' group of disorders but are characterized by the presence of lipidized histiocytes, giant cells and an admixture of other cell types. Lesions of JX occur in young infants as isolated or limited numbers of yellowish-pink nodules which eventually disappear spontaneously. In XD large numbers of papular lesions develop on all parts of the skin, and sometimes mucosae, which often persist for long periods but usually have no serious consequences.

CHAPTER

18

Disorders of hair and nails

Both hair and nails are epidermal structures that arise from invaginations of the epidermis into the skin (Figures 18.1 and 18.2). Both hair and nails may be involved in generalized skin disorders and occasionally may develop signs of disorder such as psoriasis or lichen planus in the absence of obvious skin disease. In addition there are disorders that are confined to either the hair or the nails.

Disorders of hair (Table 18.1)

Hair loss (alopecia)
Hair loss may be diffuse over the scalp or localized to one or several sites on the scalp. The process may also be destructive and cause scarring or may be nonscarring in nature.

Congenital alopecia
Congenital alopecia may occur in isolation or alongside other congenital disorders. Rarely scalp hair growth is very slow and hair shaft density is

Table 18.1 Overview of hair disorders

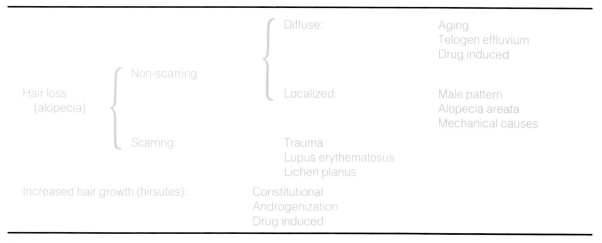

270

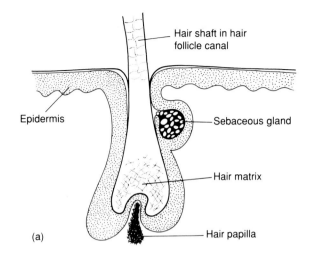

Hair shaft in hair
follicle canal

Epidermis

Sebaceous gland

Hair matrix

(a)

Hair papilla

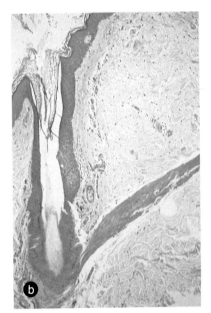

b

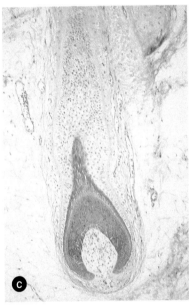

c

Figure 18.1 (a) Diagram of a hair follicle showing the relationship between the hair shaft, follicular epithelium and sebaceous glands. (b) Photomicrograph to show hair follicle on the scalp with arector pilerum muscles. (c) Photomicrograph to show hair follicle on the scalp with prominent hair matrix and hair papillae.

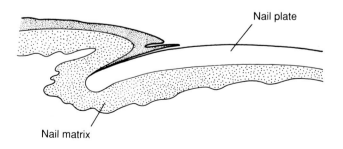

Nail plate

Nail matrix

Figure 18.2 Diagram to show nail plate and nail matrix tissue that forms it.

271

low (*congenital hypotrichosis*). A patch of scarring over the vertex with hair loss is one other uncommon type of congenital alopecia.

Diffuse hair loss sometimes accompanies the congenital disorders of keratinization, for example, lamellar ichthyosis and anhidrotic ectodermal defect.

Pattern alopecia

DEFINITION

A common, dominantly inherited, progressive form of alopecia which develops symmetrically at certain specific sites on the scalp and eventually causes almost complete scalp hair loss in some patients and which is much more common in men.

> Male pattern alopecia is a common, dominantly inherited, progressive form of alopecia which develops symmetrically at certain specific sites on the scalp and eventually causes almost complete scalp hair loss in some patients which is much more common in men.

CLINICAL FEATURES

Loss of hair starts in both temporal regions. Shortly after this bitemporal recession (Figure 18.3) thinning of the hair and then alopecia develops over the vertex (Figure 18.4). The bald area over the vertex expands to meet the triangular temporal bald areas until in the worst cases almost complete loss of hair results (Figure 18.5). A general reduction in the density of hair follicles also occurs and this may be the main feature of the disorder in women. Women do develop bitemporal recession and some vertical thinning but this is much less common than in men.

The condition may start as early as in the late 'teens but generally declares its presence in the third decade. Its rate of progress varies and

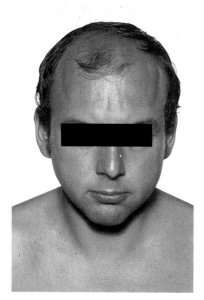

Figure 18.3 Male pattern alopecia with bitemporal recession.

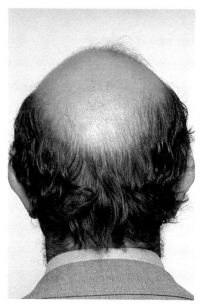

Figure 18.4 Male pattern alopecia showing typical loss over the vertex.

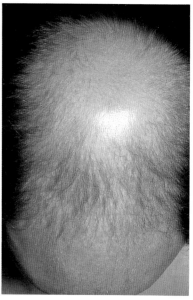

Figure 18.5 Severe male pattern alopecia.

seems uninfluenced by environmental factors. It occurs in all racial groups but may be more frequent and severe in some.

Pattern alopecia causes an enormous amount of psychological distress and patients will go to extraordinary lengths to attempt to arrest and reverse the process and/or to disguise its presence. The condition is firmly embedded in popular mythology with regard to its supposed causes that range from dietary deficiencies to sexual excesses and the supposed attributes and characteristics of its sufferers. It would be amusing if it wasn't for the genuine distress of patients with pattern alopecia.

PATHOLOGY AND PATHOGENESIS

The hair follicles in the affected areas become smaller and sparser and eventually disappear. Finally true atrophy of the skin occurs at the involved sites. The disorder is dominantly inherited but requires androgenic stimulus in the form of testosterone and the passing of the years for full phenotypic expression. The disorder can be precipitated by the administration of testosterone to female patients and is also a sign of masculinization in patients with a testosterone-secreting tumour. The molecular events responsible for the defervescence of hair follicles in particular sites on the scalp have yet to be unravelled but it is likely that the mechanism is related to the basis of hair growth as testosterone plays an important role in the normal growth and development of hair.

TREATMENT

There is no effective treatment. Its progress in men may be halted by castration, but there are few patients who would undergo (or indeed physicians who would perform) this operation for this purpose. In women 'chemical castration' with the use of an antiandrogen–prostagen combination (cyproterone acetate and ethinylestranol – Dianette) has been tried and some reduction in the rate of hair loss claimed. In recent years the antihypertensive vasodilator minoxidil has also been used topically as increased hair growth was noted as a side effect from its oral use. Although the drug may increase hair growth in 20–30% of patients, the hair is lost again when treatment stops, and the extent to which hair regrowth occurs in the relatively few in whom there is any regrowth is modest. Increased efficacy has been claimed for combinations of minoxidil with tretinoin. However, it has to be quite clearly and categorically stated that currently there is no effective medical treatment.

> It has to be quite clearly and categorically stated – currently there is no effective medical treatment for pattern alopecia.

Pattern hair loss in men may be disguised in a number of ways, including:

1. hair pieces (wigs, toupées);
2. hair weaving in which the remaining hair is woven to cover the defect;
3. plastic surgical manoeuvres in which plugs of hair-containing skin from the scalp periphery are transplanted to holes made in the bald area or flaps of skin are advanced over bald areas.

Alopeia areata

DEFINITION

Alopecia areata (AA) is an
autoimmune disorder of hair-
bearing areas of skin in which
there is perifollicular accumulation
of lymphocytes and loss of hair in
sharply defined areas of skin.

Alopecia areata (AA) is an autoimmune disorder of hair-bearing areas of the skin in which there is perifollicular accumulation of lymphocytes and loss of hair in sharply defined areas of skin.

CLINICAL FEATURES

Alopecia areata often starts quite suddenly as one or more rounded patches from which the hair is lost (Figure 18.6). The hair loss continues over some days or for several weeks, until all the hair from the affected sites has fallen. The individual areas vary in size from 1 cm^2 to involvement of the entire scalp (alopecia totalis); rarely the eyelashes and eyebrows (Figure 18.7), and all body hair is lost as well.

Affected areas may extend outwards and disease activity can be recognized by the appearance of so-called 'exclamation mark' hairs at the margin of the lesions. It occurs over a wide age range of 5 to 50 years but seems particularly frequent between the ages of 15 and 30 years.

Regrowth of AA patches occurs in most patients if the affected areas are small, limited in number, and the affected individual is 15 years old or less. When regrowth occurs the new hair is fine and nonpigmented (Figure 18.8). The outlook for regrowth worsens when large areas are affected, the patient is over 30 years old, and the subject also has atopic dermatitis.

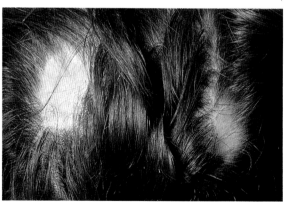

Figure 18.6 Small discrete areas of hair loss in alopecia areata.

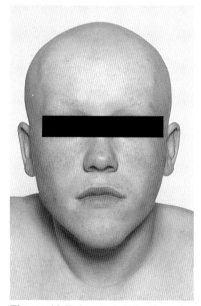

Figure 18.7 Areata totalis: there is loss of eyebrows too.

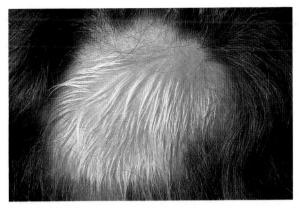

Figure 18.8 Large patch of alopecia areata showing regrowth of nonpigmented hair.

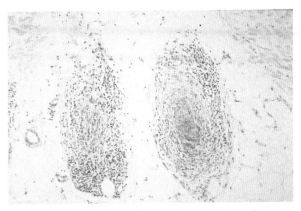

Figure 18.9 Pathology of alopecia areata showing collections of lymphocytes around hair follicle tissue.

PATHOLOGY AND PATHOGENESIS

The disorder is positively associated with autoimmune disorders including vitiligo and thyrotoxicosis, and it has been assumed that an immune attack is launched against components of the hair follicle. When biopsies are taken from an actively extending patch a dense 'bee swarm' – like cluster of lymphocytes can be seen around the follicles (Figure 18.9). When the inflammation has passed, small hairless follicles whose growth has been arrested can be seen.

> The disorder is positively associated with autoimmune disorders including vitiligo and thyrotoxicosis, and it has been assumed that an immune attack is launched against components of the hair follicle.

DIFFERENTIAL DIAGNOSIS

The main differential diagnoses are trichotillomania and tinea capitis (page 35). Patches of baldness due to trichotillomania are bizarrely shaped, are not as well demarcated as AA, and have no exclamation mark hairs at the edge. Tinea capitis is marked by broken hairs and by a degree of redness and scaling of the scalp skin. Disorders that inflame the skin and destroy hair follicles, producing scarring alopecia (page 278) may give a superficial resemblance to AA but because of the scarring can usually be easily differentiated.

TREATMENT

Patients with a solitary patch or a small number of patches usually do not need treatment. When the patches coalesce to become cosmetically a problem or when there is alopecia totalis, treatment is often demanded by patients, but is not often very effective. The following treatments have been used: topical potent or systemic steroids; photo-chemotherapy with ultraviolet radiation of the 'A' type (PUVA) to the scalp (both with systemic psoralens and topical psoralens); dithranol; allergic sensitization with diphencyprone; topical minoxidil; systemic (and topical) cyclosporin. Although each of the above have been credited by their proponents with a degree of success, they all have inconvenient side effects and usually work only while they are being given. Probably the most appropriate treatment to try for an otherwise young healthy individual with extensive AA is allergic sensitization with diphencyprone. The treatment produces an eczematous rash which is maintained by repeated application of the substance in a 1% solution. It is not known why this should 'kick' the hair follicles back into life.

Many patients, having experienced the side effects and the frustration of the lack of efficacy of one or several of the treatments, decide to cut their losses and disguise their disability with a wig. The condition is always depressing for the patient, and sympathy and support are the most useful applications.

> No treatment for AA is reliably effective but the most appropriate treatment to try is sensitization with diphencyprone.

Diffuse hair loss

This is predominantly a problem for middle-aged and elderly women although younger women and men occasionally present with this symptom. It is not a single entity and the causes include pattern alopecia and virilization; hypothyroidism; systemic illness such as systemic lupus erythematosus; and drug administration (particularly the anticancer drugs and the systemic retinoids). Diffuse hair loss is also caused by telogen effluvium (see below). Aging also results in a lesser density of hair follicles which is more obvious in some subjects than others. Having considered the possible causes listed above, there are still some patients with obvious diffuse hair loss of concern for whom there is no adequate explanation. Various deficiency states (particularly iron) have been incriminated but in the majority of instances the supposed deficiency appears to have no other sequel and attempts at its rectification fail to improve the clinical state.

Many patients become very depressed over their hair loss and need considerable sympathy and support. If there is no obvious cause for their diffuse hair loss the only medical treatment available is topical minoxidil (the antihypertensweding which has a small effect on hair growth) but this is unlikely to give substantial benefit.

> Sudden illness may precipitate hair follicles into the telogen phase of the hair cycle causing hair loss some 10–12 weeks later.

Telogen effluvium

The human hair cycle (Figure 18.10) is asynchronous but can be precipitated into a form of synchrony by childbirth, or a sudden severe systemic illness such as pneumonia or massive blood loss. The stimulus of one of the above causes all the scalp hair follicles to revert to the telogen or resting phase (see Figure 18.10). When this occurs there is a sudden and significant loss of terminal scalp hair some three months after the precipitating event which continues for a few weeks but then spontaneously stops. Hair regrowth gradually restores the scalp hair to its original state.

276

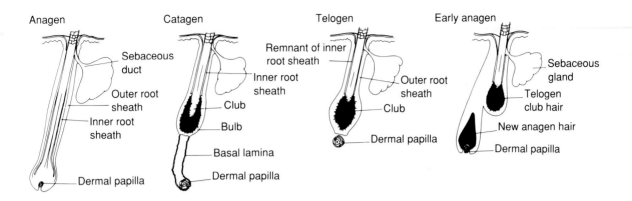

Figure 18.10 Diagram showing the various stages of the human hair cycle.

Traction alopecia

Repeated tugging and pulling on the hair shaft may produce loss of hair in the affected areas. It can result from a 'chronic pulling' as occurs when hair rollers are used (Figure 18.11). It can also develop in young children when they continually rub their scalp on their pillow. More confusingly, older children and occasionally young adults tug at their hair, producing the same effect in a bizarre distribution over the scalp (trichitillomania) (Figure 18.12). The motivation for this strange behaviour usually remains obscure but luckily the condition does not tend to persist and the hair regrows. The main differential diagnosis is alopecia areata but other disorders that cause patchy loss of scalp hair need to be considered.

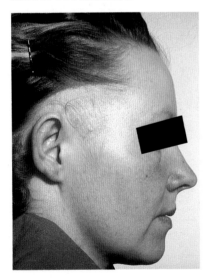

Figure 18.11 Traction alopecia due to the use of rollers.

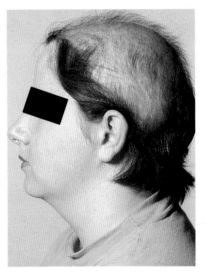

Figure 18.12 Trichotillomania. A bizarre pattern of hair loss from the scalp due to constant tugging of the hair.

Scarring alopecia

Any process that causes severe inflammation of scalp skin or traumatizes it is sufficient to cause loss of follicles and scar formation will result in permanent loss of hair in the affected area. Mechanical trauma, burns and damage from X-rays can produce scarring alopecia. Bacterial infections and severe inflammatory ringworm of the scalp can produce sufficient damage to cause permanent hair loss.

The inflammatory disorders that produce scarring alopecia include discoid lupus erythematosus (page 72) and lichen planus (page 142). In both of these diseases the scalp skin may be obviously and characteristically affected by the dermatosis concerned but it may be difficult to distinguish the two disorders, even after biopsy. Usually the affected area is scarred and there is loss of follicular orifices – the few remaining being distorted and dilated and containing tufts of hair (Figure 18.13). An odd type of scalp scarring known as '*pseudopelade*' is characterized by small rounded patches of scarring alopecia without any inflammation but is thought to be the end results of either discoid lupus erythematosus or lichen planus.

Hair shaft disorders

Hair shaft abnormalities may be either congenital or acquired. The subject has received much impetus from the use of the scanning electron microscope to characterize the disorders. Acquired abnormalities are more often seen. All long hairs tend to become 'weathered' at their ends due to climatic exposure and the usual washing and combing routines.

Twisting hairs between the fingers, and other obsessive manipulation of hair, results in a specific type of damage to the hair shafts known as

> Any process that causes severe inflammation of scalp skin or traumatizes it sufficiently to cause loss of follicles and scar formation will result in permanent loss of hair in the affected area.

> The inflammatory disorders that produce scarring alopecia include discoid lupus erythematosus and lichen planus.

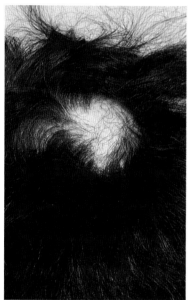

Figure 18.13 Scarring alopecia due to discoid lupus erythematosus.

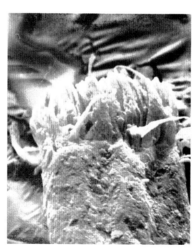

Figure 18.14 Scanning electron micrograph showing fractured hair shaft and paint brush-like end in the condition of trichorrhexis nodosa.

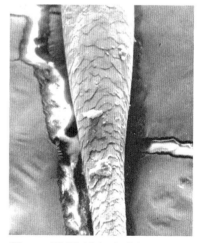

Figure 18.15 Hair shaft in monilethrix showing alternate fusiform expansions and thinning of hair shaft in this congenital disorder.

trichorrhexis nodosa (TN). In TN, expansions of the shaft (nodes) can be seen by routine light microscopy and scanning electron microscopy. These nodes rupture, and leave frayed 'paint brush' – like ends (Figure 18.14). This deformity leads to broken hairs and even to the complaint of loss of hair. Another obvious acquired change in the hair shaft is the so-called 'flag sign' of kwashiorkor in which a band at the same point on all the hairs becomes a light red in colour coinciding with times of severe protein deficiency (page 295).

Isolated congenital hair shaft disorders include the condition of *monilethrix* in which there are spindle-like expansions of the hair shaft at regular intervals (Figure 18.15) causing weakness and breaking of the scalp hair. Various abnormalities also occur as part of rare disorders of keratinization but these are outside the scope of this text.

Disorders of the nails

Psoriasis, lichen planus and eczema may each affect the nails secondarily, giving rise to characteristic clinical appearances. *Psoriasis* (page 125) characteristically causes 'thimble pitting' of the finger nails (Figure 18.16). It also causes well-defined pink-brown areas and onycholysis (separation of nail plate from the nail bed, Figure 18.17). The toe nails rarely show these changes but the nail plates may be thickened, with a yellowish brown discolouration and subungual debris (Figure 18.18), often making it difficult to distinguish from ringworm of the nails (page 35). In *lichen planus* the nail plate may develop longitudinal ridging (Figure 18.19) which in the worst cases may penetrate the whole nail. Uncommonly the inflammatory process may destroy the nail matrix and cause permanent loss of the nail. *Eczema* affecting the fingers may cause irregular deformities of the finger nails and even marked horizontal ridging at times (Figure 18.20).

> Psoriasis characteristically causes 'thimble pitting' of the finger nails. It also causes well-defined pink-brown areas and onycholysis (separation of nail plate from the nail bed).

> In lichen planus the nail plate may develop longitudinal ridging.

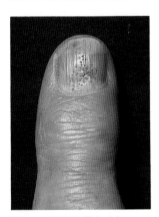

Figure 18.16 Thimble pitting of finger nail in psoriasis. There is also an area of onycholysis.

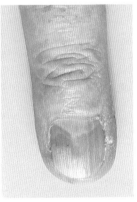

Figure 18.17 Finger nail in psoriasis showing marked onycholysis and some deformity of the nail plate.

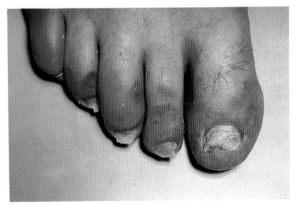

Figure 18.18 Thickened, deformed and yellowing toe nails due to psoriasis.

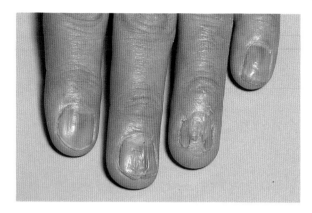

Figure 18.19 Longitudinally ridged finger nails in lichen planus.

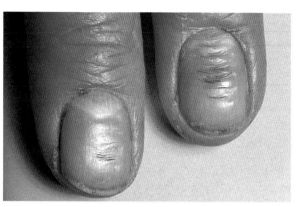

Figure 18.20 Horizontal ridging and deformity due to chronic eczema affecting the nails.

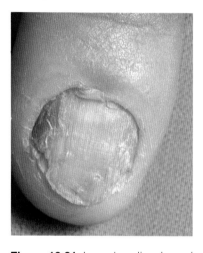

Figure 18.21 Irregular, discoloured nail plate seen in chronic paronychia.

Paronychia

This term is applied to inflammation of the tissues at the sides of the nail. In the common form of chronic paronychia the paronychial skin is thickened and reddened. It is often tender, and pus may be expressed from the space between the nail fold and the nail plate. The eponychium disappears and the nail plate is often discoloured and deformed (Figure 18.21) and may demonstrate onycholysis (see below). There is a deep recess between the nail fold and the nail plate, containing debris and micro-organisms, which is difficult to keep dry. The condition mostly occurs in women whose occupation involves frequent hand washing or other 'wet' activities (e.g. cooks, cleaners, barmaids) and it seems likely that the inability of this group of individuals to keep their hands dry contributes substantially to the condition's chronicity.

Candida micro-organisms may contribute to the recurrent inflammation to which the affected fingers are subject but they are not the cause of the disorder. The cause is compounded from mechanical trauma and overhydration resulting in microbial overgrowth in the nooks and crannies of the nail fold.

In the common form of chronic paronychia the paronychial skin is thickened and reddened. The eponychium disappears and the nail plate is often discoloured and deformed. The condition mostly occurs in women whose occupation involves frequent hand washing or other 'wet' activities.

TREATMENT

The major goals in management are keeping the fingers completely dry and the avoidance of manual work. Antimicrobial preparations in aqueous or alcoholic vehicles are also useful (e.g. povidone-iodine or an imidazole lotion). Acute exacerbations may need to be treated with systemic antibiotics.

Providing the advice is taken and the treatment used, patients usually improve within a few weeks.

Onycholysis

Onycholysis (Table 18.2) is not a disease but a physical sign in which the terminal nail plate separates from the underlying nail bed. It is observed in psoriasis, eczema, chronic paronychia, the 'yellow nail syndrome' (see below), thyrotoxicosis, from repeated mechanical trauma and for no known reason.

Brittle nails and onychorrhexis

A frequent complaint of middle-aged women is that their nails break easily and separate into horizontal strata (onychorrhexis) (Table 18.2). Various deficiencies have been incriminated without much evidence including iron deficiency and protein deficiency. Probably the single most important factor causing this problem is repeated hydration and drying as in housework, as well as mechanical and chemical trauma.

The nails in systemic disease

This is also briefly covered in Chapter 21. Onycholysis due to thyrotoxicosis has already been mentioned. In hypoalbuminaemia (as in severe liver disease) the lunulae may be lost and the nail plate turns a milky white. Beau's lines are horizontal ridges due to a sudden severe illness, trauma and/or blood loss (Figure 18.22) and presumably have the same significance as telogen effluvium. They grow outwards and are eventually lost.

Brown-black pigmentation

Pigmented linear bands along the length of the nail may be due to a mole, or if of recent onset may be caused by a malignant melanoma. Brown-black areas may be due to melanin or from haemosiderin from

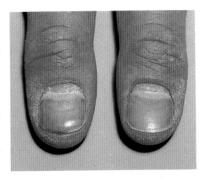

Figure 18.22 Beau's lines. These are horizontal ridges across the nail plate which occur at the time of severe systemic illness. In this patient they can be seen at the junction between the nail and the distal nail fold.

Table 18.2 Terms used to describe nail disease

Term	Meaning	Significance
Onycholysis	Separation of nail plate from nail bed	Observed in thyrotoxicosis, psoriasis, eczema, chronic paronychia, yellow nail syndrome and for no known cause
Onychorrhexis	Horizontal splitting of nail plate	Usually due to mechanical and chemical trauma or repeated hydration
Paronychia	Inflammation of paronychial tissues	

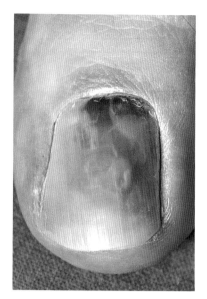

Figure 18.23 Subungual haematoma.

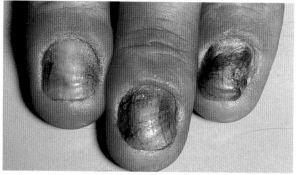

Figure 18.24 Nails in the yellow nail syndrome. The nails are discoloured a yellowish green and show increased curvature. There is also longitudinal eponychium.

trauma, and the two may be very difficult to tell apart (Figure 18.23). Uncommonly, Pseudomonas infection of the nail plate produces a diffuse black or black-green pigmentation. A blackish, yellow-green discolouration is also seen in the *yellow nail syndrome* (Figure 18.24). In this rare disease it is notable that nail growth is greatly slowed and apart from the altered colour, the nails are thickened and show increased curvature. In addition ankle and facial oedema, as well as sinusitis and pleural effusion, often accompany the condition. Unfortunately there is no adequate treatment.

Ringworm of the nails (tinea unguium) (page 35)

Ringworm of the toe nails is quite common but infection of the finger nails is quite uncommon. The affected nails are thickened and crumbly and are discoloured yellow or irregular yellowish white, or yellowish black or green (Figure 18.25). Subungual debris is often present. Affected finger nails show some thickening and discolouration only. Differential diagnosis includes psoriasis and paronychia as well as the rare yellow nail syndrome.

TREATMENT
Treatment is dealt with on page 36.

Figure 18.25 (a) Deformity, discolouration and subungal debris in a big toe nail due to ringworm infection (tinea unguium). (b) Here, the second toe is also affected.

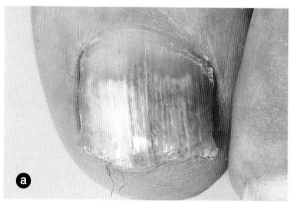

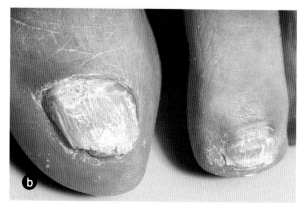

Systemic disease and the skin

Skin markers of malignant disease

There are a number of skin disorders which are sometimes precipitated by an underlying malignancy and there are others that almost always indicate a visceral neoplasm. Clearly it is important to recognize these conditions and deal with the underlying neoplastic disease as quickly as possible (Table 19.1).

Disorders with a strong association with underlying malignancy

Necrolytic migratory erythema
This is usually caused by a tumour of the pancreatic islet alpha cells

Table 19.1   Skin markers of malignant disease

Acquired ichthyosis	See Table 16.1
Acanthosis nigricans	Distinguish from pseudo-acanthosis nigricans; mostly associated with gastrointestinal adenocarcinoma
Dermatomyositis	Associated with several neoplastic diseases but particularly of the genital system in women over 40
Erythema gyratum repens	Very rare; strong association with underlying carcinoma
Necrolytic migratory erythema	Strong association with pancreatic alpha cell tumour – diabetes and low plasma amino acids accompany
Bullous pemphigoid	May be a weak association with malignancy, but not certain
Skin metastases	6% of all metastases; metastases from carcinomas of lung, prostate, breast, kidney and stomach

that secrete glucagon but it is sometimes caused by hyperplasia or benign adenomatosis of these cells, and rarely no underlying abnormality can be found at all.

CLINICAL FEATURES

Areas of erythema which become eroded and crusted (Figure 19.1) develop around the groins, on the lower trunk, around the flexures and at the sides of the mouths. They do not respond to treatment with topical agents but may temporarily remit at one site to appear elsewhere. The skin disorder responds to removal of the underlying tumour but mostly complete removal is not possible as the disorder is usually too advanced at the time of diagnosis.

PATHOLOGY AND PATHOGENESIS

Biopsy reveals a characteristic picture with degenerative change in the upper epidermis (Figure 19.2). Blood tests reveal increased circulating glucagon, hyperglycaemia and hypoaminoacidaemia and it is the latter that may be responsible for the curious skin disorder.

Acanthosis nigricans

Acanthosis nigricans may occur in association with endocrine disease and may also rarely accompanies lipodystrophies. A very similar clinical picture (if not identical) also accompanies obesity and is then known as pseudoacanthosis nigricans. When the condition occurs in an adult unaccompanied by obesity or endocrine disease an underlying neoplasm is usually the cause. The neoplasm involved is for the most part a gastrointestinal adenocarcinoma.

CLINICAL FEATURES

There is a velvety thickening and increased rugosity of the skin of the flexures – the axillae and groins in particular (Figure 19.3). The sides and back of the neck and the sides of the mouth are other affected sites.

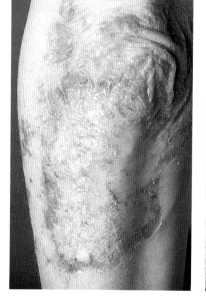

Figure 19.1 Necrolytic migratory erythema: area of erythema and erosion on the forearm.

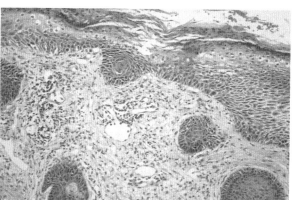

Figure 19.2 Pathology of necrolytic migratory erythema showing degenerative change in upper epidermis with crusting and parakeratosis.

The thickened areas are also pigmented and bear skin tags and seborrhoeic warts (Figure 19.4). There may also be some generalized increase in pigmentation as well as thickening and increased rugosity of the buccal mucosa and the palmar skin.

PATHOLOGY AND PATHOGENESIS
There is overall hypertrophy of all components of the skin of the affected areas. Insulin-like growth factors may be involved.

Erythema gyratum repens
This is probably the rarest of the specific skin markers of visceral malignancy. This odd disorder is almost always a marker of a neoplasm, often carcinoma of the bronchus.

> The conditions of necrolytic migratory erythema, acquired ichthyosis acanthosis nigricans and erythema gyratum repens are strongly associated with an underlying visceral malignancy.

CLINICAL FEATURES
Large rings composed of reddened polycyclic bands are seen, the rings contain concentric rings within, giving a wood grain effect (Figure 19.5). The rings gradually enlarge and change shape.

Rarely, other less dramatic types of annular erythema may be a sign of an internal malignancy.

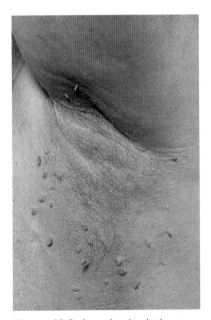

Figure 19.3 Acanthosis nigricans. Increased pigmentation and rugosity with skin tags in axilla.

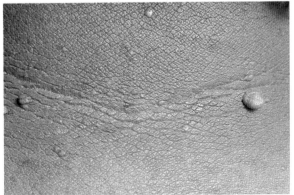

Figure 19.4 Acanthosis nigricans. Increased pigmentation, rugosity and skin tags around neck.

285

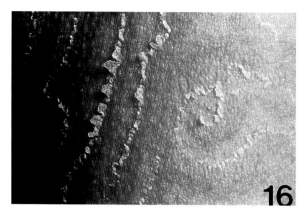

Figure 19.5 Erythema gyratum repens in a patient with carcinoma of the lung. Note the concentric areas of scaling.

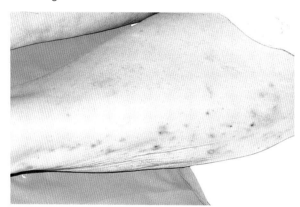

Figure 19.6 Numerous small metastases from carcinoma of the vulva.

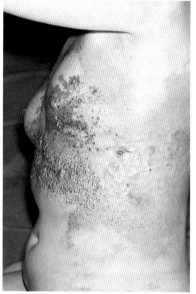

Figure 19.7 Numerous metastases affecting chest wall from carcinoma of the breast.

Skin metastases

Carcinoma of the breast, bronchus, stomach, kidney and prostate are the most frequent visceral neoplasms to metastasize to the skin. Secondary deposits on the skin may be the first sign of the underlying visceral cancer. The lesions themselves are usually smooth nodules which are pink or skin coloured (Figure 19.6) (but may be pigmented in deposits of melanoma). Secondary deposits may also be the result of spread from a lesion in the same region of the body, for example, from carcinoma of the breast (Figure 19.7).

Acquired ichthyosis (page 257)

When generalized scaling without erythema starts for the first time in adult life there is a strong likelihood of there being an underlying neoplasm. It has to be distinguished from mild dryness of the skin and slight irritation seen in many chronic disorders, known as xeroderma.

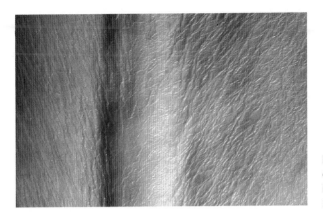

Figure 19.8 This woman suddenly developed 'dry and itchy' skin. On investigation she was found to have Hodgkin's disease.

Other causes of acquired ichthyosis include acquired immune deficiency syndrome (AIDS), some lipid lowering drugs (such as nicotinic acid and butyrophenones), sarcoidosis and leprosy, but if these can be excluded then a neoplastic cause is by far the most likely explanation (Figure 19.8).

Disorders that are sometimes associated with underlying malignant disease

Bullous pemphigoid (page 83)
This subepidermal blistering disorder occurs mainly in those over 60 years of age who are anyway more likely to be affected by a neoplasm. Notwithstanding this, there does appear to be a small cohort of patients with pemphigoid whose skin disorder is provoked by the malignancy and which remits after the neoplasm has been removed.

> Dermatomyositis is occasionally and bullous pemphigoid rarely associated with underlying malignant disease.

Dermatomyositis (page 78)
Without the cutaneous component this disorder is known as polymyositis. The association with malignant disease is real but uncertain in magnitude as in some groups the association is closer than in others. Women over the age of 40 years with dermatomyositis may have a 50% chance of a malignant tumour of the genitourinary tract but infants with the disease have no greater risk than a control group. Overall, even in adults, the association is not common and most cases of dermatomyositis occur without an identifiable cause. There is the clinical impression that dermatomyositis provoked by malignant disease is more severe than 'nonmalignant' varieties.

Figurate erythemas
Rarely, annular erythema and erythema multiforme (page 69) seem to be caused by underlying malignant disease.

Endocrine disease, diabetes and the skin

The skin is responsive to many endocrine stimuli and in endocrine disease the skin's reactions to the abnormal hormone environment may result in symptoms and signs.

Thyroid disease

The most notorious of the thyroid-skin associations is the condition known as *pretibial myxoedema*. This disorder is characterized by reddened elevated plaques, often with a *peau d'orange* appearance on the surface (Figure 19.9). Histologically they can be seen to consist of a cellular connective tissue with deposition of mucinous material. The serum from such patients contains substances that can be shown to stimulate growth and activity of fibroblasts.

The condition is almost always a sign of thyrotoxicosis and is accompanied by exophthalmos. It has been found to occur in 5% of patients with thyrotoxicosis. It is quite persistent and difficult to treat although treatment with photochemotherapy with ultraviolet radiation of the 'A' type (PUVA) seems to be successful on some occasions. Rarely there is diffuse infiltration with similar mucinous connective tissue of the hands and feet and finger clubbing in the condition of *thyroid acropachy*. Patients with thyrotoxicosis have warm, sweaty skin, and a proportion complain of pruritus. Thyroid hormone is stimulatory to epidermal growth and metabolism but it is not known whether this is responsible for the clinical changes observed.

In myxoedema the skin often feels dry and rough and may have a

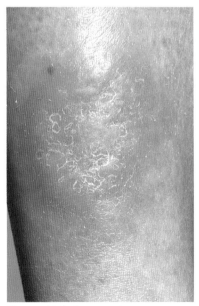

Figure 19.9 Plaque of pretibial myxoedema.

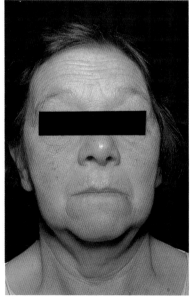

Figure 19.10 Myxoedema demonstrating thickened skin and 'peaches and cream' appearance.

yellowish orange tint as carotenaemia may accompany the disorder. In addition there may be coarsening of the scalp hair with some hair loss. Characteristically there is loss of the outer third of the eyebrows, some puffiness of the face with pinkish cheeks but a yellowish background colour – the so-called peaches and cream complexion (Figure 19.10).

> In myxoedema the skin often feels dry and rough and may have a yellowish orange tint as carotenaemia may accompany the disorder.

> Pretibial myxoedema and thyroid acropachy are conditions associated with thyrotoxicosis in which there is infiltration of dermal connective tissue with mucinous substances.

Parathyroid disease

Disturbances of calcium metabolism certainly affect the skin. Calcium plays an important part in epidermal growth and differentiation and it is not surprising that clinical changes occur when calcium balance is disturbed. Acute attacks of pustular psoriasis may be precipitated by hypocalcaemia. In hyperparathyroidism there is sometimes intractable pruritus and in both hypo- and hyperparathyroidism the skin may feel dry and rough.

Diabetes

Necrobiosis lipoidica

The skin manifestations of diabetes are summarized in Table 19.2. The most specific is necrobiosis lipoidica. Of individuals who present with this disorder, more than 50% will already have insulin-dependent diabetes. A substantial number of those who do not have diabetes when they present with their skin disorder will develop diabetes or have a first degree relative with diabetes.

Table 19.2   Skin manifestations of diabetes

Necrobiosis lipoidica	Majority of patients with this disorder eventually have diabetes
Diffuse granuloma annulare	Rare type of granuloma annulare with strong association with diabetes
Xanthomas	Eruptive xanthomas seen in uncontrolled diabetes
Neuropathic ulceration	Due to neuropathy; perforating ulcers on sole of foot may occur
Ischaemic changes and infection	Increased incidence and severity of atherosclerosis and microvascular disease may lead to ischaemic necrosis and increased incidence of skin infection

Clinical features

Typically, irregular yellowish-pink plaques occur on the lower legs and around the ankles (Figure 19.11). Uncommonly lesions may occur elsewhere. Areas of atrophy and ulceration may occur. These plaques are persistent and quite resistant to treatment.

PATHOLOGY

Histologically there is a central area of altered and damaged collagen in the mid dermis surrounded by inflammatory cells, including giant cells (Figure 19.12).

Granuloma annulare

This disorder has some superficial resemblance to necrobiosis lipoidica, both clinically and histologically, but in its common form has no association with diabetes. However, there is a rare generalized and 'diffuse' form that is strongly related to diabetes.

Diabetic dermopathy (Binkley's spots)

These are allegedly more common in diabetics but are not specific to the disorder. The term is used to describe multiple small (1 cm diameter) brownish, slightly atrophic spots on the front of the shins of diabetics. They are more common in males (Figure 19.13).

Ulceration of the skin in diabetics

The neuropathy of diabetes can result in neuropathic ulceration due to failure of the so-called nocioceptive reflex in which the limb is rapidly withdrawn from a painful stimulus. Deep 'perforating ulcers' may develop on the soles and elsewhere around the feet (Figure 19.14).

Atherosclerotic vascular disease is more common in diabetics and the resulting ischaemia may also contribute substantially to the ulceration of the skin of the feet or lower legs. There is also a depressed ability to

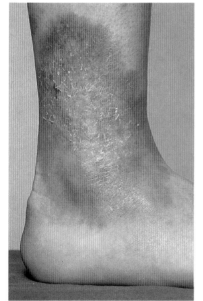

Figure 19.11 Necrobiosis lipoidica on ankle.

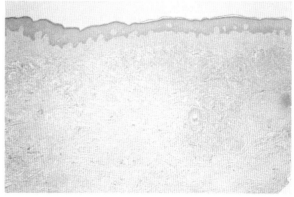

Figure 19.12 Pathology of necrobiosis lipoidica. There is an area of central degenerative change surrounded by a dense inflammatory cell infiltrate composed of lymphocytes, histiocytes and giant cells.

cope with infections and infection of the ulcerated area usually complicates such lesions in diabetics. The resulting ulcerating areas tend to be moist, sloughly and purulent. They tend to spread rapidly and result in gangrene.

Wounds in diabetics also tend to heal more slowly, compounding the problem and turning any minor injury of the foot or ankle into a serious health risk.

Xanthoma (page 265)

Xanthomata are nodular (or rarely plane) deposits of lipid within histiocytes in the dermis. The particular composition of their lipid content and their clinical appearance depend on the type of lipid abnormality. In diabetes it is most frequently accompanied by a mixed hyperlipidaemia in which both cholesterol and triglycerides are elevated. When the lipid levels are very elevated, eruptive xanthomas may develop in which numerous, small, yellow-pink papules appear anywhere on the skin but more especially on extensor surfaces (Figure 19.15).

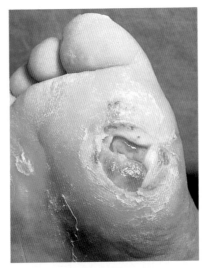

Figure 19.14 Perforating ulcer on the sole of a patient with diabetes.

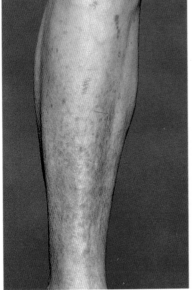

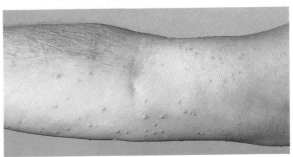

Figure 19.13 Brown spots on the shin of a diabetic patient in 'diabetic dermopathy'.

Figure 19.15 Numerous yellow pink papules due to eruptive xanthoma in a patient with diabetes.

Skin infection and pruritus

As mentioned above, diabetics appear particularly susceptible to skin infections. Monilial infection seems to be a particular problem for them and monilial vulvovaginitis and balanoposthitis are not uncommon. These are 'itchy disorders' and it may be that this is how it came to be believed that diabetics may develop generalized itch. In fact there is very little evidence that diabetes is responsible for generalized itch. If a diabetic complains of generalized itch it is more likely that scabies is the cause of the problem than the patient's diabetes!

> Skin manifestations of diabetes include necrobiosis lipoidica, eruptive xanthoma, neuropathic ulcers and susceptibility to skin infection.

Cushing's syndrome

The cutaneous signs of Cushing's syndrome are the same regardless of whether they are caused by an adrenal cortical tumour, hyperplasia or the responsible glucocorticoids given orally (or topically page 310) in the course of treatment.

CLINICAL FEATURES

1. The most consistent clinical feature is *skin thinning* so that the underlying veins can be easily seen and the skin has a 'transparent' quality (Figure 19.16). The thinning is mostly due to the suppressive action of glucocorticoids on the growth and synthetic activity of dermal fibroblasts although these agents also 'thin' the epidermis.
2. The dermal thinning also results in rupture of the elastic fibres and *striae distensae* (Figure 19.17). These are band-like atrophic areas that develop in areas of maximal stress on the skin. A certain

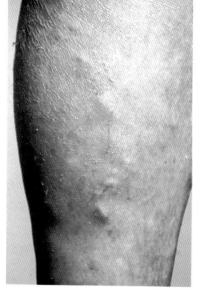

Figure 19.16 Skin thinning in Cushing's syndrome.

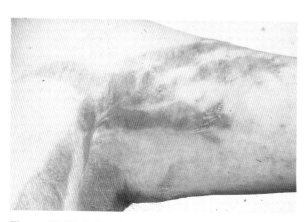

Figure 19.17 Striae distensae of anterior axillary fold in iatrogenic Cushing's syndrome.

number are found on the upper arm, the anterior axillary fold, the lower back and occasionally elsewhere in normal adolescents. They are also evident in most pregnant women on the thighs, breasts, anterior axillary folds and over the flanks and lower abdomen. It is thought that both tissue tension and the level of circulating glucocorticoids are important in the production of striae.

Striae due to corticosteroids used in treatment, either oral or topical, or due to Cushing's syndrome, are broader, more prolific and more vivid in colour than 'normal' striae.

3. *Acne* papules occur on the chest, back and face in most patients with Cushing's syndrome though it is uncertain why this should be the case as cortisone does not appear to increase the rate of sebum excretion (page 154). Steroid acne differs from ordinary adolescent acne in that it is more uniform in the appearance of its lesions and consists predominantly of small papules with few comedones. It is more resistant to treatment than ordinary acne.

4. *Skin infections* are also more common and more severe in patients with Cushing's syndrome. Pityriasis versicolor is often present and is often very extensive.

> Skin thinning, striae distensae, acne and susceptibility to skin infection are characteristics of Cushing's syndrome.

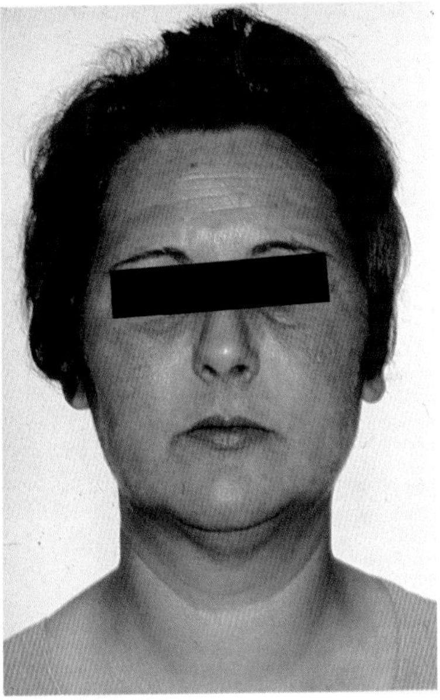

Addison's disease

This disorder, due to destruction of the adrenal cortex from autoimmune influences, tuberculosis, amyloidosis or metastatic neoplastic disease, results in weakness, hypotension and generalized hyperpigmentation (Figure 19.18). The increased pigmentation may be particularly evident on the buccal mucosa and in the palmar creases.

Nelson's disease

This is generalized deep hyperpigmentation following adrenalectomy for Cushing's syndrome.

Figure 19.18 Hyperpigmentation of facial skin in Addison's syndrome.

Androgenization (virilization)

This is predominantly a problem of women and may occur due to androgen-secreting tumours of the ovaries or of the adrenal cortex, but in practice is most often seen in the condition of polycystic ovaries in which there is an abnormality of steroid metabolism leading to an accumulation of androgens. Patients with such a disorder often present with acne and an increase in greasiness of the skin.

Increased hair growth is also often a major complaint of patients with androgenization. Vellus hair on forearms, thighs and trunk is transformed to pigmented, thick, terminal hairs. A masculine distribution of body and limb hair develops. Although these changes are upsetting, of

> Virilization is most often seen in the condition of polycystic ovaries in which there is an abnormality of steroid metabolism leading to an accumulation of androgens.

even greater distress is the appearance of beard hair, and this is usually the reason for the patient attending the clinic (Figure 19.19). In clinical practice the most frequent problem in this area is to distinguish hirsutes due to androgenization from hirsutes due to nonendocrine causes. It is not generally recognized that the presence of some terminal hair on the face or limbs of otherwise healthy women is not uncommon. This is particularly the case in dark complexioned women of Arab or Asian descent or who stem from the Mediterranean area. The tendency for 'excess hair' is also familial. Thinning of the scalp hair and pattern alopecia is also quite common and very distressing to women with virilization.

In authentic virilization the following features help distinguish the condition from 'nonendocrine' hirsutes:

1. the excess hair is recent in onset and progressively becoming more noticeable;
2. the hirsutes is accompanied by other physical signs including acne and seborrhoea;
3. there is a significant menstrual disturbance.

In most cases extensive investigation is not appropriate and plasma testosterone and abdominal ultrasound are all that are required.

> In authentic virilization the following features help distinguish the condition from 'non-endocrine' hirsutes: (1) the excess hair is recent in onset and progressively becoming more noticeable; (2) the hirsutes is accompanied by other physical signs including acne and seborrhoea; (3) there is a significant menstrual disturbance.

Nutrition and the skin

Vitamin A (retinol)

Retinol is a vital lipid-soluble vitamin found in dairy produce and liver and is also obtainable in the form of beta-carotene from carrots, tomatoes and other vegetables. It is essential for growth and development, resistance to infection, reproduction and visual function. Amongst its many important functions in growth and development is its role in epidermal differentiation. In deficiency states it causes follicular hyperkeratosis and roughening of the skin (phrynoderma). When excessive amounts are ingested, (as has happened when Arctic explorers have eaten polar bear liver), pruritus, widespread erythema and peeling of the palms and soles occurs. These symptoms and signs are similar to those of retinoid toxicity (page 316).

> In hypervitaminosis A, pruritus, widespread erythema and peeling of the palms and soles occurs.

Nicotinic acid

This is a water-soluble B vitamin found in grains and vegetables. Deficiency causes the condition of pellagra, resulting in diarrhoea, dementia and a photosensitivity dermatitis. The latter develops a characteristic postinflammatory hyperpigmentation and is often very marked around the neck (Figure 19.20).

Vitamin C (ascorbic acid)

Vitamin C is a water-soluble vitamin found in fruit and vegetables. Deficiency results in scurvy, which causes a clotting defect and poor

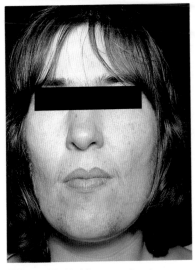

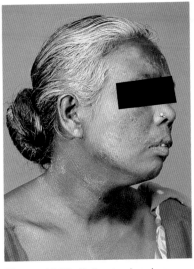

Figure 19.19 Hirsutes due to androgenization.

Figure 19.20 Pellagra showing pigmented scaling dermatosis.

wound healing. A characteristic rash seen in patients with scurvy consists of numerous tiny haemorrhages around hair follicles.

Deficiency of nicotinic acid causes pellagra and deficiency of ascorbic acid causes scurvy.

Kwashiorkor
This is due to severe protein deficiency in children and is seen in the poorer underprivileged parts of the world including areas in Africa and India. Generalized oedema develops and the degree of skin pigmentation decreases. In addition the hair becomes reddish during the time of the deficiency – the so-called flag sign.

Senile osteoporosis
In this disorder of faulty bone mineralization due to vitamin D

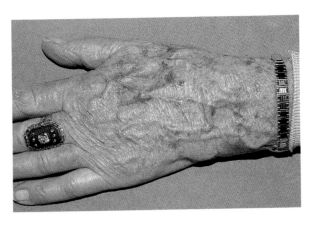

Figure 19.21 Thin fragile skin of back of hand due to osteoporosis.

deficiency, bone thinning and multiple fractures, the skin becomes 'thinner'. This can be demonstrated and measured using callipers or ultrasound. Clinically the skin looks smooth and is almost transparent, with the veins being abnormally prominent (Figure 19.21).

Skin and the gastrointestinal tract

There are numerous interrelationships between the skin and the gastrointestinal tract, and only the more obvious ones fall within the scope of a book of this size.

Dermatitis herpetiformis (page 85)

Dermatitis herpetiformis is strongly associated with an absorptive defect of the small bowel. Small bowel mucosal biopsy demonstrates partial villous atrophy in some 70–80% of patients with DH.

This itchy blistering disorder is strongly associated with an absorptive defect of the small bowel. Small bowel mucosal biopsy demonstrates partial villous atrophy in some 70–80% of patients with dermatitis herpetiformis (DH). Apart from this structural abnormality there are also some minor functional absorptive abnormalities in most patients. This gut disorder is in fact a form of gluten enteropathy (as is coeliac disease) and can be improved by a gluten-free diet.

Peutz-Jeghers syndrome

This is a rare autosomal dominant disorder in which perioral and labial pigmented macules occur in association with jejunal polyps. Pigmented macules also occur over the fingers.

Gardener's syndrome

In this dominant disorder epidermoid cysts and benign epidermal tumours occur in association with colonic polyposis.

Hepatic disease

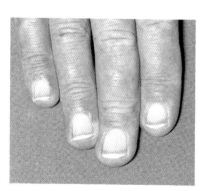

Figure 19.22 White finger nails due to liver disease.

In severe chronic hepatocellular liver failure, hypoalbuminaemia occurs which results in the curious sign of whitening of the finger nails (Figure 19.22). Severe liver failure may also cause multiple spider naevi to occur over the arms, upper trunk and face (Figure 19.23). These vascular anomalies consist of a central 'feeding' blood vessel with numerous fine radiating legs emanating from the central body. Their cause is uncertain but may be related to the plasma levels of unconjugated oestrogens.

In biliary cirrhosis, severe pruritus develops, resulting in excoriations and prurigo papules. There is also a degree of jaundice and in long-standing cases a generalized dusky pigmentation is seen in addition.

In chronic active hepatitis a faint pink macular rash has been described which may have a capillaritis as its basis.

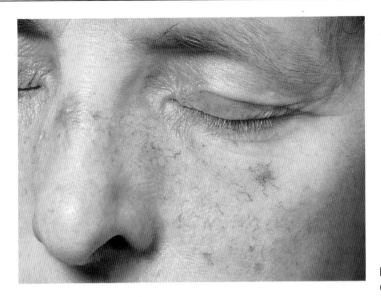

Figure 19.23 Multiple spider naevi due to liver disease.

Pancreatic disease

The effects of diabetes and of alpha cell tumours on the skin have already been discussed earlier in this chapter. Pancreatitis may result in the liberation of digestive enzymes into the blood and the onset of deep inflammatory nodules of panniculitis as a result of the liberation of lipase.

Systemic causes of pruritus

1. End-stage renal failure (uraemia) often causes persistent severe itch. The itch is accompanied by a dusky grey-brown pigmentation.
2. Obstructive jaundice from any cause results in intolerable itching.
3. Thyrotoxicosis sometimes causes itching but does not seem due to the sweatiness or increased warmth of the skin experienced by such patients.
4. Itching is sometimes a complaint of patients with hyperparathyroidism.
5. The symptom of itch is occasionally a sign of Hodgkin's disease or less often of another type of lymphoma. Rarely the itch is a presenting symptom of the neoplasm.
6. Itch is a well-known disabling complaint of patients with polycythaemia rubra vera. For some curious reason the itch may be a particular problem when these patients take a bath.
7. It has often been claimed that patients with diabetes have pruritus but if this is the case it must be extremely rare. Diabetics are prone to candidiasis which causes perigenital itch and it is possible that this is how the idea began.

CHAPTER

20

Disorders of pigmentation

> The degree of racial pigmentation does not depend on the number of melanocytes present but on their metabolic activity and the size and shape of their melanin producing organelles – the melanosomes.

Melanin pigment is produced in melanocytes in the basal layer of the epidermis. The degree of racial pigmentation does not depend on the number of melanocytes present but on their metabolic activity and the size and shape of their melanin-producing organelles – the melanosomes. Melanocytes are found in the basal layer of the epidermis where they account for 5–10% of the cells present. They are dendritic in nature (Figure 20.1) but appear as 'clear cells' in formalin fixed sections (Figure 20.2).

Melanin synthesis is under pituitary control (melanocyte-stimulating hormone) and is also influenced by other endocrine secretions including oestrogens and androgens. Melanocytes are also stimulated by ultraviolet radiation (UVR) and by mechanical and other irritative stimuli.

> Melanin is a complex black brown polymer synthesized from the amino acid L-DOPA (dihydroxyphenyl alanine).

Melanin is a complex black-brown polymer synthesized from the amino acid dihydroxyphenyl alanine (L-DOPA) (Figure 20.3). Two forms of melanin exist: 'ordinary' melanin known as eumelanin and a melanin synthesized from cysteinyl DOPA with a more reddish hue, known as phaeomelanin. The initial part of melanin synthesis is catalysed by a copper-containing enzyme complex known as tyrosinase, which also catalyses the transformation of L-DOPA to tyrosine.

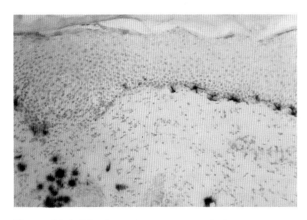

Figure 20.1 Dihydroxyphenyl alanine (DOPA) oxidase reaction to reveal melanocytes in the basal layer of the epidermis as blackened cells with dendritic processes.

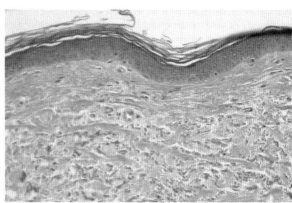

Figure 20.2 Formalin fixed histological section of normal skin showing several 'clear cells' at the base representing melanocytes.

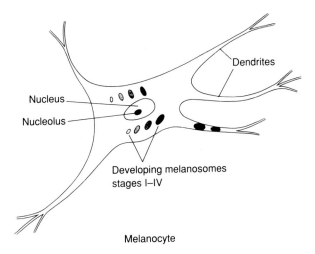

Melanocyte

Figure 20.3 Diagram of a melanocyte showing dendrites and different stages of melanosomes.

Melanin is produced in melanocytes but 'donated' by their dendrites to the keratinocytes in the immediate vicinity. The melanin granules then ascend through the epidermis in the keratinocytes. The melanin is synthesized in melanosomes which can be seen to go through a number of stages during their melaninization (stages I–IV). Figure 22.3a demonstrates that the mature melanosomes aggregate into melanin granules and these are injected via the melanocyte dendritic processes into the keratinocytes. It is these granular particles within keratinocytes that are responsible for their protective function against damage from UVR.

Melanin in keratinocytes is black and absorbs all visible light, UVR and infrared radiation. It is also a powerful electron acceptor and may have other protective functions which as yet have been poorly characterized.

> Melanin in keratinocytes is black and absorbs all visible light, UVR and infra red radiation. It is also a powerful electron acceptor and may have other protective functions which as yet have been poorly characterized.

Types of pigmentary disorder

Excessive pigmentation is known as hyperpigmentation and decreased pigmentation is known as hypopigmentation. Both may be localized or generalized. In addition, increased pigmentation may result from deposits of abnormal nonmelanin pigments in the skin.

Generalized hypopigmentation

Oculocutaneous albinism

There are several varieties of genetically determined defects in melanin synthesis. The common variety is recessively inherited oculocutaneous albinism.

> There are several varieties of genetically determined defects in melanin synthesis. The common variety is recessively inherited oculocutaneous albinism.

CLINICAL FEATURES

Affected individuals have a very pale or even pinkish complexion with flaxen, white or slightly yellowish hair and very light blue or even pink eyes. Albinos are also subject to nystagmus, either horizontal or rotatory. In addition they are photophobic and frequently have serious refractive errors. They are extremely sensitive to the harmful effects of solar irradiation and in sunny climates often develop skin cancers.

PATHOGENESIS

> Albinos have a normal number of melanocytes in the basal layer of the epidermis but they lack tyrosinase and are unable to synthesize melanin.

Albinos have a normal number of melanocytes in the basal layer of the epidermis but they lack tyrosinase and are unable to synthesize melanin. If hair is plucked and incubated in a medium containing L-DOPA the hair bulb does not turn black as it does normally.

MANAGEMENT

Albino patients must be instructed on ways of protecting themselves against solar UVR, including the regular use of sunscreens and the total avoidance of the sun one hour either side of noon. Regular checking to detect early changes of skin cancer is also important.

Other forms of albinism

There are several other types of albinism, most of which are inherited as recessive characteristics. One of these is the Hermanski-Pudlak syndrome in which there is an associated clotting defect due to a platelet abnormality. This condition is 'tyrosinase positive', so that hair bulbs turn black after they are incubated in medium containing L-DOPA.

There are also several types of albinism where the abnormality of melanin synthesis is confined to the eyes.

Localized hypopigmentation

Piebaldism

In this condition there is a white forelock and white patches on the skin surface. In Waardenburg's syndrome the condition is associated with sensory deafness.

Hypopituitarism

Generalized hypopigmentation is seen in pituitary failure as in Simmond's disease and is due to decreased levels of melanocyte-stimulating hormone.

Vitiligo

> In vitiligo there is focal failure of pigmentation due to destruction of melanocytes which is thought to be mediated by immunological mechanisms causing sharply defined areas of depigmentation.

DEFINITION

A common skin disorder in which there is focal failure of pigmentation due to destruction of melanocytes which is thought to be mediated by immunological mechanisms.

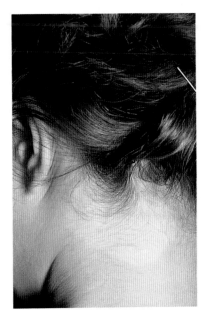

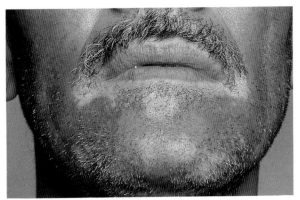

Figure 20.4 (a) Sharply defined patch of vitiligo on the neck. (b) Vitiligo in dark-skinned patient.

CLINICAL FEATURES

Sharply defined areas of depigmentation appear (Figure 20.4). Occasionally the depigmented areas are slightly pink at the start of the disorder. Often the depigmented patches are symmetrical, especially when the disorder is distributed over the peripheral parts of the limbs and the face. Odd patterns are sometimes noted as, for example, when the depigmentation occurs over the front of the neck over the thyroid gland or on the abdomen over the site of the pancreas or on the flanks over the sites of the adrenal glands.

It is much more noticeable in the summer time when the surrounding skin has become slightly sunburnt. It is a serious cosmetic problem for darkly pigmented peoples.

The condition often starts in childhood, and either spreads, over the years, so that ultimately the skin is totally depigmented, or persists with irregular remissions and relapses.

Halo naevus (Sutton's naevus) is a related disorder in which the depigmentation begins around one or a few compound naevi (Figure 20.5). Ordinary vitiligo may occur alongside.

PATHOGENESIS AND EPIDEMIOLOGY

Vitiligo occurs in 1–2% of the population and is more common when it has occurred in other members of the family. It is more common in diabetes, thyroid disease and alopecia areata, and appears to be due to an immunological attack on the melanocytes. This would suggest that it is an autoimmune disorder.

TREATMENT

The condition is relatively resistant to treatment and if the disorder is limited in extent the best approach is to offer firm reassurance and if

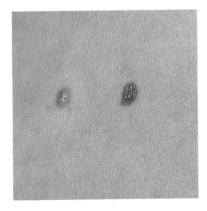

Figure 20.5 There is a white 'halo' around this naevus on the neck.

necessary advice concerning cosmetic camouflage. Staining the skin with 2% hydroxyacetone may be helpful.

Treatments with topical corticosteroids, PUVA or topical PUVA (pages 139–140) are sometimes effective in stimulating repigmentation but the irregularity of a response and the long period over which the treatments have to be administered greatly detract from the acceptability of the treatment.

Other causes of localized depigmentation of skin

In many countries the fear of leprosy makes differential diagnosis of a 'white patch' an urgent and vitally important issue. The causes of localized hypopigmentation are summarized in Table 20.1. Examination of the skin in long wave UVR helps distinguish whether there is total depigmentation (as in vitiligo) or not. It may also detect areas of depigmentation not easily seen in ordinary daylight as well as detecting a lemon-yellow fluorescence seen in some cases of pityriasis versicolor.

> Examination of the skin in long-wave UVR helps distinguish whether there is total depigmentation (as in vitiligo) or not. It may also detect areas of depigmentation not easily seen in ordinary daylight.

Table 20.1 Causes of localized hypopigmentation

Vitiligo	Destruction of melanocytes; common; acquired; multiple sharply defined nonpigmented patches anywhere
Pityriasis versicolor	Superficial fungus infection leading to disturbance in pigment production; common; multiple pale scaling patches on trunk
Pityriasis alba	Mild patchy eczema of the face in children causing a disturbance in pigment production
Leprosy	One or several paler macules on trunk or limbs that are hypoaesthetic
White macules of tuberous sclerosis	Uncommon development of anomaly affecting CNS connective tissue and skin; several 'maple leaf'-shaped hypopigmented macules
Postinflammatory hypopigmentation	After inflammatory skin disease (often eczema) or trauma to the skin; irregular in shape and in depth of pallor
Naevus anaemicus	Rare developmental solitary white patch usually on trunk; thought to have a vascular basis
Chemical toxicity	May look very like vitiligo; seen in workers in the rubber industry exposed to paratertiary benzyltoluene

Hyperpigmentation

Whenever increased pigmentation of the skin is observed the decision has to be taken as to whether the increased pigment is due to increased melanin content or due to some other pigment. The other pigments that may give rise to a dark brown-black discolouration are set out in Table 20.2

Generalized melanin hyperpigmentation is seen in *Addison's disease* due to destruction of the adrenal cortex caused by tuberculosis, autoimmune influences, secondary deposits of carcinoma or amyloidosis. Pigmentation is most marked in the flexures and the light-exposed areas (Figure 20.6) but mucosae and nails are also distinctively hyperpigmented. The diagnosis is supported by hypotension, hyponatraemia and extreme weakness. The hyperpigmentation is due to the excess of pituitary peptides resulting from the lack of adrenal steroids. After bilateral adrenalectomy the degree of pigmentation may be extreme (**Nelson's syndrome**).

Some generalized darkening of the skin is seen in pregnancy (page 241), although this is more marked on the face, the nipples and the midline of the abdomen. Generalized hyperpigmentation may also be part of *acanthosis nigricans* (page 284) although the hyperpigmentation is much more marked in the flexures and is accompanied by increased skin markings and skin tags.

A 'bronzed appearance' is seen in *primary haemochromatosis* (bronzed diabetes) in which iron is deposited in the viscera including the pancreas, giving rise to diabetes, and the liver, causing cirrhosis. The increased skin pigmentation is caused both by iron and excess melaninization in the skin. Increased skin pigment is also evident in secondary haemosiderosis. Other causes of generalized hyperpigmentation include hepatic cirrhosis, particularly biliary cirrhosis, chronic renal failure, glycogen storage disease and Gaucher's disease. Biliary cirrhosis and renal failure are usually accompanied by severe pruritus.

> Generalized melanin hyperpigmentation is seen in *Addison's disease*.

> Generalized hyperpigmentation may also be part of *acanthosis nigricans*.

> A 'bronzed appearance' is seen in *primary haemochromatosis*.

> Other causes of generalized hyperpigmentation include hepatic cirrhosis – particularly biliary cirrhosis, chronic renal failure, glycogen storage disease and Gaucher's disease.

Table 20.2 Nonmelanin causes of brown-black discolouration

Haemosiderin – from broken down haem pigment in extravasated blood

Homogentisic acid – deposited in cartilage in particular in the inherited metabolic defect known as alkaptonuria

Unknown pigment in thickened stratum corneum of severe disorders of keratinization such as lamellar ichthyosis and epidermolytic hyperkeratosis

Drugs and heavy metal toxicity. Dark pigmentation of skin and mucosae seen in silver, gold, mercury and arsenic poisoning. Amiodarone and phenothiazines cause slate grey, dusky skin pigmentation in exposed sites. Minocycline may cause patchy pigmentation in exposed or other sites

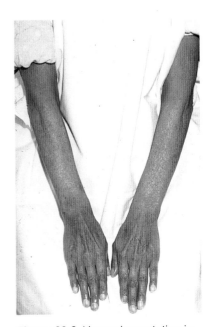

Figure 20.6 Hyperpigmentation in Addison's disease.

Dusky irregular pigmentation may also be seen in the disorder known colourfully as 'vagabond's disease'. Dirt and perpetual rubbing and scratching from infestations are the cause of this discolouration.

> Drugs can cause generalized diffuse hyperpigmentation, patchy generalized or localized hyperpigmentation.

Drugs can cause generalized diffuse hyperpigmentation, patchy generalized or localized hyperpigmentation. The classic examples of this are due to heavy metal intoxications, but are now quite rare. Arsenic ingestion causes a generalized 'raindrop' pattern of hyperpigmentation and the use of silver preparations topically caused 'argyria' producing a dusky greyish discolouration of the skin and mucosae. Bismuth and gold can also cause hyperpigmentation.

Modern drugs can also produce darkening. *Minoxycycline* (Minocin) can cause darkening of the scarred acne for which it is given; it can also produce dark patches on exposed areas. The pigment is a complex of iron, the drug and melanin and the condition is only partially reversible. *Amiodarone*, the antiarrhythmic drug, causes a characteristic greyish colour on the exposed areas of skin. The *phenothiazines*, in high doses given over long periods, produce a purplish discolouration in the exposed areas due to the deposition of a drug–melanin complex in the skin. *Chlorpromazine* is particularly prone to do this and when it was first used in long-stay psychiatric hospitals many 'purple people' were produced by giving too high a dose for too long.

Carotenaemia produces an orange-yellow golden hue due to the deposition of beta-carotene in the skin. It is seen in food faddists who eat large numbers of carrots and other red vegetables. Beta-carotene is also given for the condition of eyrthropoietic protoporphyria (page 264).

Canthexanthin is another carotenoid that produces a similar skin colour and was sold for this purpose to simulate a 'bronzed' sun tan. Pigment crystals were found in the retina of patients taking the drug and it has been withdrawn for this reason.

Transient skin discolouration is seen in methaemoglobinaemia and sulphaemoglobinaemia due to **dapsone** administration.

Localized hyperpigmentation

All the melanocytic naevi produce small dark nodules or macules (pages 189–194) and are easily recognized. However, Mongolian spots, and the naevus of Ota and the naevus of Ito, are large flat grey brown

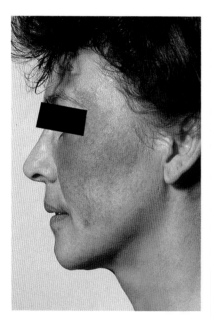

Figure 20.7 Macular grey-brown pigmentation in naevus of Ota.

Figure 20.8 Light brown macule (*café au lait* patch) due to Von Recklinghausen's disease.

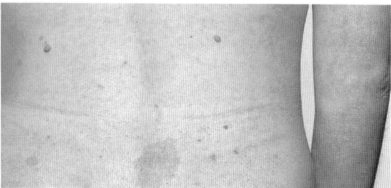

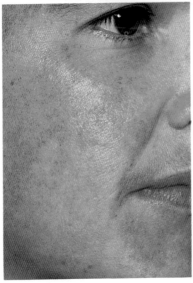

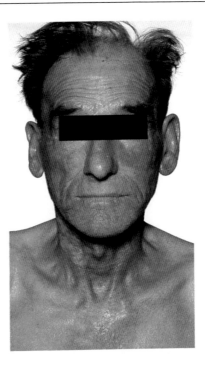

Figure 20.10 Diffuse dusky brown pigmentation due to perpetual rubbing and scratching in atopic dermatitis.

Figure 20.9 Diffuse brown pigmentation of the cheek in chloasma.

patches and can be confused with bruising and other conditions (Figure 20.7). *Café au lait* patches are part of the dominantly inherited condition of neurofibromatosis (Von Recklinghausen's disease) (page 210). Numerous flat light brown macules which vary from 0.5 to 4 cm^2 are present all over the skin surface – the trunk in particular and consistently in the axillae. They occur alongside the neurofibromata together producing a characteristic clinical picture (Figure 20.8).

Not dissimilar brown macules are found on the lips and around the mouth and on the fingers in Peutz-Jegher's syndrome accompanied by small bowel polyps, and in Albright's syndrome, in which there are associated bone abnormalities.

Probably the commonest type of localized hyperpigmentation not of naevoid origin is patterned chloasma. This facial pigmentation may be part of the increased pigmentation of pregnancy or may occur independently. There is increased epidermal pigment due to increased melanocyte activity. The cheeks, periocular regions, forehead and neck may be affected in this so-called 'mask of pregnancy' (Figure 20.9).

Another common cause of localized hyperpigmentation is post-inflammatory hyperpigmentation. This may be due to melanocytic hyperplasia occurring as part of epidermal thickening following inflammation. Commonly this is seen in eczema, particularly atopic eczema (Figure 20.10). This is transient and of no real consequence.

It may also be due to the shedding of melanin from the damaged epidermis into the dermis where it is engulfed by macrophages. This 'tattooing' is quite long lasting (maybe many months). It is seen in lichen planus (page 142) (Figure 20.11) and in fixed drug eruption (page 91).

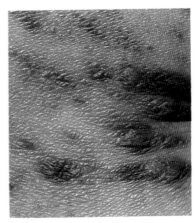

Figure 20.11 Dark patches following resolution of lichen planus.

> Localized hyperpigmentation may also be due to the shedding of melanin from the damaged epidermis into the dermis where it is engulfed by macrophages.

21

Management of skin disease

Psychological aspects of skin disorder

Does skin disorder affect the psyche?

The skin is vital to interpersonal relationships. It is a vital part of our communications system. If it is destroyed or deranged in any way, 'unfriendly messages' are transmitted. Instead of the message, 'Here is a healthy harmless member of the human race', the signal from an abnormal skin is interpreted as announcing, 'Beware of the contagion'.

> There is a primitive dislike and distrust of individuals with skin disease or skin deformity.

There is a primitive dislike and distrust of individuals with skin disease or skin deformity. It is not merely that skin disease makes people look different, but more that the problem seems to engender genuine fear and revulsion. It has been suggested that this is a hangover from primitive stages of human development when avoidance of people with infected or infested skin had a survival advantage.

Interestingly, the patient's own view of their abnormal skin is not dissimilar to that of observers. Often patients with obvious skin disease are very disturbed by its appearance and tend to shun the company of others and become quite isolated. These attitudes are known collectively as 'the leper complex' and are important to understand. Wherever possible, patients with skin disease should receive sympathy and reassurance. The use of prostheses, hair pieces and cosmetic camouflage should be encouraged rather than sneered at.

> Patients with deformities, obvious disease of the exposed areas, widespread skin disease and persistently itchy skin disorder become depressed.

Patients with deformities, obvious disease of the exposed areas, widespread skin disease and persistently itchy skin disorder become depressed. Recognition of this is important. Often all that is required is sympathy and general support, but some patients may need psychotropic drugs and skilled help from a psychiatrist.

Does the psyche affect the skin?

A frequent question from patients is, 'Is it my nerves, doctor?'. It has become an engrained part of popular mythology that skin disease is caused by psychological disturbance. It has to be said that for the most part there is no truth to this assertion. There is no doubt that 'stress' of all kinds can precipitate or aggravate all kinds of disease, including cardiovascular disease, endocrine disease, gastrointestinal disease and

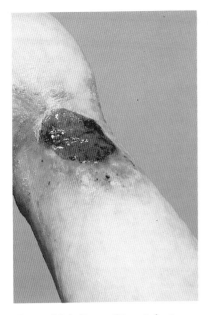

Figure 21.1 Dermatitis artefacta. Eroded area on the arm with scars due to self-mutilation.

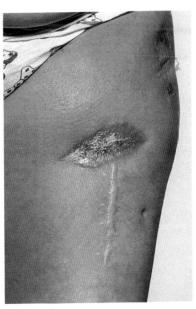

Figure 21.2 Dermatitis artefacta. Scarred area on the thigh from self-induced injury.

skin disease. But there is very little evidence that psychological abnormality causes skin disorder.

There is one major exception to this – that is the disorder known as *dermatitis artefacta*. The skin disorder in these patients is entirely self induced. The degree of insight possessed concerning the causation of their problems varies. Some admit scratching, picking or rubbing but say they can't stop doing it. Others hotly deny producing the injury to the skin.

The extent of the injury is itself varied. Clearly in some patients the problem is hysterical in the psychiatric sense. At one end of the scale the condition of nodular prurigo (page 117) can be said to be a form of dermatitis artefacta. At the other end of the scale there is a devastating injury resulting in serious permanent disability (Figure 21.1). In some cases the artefactual injury is frank malingering for obvious gain (Figure 21.2).

Regrettably, recognition of the problem is the nearest that the doctor can get to helping patients with dermatitis artefacta. Psychotherapy and psychotropic drugs appear to offer very little and their artefacts may persist for years.

Delusions of parasitosis

This is a rare psychosis in which the individual believes that his skin is infested with some type of insect or worm. Often the person who holds this irrational belief will bring to the doctor rolled up horn or other skin debris and point proudly to the 'infesting insect'. They may point to specks or blemishes on the skin as evidence of their problem. Unfortunately these patients' beliefs are quite unshakeable, and psychiatrists throw up their hands in despair at the prospect of dealing with them. The drug pimozide has been said to be helpful for patients with delusional parasitosis.

Body image

We all have a particular 'view' of ourselves and a special 'conceit' over our own visual worth. For reasons that are not well understood, some individuals have a distorted body image that at times amounts to a delusional belief. Too much hair, too little hair, discolourations, minor blemishes – all can become a major focal point of complaint. Sympathy is required for this type of problem as we are all prone to it in one degree or another. Dysmorphophobia is a term that has been used to describe individuals with a severely distorted body image.

> Dysmorphophobia is a term that has been used to describe individuals with a severely distorted body image.

Skin disability

> Skin disease can be as much if not more disabling than disease of other organ systems.

Skin disease can be as much if not more disabling than disease of other organ systems. Disability from skin disease can be thought of as consisting of physical, emotional and social components. The physical disability derives from decreased mobility from the abnormal stratum corneum present in eczema, psoriasis or the ichthyotic disorders. The abnormal horn lacks extensibility and cracks when stretched. The abnormally stiff dermis as occurs in scleroderma or scarring also affects mobility. The emotional disability stems from the psychological problems discussed above and can lead to serious depression and its consequences. The social disability stems from the 'isolation' imposed both by the patients themselves and society at large. It results in domestic and occupational problems.

Increasing awareness of the serious disability caused by skin disease will lead to improvement in the general 'lot' of patients with skin disease in a host of different ways, from assistance with domestic arrangements to advice concerning occupation.

Topical treatments for skin disease

Only general comments and advice concerning certain medicaments is given here as specific treatment is given in each section.

Drugs for use topically are incorporated into vehicles. These are either greasy single-phase ointments, creams which are mostly oil in water, or water in oil emulsions or aqueous lotions. Pastes are thick substances containing a particulate solid phase and are now not much used; alcoholic lotions have some limited use, for example, for scalp treatments; gels are semisolid translucent water – or alcohol-filled matrices and although not extensively used are quite useful at times, for example, for scalp disorders; paints, varnishes and powders are only occasionally used.

In general, ointments are prescribed for chronic scaling conditions, including psoriasis and persistent eczema, while creams and lotions are prescribed for acute and exudative disorders. This is not a hard and fast rule and, for example, creams are appreciated by many of those with chronic dermatoses. When the disorder is weeping and very exudative, bathing and wet dressings are required. Gauze dressings kept moist with saline or dilute potassium permanganate solution (1: 8000) or aluminium subacetate solution (8%) should be used.

Shampoos are helpful for psoriasis and seborrhoeic dermatitis of the scalp but should not be the sole treatment.

How much to prescribe?

It takes about 25 g to cover the body completely with a cream or ointment and it is silly to prescribe one 30 g tube for someone who has to treat extensive areas of skin twice daily for a month. Enough medication should be prescribed. Fifty grams would be sufficient for a topical treatment for a bilateral hand dermatitis for a month. Clearly, 100 g would be needed for hands and feet. Emollients and cleansing preparations need to be prescribed in much larger quantities.

> It takes about 25 g to cover the body completely with a cream or ointment.

Adverse side effects from topical preparations (Table 21.1).

If a patient does not improve with the topical medicine prescribed, it may be because:

Table 21.1   Adverse side effects to topical medications

Effect	Sign/cause
Allergic contact dermatitis (dermatitis medicamentosa) to the drug or a component of the vehicle	Eczematous rash at site of application, e.g. from neomycin
Irritation of the skin	Eczematous rash at site of application, e.g. from benzoyl peroxide
Photosensitivity	Erythematous or eczematous rash at exposed site of application, e.g. from a halogenated salicylanilide antimicrobial
Acneiform folliculitis	Acneiform rash at site of application, particularly in acne-prone areas
Absorption of drug or component of the preparation	Systemic toxicities, dependent on particular preparation

1. there is an adverse effect from use of the preparation (e.g. contact allergy);
2. the condition has been wrongly diagnosed;
3. the patient hasn't used the medication;
4. the condition is resistant to the treatment prescribed.

The use of emollients

Emollients (moisturizers) act by occluding the skin surface with a greasy film which prevents evaporation of water from the surface, allowing it to accumulate within the stratum corneum. Emollients may be single-phase oils or greasy ointments, oil in water or water in oil emulsions, either as creams or lotions. An emollient effect can be obtained by using a bath oil or a cleanser that deposits an oil film on the skin surface.

Emollients have important effects:

1. They make the stratum corneum swell and flatten out the surface irregularities so that the skin looks and feels smoother.
2. They increase the extensibility of skin so that it cracks less.
3. They decrease binding forces between the horn cells and decrease the tendency to scaling.
4. Itch decreases when they are used.
5. They have some anti-inflammatory properties in their own right, possibly because they decrease mitotic activity as well as possessing antiprostaglandin synthetase activity.

Uses

1. Emollients may be all that is required for patients with mild ichthyotic disorders.
2. They are also useful for patients with eczematous rashes – particularly those with atopic dermatitis.
3. Emollients are helpful for patients with psoriasis and other chronic scaling dermatoses.

Topical corticosteroids

There are numerous preparations containing topical corticosteroids, with different potencies (Table 21.2). Apart from the different compounds, preparations are also available with antimicrobial agents. Their predominant use is for eczematous dermatoses but in some situations they are also useful in the treatment of psoriasis. They have marked anti-inflammatory and antiproliferative effects. A major part of their action is in inducing lipocortin – the endogenous inhibitor of prostaglandin synthetase – important in the generation of eicosanoid compounds involved in the inflammatory process.

Adverse side effects from topical corticosteroids (Table 21.3)

The most important of these results from the absorption of the corticosteroid agent. If enough is absorbed there is suppression of the pituitary–adrenal axis and adrenal atrophy. If even more is absorbed a

> Emollients make the stratum corneum swell and flatten out the surface irregularities so that the skin looks and feels smoother, increase the extensibility of skin so that it cracks less, decrease binding forces between the horn cells and decrease the tendency to scaling, have some anti-inflammatory properties and decreases itch.

> Corticosteroids should mainly be used for eczema. They induce an endogenous inhibitor of prostaglandin synthetase known as lipocortin.

Table 21.2   Classification of corticosteroids according to potency

Category	Activity	Examples
1.	Mild (weak)	Hydrocortisone Clobetasone butyrate
2.	Moderately potent	Flurandrenolone Desoxymetasone
3.	Potent	Betamethasone-17-valerate Fluocinolone acetonide
4.	Very potent	Clobetasol-17-propionate Halcinonide Ulobetasol

Table 21.3   Side effects of topical corticosteroids

Absorption and pituitary–adrenal axis suppression and
  hypercortisonism

Skin thinning effects causing telangiectasia, striae and fragility

Depressed wound healing

Masked infection, particularly ringworm (tinea incognito)

Miscellaneous, including acne, hirsutes and depigmentation

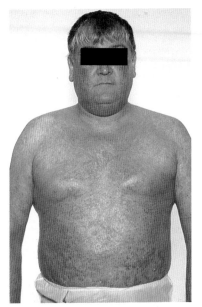

Figure 21.3 Iatrogenic Cushing's syndrome due to the use of large amounts of potent topical corticosteroid (fluocinolone acetonide) over a three-year period.

Cushingoid-like state can develop (Figure 21.3). These effects are potentially life-threatening. A general guideline is that not more than 50g 0.1% betamethasone 17-valerate ointment or cream should be used per week, or not more than 30g 0.1% clobetasol 17-propionate.

Effects on the skin:

1. Skin thinning and striae (Figure 21.4). These result from the wasting action of corticosteroids on the dermal connective tissue.
2. Masked infection, particularly ringworm, resulting in extensive and unusual appearing ringworm (tinea incognito).

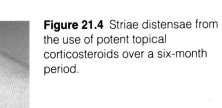

Not more than 50 g of 0.1% betamethasone 17-valerate ointment or cream should be used per week, or not more than 30 g of 0.1% clobetasol 17-propionate to avoid pituitary-adrenal axis suppression.

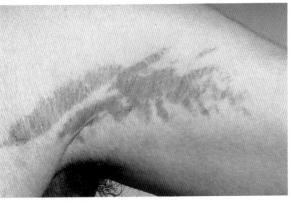

Figure 21.4 Striae distensae from the use of potent topical corticosteroids over a six-month period.

311

Note: dilution of proprietary preparations is NOT advised because the formulations are complex and the important excipients are also diluted and may be ineffective when the dilution is made. In addition, it must not be thought that dilution necessarily decreases the effect proportionately.

Topical antimicrobial agents

Topical antimicrobial agents are required to treat ringworm, erythrasma moniliasis, impetigo, wound infections, infected eczema, herpes simplex and herpes zoster. Several points should be borne in mind before prescribing treatment with a topical antimicrobial agent.

1. All that weeps and contains pus is not infected. Many inflamed skin disorders are exudative but are not due to an infection.
2. Some antimicrobial agents are irritating while others are sensitizing and may cause allergic contact dermatitis. Some imidazoles and older halogenated phenolic compounds may irritate. Some antibiotics (e.g. neomycin, chloramphenicol) sensitize.
3. Different infections respond differently to different antimicrobial agents.
4. It is quite easy to induce bacterial resistance and agents that may be used systemically should not be used topically.

> Amongst the safest and most useful compounds for bacterial and fungal infections are the imidazoles (e.g. econazole, miconazole, isoconazole), the triazoles (naftifine, terbinafine) and povidone iodine.

Amongst the safest and most useful compounds for bacterial and fungal infections are the imidazoles (e.g. econazole, miconazole, isoconazole), the triazoles (naftifine, terbinafine) and povidone iodine. The antibiotic mupiricin is also of considerable usefulness. Acyclovir and idoxuridine are antiviral preparations used for herpes simplex, the former also being used for herpes zoster.

Surgical aspects of the management of skin disease

Surgical aspects of dermatology are an increasingly important aspect of dermatological practice. This is partially because:

5. there is a growing demand for the removal of moles, seborrhoeic warts and similar benign lesions;
6. the incidence of skin cancers of all types is increasing;
7. there is a growing realization that a knowledge of skin biology and skin disease are helpful in the surgical management of these lesions.

Biopsy

Removal of a small fragment of skin tissue is a routine diagnostic procedure. Mostly such tissue is for routine histological preparation and light microscopy, but tissue for electron microscopy, immunofluorescence or other immunolocalization studies, or microbial culture, may also be required.

If biopsy only is required, rather than excision and subsequent histological examination, trephine (punch biopsy) is usually adequate.

Sharp disposable trephines are available of 2–6 mm in diameter. Sutures are not necessary for biopsies of less than 4 mm diameter taken this way, and only occasionally for 4 mm trephines. Useful tips in taking biopsies:

1. Choose a new and typical lesion or the edge of an established lesion.
2. It may be necessary to biopsy a disorder at several points in time or to sample different types of lesions.
3. Handle the biopsy as little and as gently as possible.
4. Especial precautions need to be taken when biopsying HIV positive and hepatitis B positive patients and the laboratories need to be notified beforehand.
5. Patients with bleeding diatheses and valvular disease of the heart may need prophylactic treatment beforehand.

Ablative procedures

These are mainly used to treat seborrhoeic and viral warts and solar keratoses but may also be used for other minor benign localized lesions.

Laser treatment

Lasers are high-intensity coherent light sorurces of particular wavelengths, and are employed for their destructive capacity. The particular tissue effect is influenced by the energy, the wavelength and the pulse duration of the emission, as well as the colour of the tissue. They are particularly useful for the destruction of vascular birthmarks, but other kinds of lesion can also be tackled.

Special equipment and skills are required for their use.

Curettage and cautery

This is performed using sharp spoon-shaped curettes or disposable ring curettes. After the curettage the base of the lesion is carefully and lightly touched with the tip of an electrocautery loop. Infiltration of the area with a local anaesthetic is required beforehand. In many ways it is preferable to other ablative techniques as tissue is available for histological examination.

> Cryotherapy is especially useful for viral warts and solar keratoses.

Cryotherapy

This is especially useful for viral warts and solar keratoses. Various instruments and methods are available. An often used method is one employing a device supplying a fine spray of liquid nitrogen. The frozen skin turns snow white and needs to stay this colour for 15–20 seconds before tissue destruction is complete.

> Patients must be warned to expect pain and blistering at the frozen site.

Caution is required when treating lesions on the fingers as although the tissue damage is superficial with cryotherapy, the digital nerves can be damaged. Patients **must** be warned to expect pain and blistering at the frozen site and told to keep the treated area clean and covered for the next few days.

313

Shave excisions

This procedure is only suitable for raised dome-shaped lesions which are believed to be benign, such as stable melanocytic naevi, as some abnormal tissue is left behind. After local anaesthesia the lesion is shaved off flush with the skin surface with a sharp disposable scalpel. The raw base is then lightly cauterized with an electrocautery loop. The tissue removed is sent for histological examination.

Excision of small tumours

Benign moles, dermatofibroma, and small basal cell carcinoma are examples of lesions that can be easily removed by elliptical incisions around the lesion. At least 3 mm margins need to be left at the sides of the lesion. The margins of the excision are then sutured **without tension** using a silk or a synthetic suture material. The axis of the incision should be parallel to Langer's lines on the limbs and trunk but in the 'crease' lines on the face. Providing this advice is followed, scarring should be minimal. Hypertrophic or even keloid scars tend to develop in patients aged 12–30 years with excisions over the shoulders, upper arms and the front of the chest.

'Flaps' and grafting procedures

These are beyond the scope of this text and one of the many dermatological surgical texts should be consulted.

Systemic therapy

Systemic therapy is available for psoriasis, atopic dermatitis, congenital disorders of keratinization, autoimmune disorders, hypersensitivity conditions and skin infections. In many cases topical treatments are also available and decisions as to whether to use a topical or a systemic agent need to be made. Some of the considerations are as follows:

1. Systemic agents usually carry a considerably greater risk of adverse side effects than topical agents.
2. Systemic agents tend to have more potent therapeutic effects than topical agents.
3. Many patients prefer a topical agent because they fear the side effects of systemic treatment – although it is not rare to absorb sufficient of a drug applied topically to cause systemic side effects.
4. Some patients dislike putting ointments and creams on their skin and would prefer to take the risk of side effects.
5. Topical treatment may be impracticable in (a) patients with widespread skin disease, and (b) the elderly and infirm.

It is important to discuss these issues with the patient. If patients don't like, distrust or have no confidence in the treatment prescribed, the drugs will remain unused and cannot help the patient. Details of the undermentioned drugs are given in Table 21.4.

Table 21.4   Details of systemic drugs

Drug	Usual dose	Main indications	Main side effects	Comments
Cortico-steroids	5–50mg daily (prednisol-one equivalent)	Severe eczema, severe drug reactions, severe autoimmune disease and hypersensitivity disorders, bullous diseases	Hypertension, diabetes, osteoperosis, psychosis, infections, gastrointestinal bleeding, skin thinning and striae, adrenocorticol suppression	Lowest dose possible is needed; monitoring four-weekly when 'stabilized', more frequently early in treatment; caution is needed on stopping treatment because of adrenocortical suppression – gradual reduction in dose is necessary; dose needs to increase during intercurrent illness
Retinoids Etretinate/ Acitretin	0.5–1.0 mg/kg body weight daily	Severe psoriasis and disorders of keratinization, multiple nonmelanoma skin cancers	**Minor**: cheilitis, drying of oral/nasal/ ocular mucosae, diffuse hair loss, paronychiae, pruritus **Major**: teratogenicity, hepatotoxicity, rise in serum lipids, bone toxicity – hyperostosis and ossification of ligaments	Effects start after four weeks; relapse is usual after stopping; careful monitoring is required every 4–8 weeks
Isotretinoin	0.5–1.0 mg/kg body weight daily	Severe acne (cystic)	As above	Effects start after four weeks; initial aggragation is common; relapse after stopping is unusual; careful monitoring is required monthly over a four month course of treatment
Metho-trexate	5–25 mg weekly	Severe psoriasis (pustular, erythrodermic, arthropathic and severe recalcitrant plaque type), pemphigus/ pemphigoid	Hepatotoxicity with eventual fibrosis, myelotoxicity; nausea and mucositis may occur as acute effects	Regular monitoring is required (4–8 week intervals); liver biopsies are required after a cumulative dose of 1.5 g; may be given in combination with steroids for bullous disease
Azathio-prine	50–150 mg daily	Lupus erythematosus and other autoimmune disorders, pemphigus/ pemphigoid	Nausea, myelosuppression	Often used in combination with corticosteroids; monitoring is required to check on blood picture every 4–8 weeks

Drug	Usual dose	Main indications	Main side effects	Comments
Cyclosporin	2–5 mg/kg body weight daily	Severe psoriasis (erythrodermic or recalcitrant plaque type), severe atopic dermatitis	Renal toxicity and hypertension; nausea and hirsutes are sometimes a problem; over the long-term, development of neoplastic disease is a possibility	Potent immunosuppressive agent; interactions with ketoconazole may occur; monitoring 4–6 weekly is advised
Dapsone	25–150 mg daily	Leprosy, dermatitis herpetiformis	Haemolysis, methaemoglobinae-mia, sulphaemoglobinae-mia, fixed drug eruption; a granulocytosis is recorded	Monitoring every 4–8 weeks is advised

Systemic corticosteroids

> Systemic corticosteroids are needed because of the severity of the dermatosis they must be given with both the doctor's and the patient's understanding of both the risks and the benefits of such treatment.

If these are needed because of the severity of the dermatosis they must be given with both the doctor's and the patient's understanding of both the risks and the benefits of such treatment. Provision should also be made for monitoring the response as well as the side effects. Their action is predominantly suppressive by virtue of their anti-inflammatory properties. There are particular dangers in using corticosteroids for psoriasis and they should not be used in this disease.

Retinoids

> Oral retinoids carry a serious danger of teratogenicity if the drug is given to a woman in the reproductive age group, and contraception is important.

These drugs are potent agents that require monitoring by dermatologists or by other physicians with experience in their use. Although the usage of isotretinoin and etretinate (or acitretin) differs, the precautions and side effects are quite similar. There is a serious danger of teratogenicity if the drug is given to a woman in the reproductive age group, and contraception is important. Etretinate is stored in body fat and continues to be detectable in the tissues for up to two years after administration, and contraception must be practiced during this period. Acitretin is mostly excreted quite quickly but in some patients a small proportion is 'back metabolized' to etretinate, so that the risks are similar. It is expected that etretinate will gradually be withdrawn by the manufacturers. Particular care must be taken with isotretinoin as this drug is given for severe acne and many young women are exposed to it. The mode of action of the retinoid drugs is uncertain as these agents have so many clinical effects. They appear to have fundamental effects on cellular differentiation.

Patients on retinoids require monitoring for hepatotoxicity, elevation of serum lipids every four to eight weeks, and bone toxicity annually.

Methotrexate

This is an antimetabolite that effectively stops cell division by blocking DNA synthesis. It also has many other metabolic effects. It is used in dermatology both for its antiproliferative actions and for its immuno-suppressive effects. Patients require regular monitoring for myelotoxic-ity and hepatotoxicity when on the drug (every four to eight weeks) and may need liver biopsies after a cumulative dose of more than 1.5 g because of the frequency of serious liver toxicity, particularly in those who abuse alcohol.

Azathioprine

This is an antimetabolite that also blocks DNA synthesis whose prime use in dermatology is its immunosuppressive activity. As with methotr-exate, patients on azathioprine require regular monitoring for myelo-toxicity.

Cyclosporin

This drug blocks lymphokine synthesis by lymphocytes of the T-helper phenotype. It is a very potent immunosuppressive agent. Patients on the drug should be monitored for drug levels, renal toxicity and hypertension every four to eight weeks.

Dapsone (diaminosulphone)

The mode of action of this drug is unclear. It somehow interferes with polymorphonuclear cell involvement in inflammatory disease and also may be involved in complement-mediated disorders. Its antimicrobial effects may be unrelated to its anti-inflammatory activity. It is myelo-toxic and patients on the drug need monitoring every four to twelve weeks.

Other systemic drugs in frequent use

Antihistamines

Antihistamines are either blockers of the H1 receptor or of the H2 receptor. H1 blockers are mainly of use in urticaria. They do not have an independent antipruritic action.

> Antihistamines do not have an independent antipruritic action.

Antibiotics

These are used both for primary skin infections such as cellulitis, erysipelas and impetigo and secondarily infected skin disorders such as eczema and venous ulcers. Some antibiotics are used for acne and rosacea where their action may not depend on antimicrobial effects but on anti-inflammatory activity. Each antibiotic has its own particular doses and toxicities for which appropriate formularies should be consulted.

Antifungal agents

Griseofulvin, terbinafine and itraconazole are effective against dermato-phyte infections. Itraconazole, fluconazone and ketoconazole are effec-

Table 21.5   Doses and side effects of antifungal agents

Drug	Dose	Indication	Side effects
Griseofulvin	0.5–1.0 g daily	Ringworm infection only	Headaches, photosensitivities
Ketoconazole	200 mg daily	Systemic mycoses, severe ringworm and yeast infections	Nausea, rashes, headaches, liver damage
Amphotericin	250 µg per kg daily by IV infusion	Systemic candidiasis	Multiple toxicities including renal, neurological and hepatic
Fluconazole	50 mg daily	Candidiasis, especially in immunosuppressed patients	Nausea, rash
Itraconazole	1–200 mg daily	Ringworm and yeast infections	Nausea
Terbinafine	250 mg daily	Ringworm and onychomycosis	Nausea, rash

tive against infections with yeast-like micro-organisms. The doses and side effects are seen in Table 21.5.

Phototherapy for skin disease

Many patients say that their psoriasis improves in the summer time after being out in the sun. The same is true for patients with acne and even some patients with atopic dermatitis. It is the ultraviolet portion of the solar spectrum (page 21) that seems to aid these patients and artificial sources of ultraviolet radiation (UVR) are now often used in treatment.

Natural sunshine can also be used if the local weather conditions permit. Special 'spas' have been established at the Dead Sea in Israel, around the Black Sea and in the Canary islands for the treatment of psoriasis.

Treatment with the 'sunburn' part of the UV spectrum (UVB 280–320 nm) from arrays of special tubes is sometimes used to treat patients with acne and psoriasis. Caution is necessary to prevent burning in the short term and chronic photodamage and skin cancers in the long term by giving the minimum dose of UVR necessary to clear the patients' problems.

> Treatment with the 'sun-burn' part of the UV spectrum (UVB) from arrays of special tubes is sometimes used to treat patients with acne and psoriasis.

> In PUVA the skin is photosensitized with psoralen drugs given either orally two hours before irradiation or topically (in a bath) immediately before the UVR.

PUVA treatment

A more usual form of phototherapy in recent years is photochemotherapy with long wave UVR (UVA) known as PUVA. In this treatment the skin is photosensitized with psoralen drugs given either orally two hours before irradiation or topically (in a bath) immediately before the UVR. Most patients are given the drugs orally and mostly this is 8-methoxy psoralen given in a dose of approximately 0.6 mg/kg body weight/day. Photochemotherapy with UVA has become a standard treatment for patients with severe and generalized psoriasis and is successful in 70–80% patients within six to eight weeks. Usually treatment is given two or three times per week starting at a low dose and gradually increasing the dose until a good effect is obtained.

Other types of patient may benefit, especially patients with T-cell lymphoma of the skin (mycosis fungoides, Sèzary syndrome) and some patients with atopic eczema.

Burning is a danger, and sun-sensitive patients must be treated very carefully with low doses. Nausea is common and due to the psoralen. Dry skin is also a side effect in the short term. Unfortunately it has been found that some eight to ten years after 'high-dose' PUVA treatment there is a greatly increased incidence of skin cancers – particularly squamous cell carcinoma. Other forms of skin cancer and chronic photodamage also seem increased after UVA.

Goggles or glasses that block UVA must be used during treatment and for 24 hours afterwards to prevent cataracts. The UVA is given in specially constructed cabinets or under arrays of lights arranged to irradiate particular parts of the body.

> It has been found that some eight to ten years after 'high dose' PUVA treatment there is a greatly increased incidence of skin cancers – particularly squamous cell carcinoma.

Further reading

Recommended reading

Adler, M.W. (1990) *ABC of Sexually Transmitted Diseases*, British Medical Journal.

Adler, M.W. (1991) *ABC of AIDS*, British Medical Journal.

Ashton, R.E. (1992) *Differential Diagnosis in Dermatology*, 2nd edn, Radcliffe Medical Press.

Basset, A., Liautaud, B. and Ndioye, B. (1986) *Dermatology of Black Skin*, Oxford University Press.

Burge, S. and Rayment, R. (1986) *Simple Skin Surgery*, Blackwell Scientific.

Cunliffe, W.J. (1988) *A Pocket Guide to Acne*, Science Press.

Harper, J. (1990) *Handbook of Paediatric Dermatology*, Butterworths.

Levene, G.M. and Goolamali, S.K. (1986) *Diagnostic Picture Tests in Dermatology*, Wolfe Medical Publications.

MacKie, R. (1989) *Skin Cancer*, Martin Dunitz.

Marks, R. (1981) *Psoriasis*, Macdonald Optima.

Marks. R. (1987) *Skin Disease in Old Age*, Martin Dunitz.

Marks, R. (1992) *Sun Damaged Skin*, Martin Dunitz.

Marks, R. (ed.) (1992) *Eczema*, Martin Dunitz.

McKee, P.H. (1989) *Pathology of the Skin*, Lippincott.

Meneghini, C.E. and Bonifizi, E. (translated and edited by Marks, H. and Marks, R.) (1986) *An Atlas of Paediatric Dermatology*.

Ryan T.J. (1987) *The Management of Leg Ulcers*, Oxford Medical Publications.

Sharvill, D.E. (1988) *Skin Signs of Systemic Disease*, Pocket Picture Guides.

Wisdom, A. (1989) *A Colour Atlas of Sexually Transmitted Disease*, Wolfe Medical Publications.

Zachary, C.B. (1991) *Basic Cutaneous Surgery*, Churchill Livingstone.

Reference books

Braun-Falco, O., Plewig, G. *et ak* (1991) *Dermatology*, Springer-Verlag.

Goldsmith, L.A. (ed.) (1991) *Physiology, Biochemistry and Molecular Biology of the Skin*, 2nd edn, Oxford University Press.

Rook, Wilkinson *et al* (eds) (1992) *Textbook of Dermatology*, Blackwell Scientific (in three volumes).

Sams, W.M. and Lynch, P.J. (1990) *Principles and Practice of Dermatology*, Churchill Livingstone.

Index

Page numbers appearing in **bold** refer to figures and page numbers appearing in *italic* refer to tables.